TEXTBOOK OF COMMUNITY MEDICINE
(Preventive & Social)

TEXTBOOK OF COMMUNITY MEDICINE

(PREVENTIVE & SOCIAL)

by the Editors of
B. Jain Publishers

Taru Bhagat, BHMS
Rohit Jain, BHMS
Amina Khatoon, BHMS

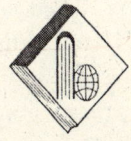

B. JAIN PUBLISHERS (P) LTD.
An ISO 9001 : 2000 Certified Company

TEXTBOOK OF COMMUNITY MEDICINE
(Preventive & Social)

© All rights are reserved

No part of this publication may be reproduced, stored in a retrieval system or transmitted, in any form or by any means, mechanical, photocopying, recording or otherwise, without prior written permission of the publishers.

First Edition : 2005

Price: Rs. 250.00

Published by
Kuldeep Jain
for
B. Jain Publishers (P) Ltd.
1921, Chuna Mandi, St. 10th Paharganj,
New Delhi-110 055
Ph: 91-011-23580800, 23581100, 23581300, 23583100
Fax: 91-011-23580471
Email: bjain@vsnl.com, Website: www.bjainbooks.com

PRINTED IN INDIA
by
J.J. Offset Printers
522, FIE, Patpar Ganj, Delhi-110 092

ISBN: 81-8056-669-2
BOOK CODE: BB-5898

PUBLISHER'S NOTE

Community medicine is one of the most important aspect of the medical system. It deals with various facets of health and health-related problems. Though the basic pattern of community medicine remains same but there are day-to-day changes in datas, technology as well as health hazards which lead to rapid evolvement in the arena of community medicine. Thus, in this book, it has been tried to make the study of community medicine comprehensive along with homoeopathic approach on each aspect.

Following are the highlights of "Textbook of Community Medicine" :

- *Health, Illness & Medicine : History & Evolution* deals with evolution of medicine from ancient time till date along with emergence of Hahnemann and his principle "Let likes be treated by likes."
- *Concept of Health & Diseases* deals with various dimensions of health & different concepts of diseases like germ, miasms, etc.
- *Principles of Epidemiology and Epidemiologic Methods* is concerned with history of principles, measurement and methods of epidemiology.
- Communicable diseases are taken up under *Respiratory Infections, Intestinal Infections, Arthropod Borne Diseases* and *Contact Infections* where each disease state is discussed with its epidemiology, mode of transmission, clinical features, Laboratory diagnosis, management & homoeopathic treatment.
- *Epidemiology of Non-Communicable Diseases* is concerned with the subject like Accidents & Blindness where the topics like magnitude of problem, causative factors and prevention has been dealt in detail.
- The chapter *Demography and Family Planning* covers the various aspect of scientific study of human population like fertility, sex ratio etc., along with family planning services, methods and various family welfare programmes in India. It includes National Health Policy too.
- *Maternal & Child Health* includes the promotive, preventive, curative & rehabilitative care for mothers and children.
- *Nutrition & Health* deals with classification of food, nutritional requirements, nutritional problems and their control programme as well as various assessing components of nutritional status.

- *Environment & Health* is concerned with various environmental factors affecting health.
- Occupation is also leading to various health problems which have been dealt in detail with homoeopathic efficacy and legislative measures in *Occupational Health*.
- *Genetics & Health* deals with incidence, prevalence, categories, preventive measures of genetic diseases as well as genetic counselling.
- Social science plays an important role in maintaining health which has been discussed in *Social Science & Medicine*.
- Mental aspect is one of the most important dimension of health which has been elaborated with homoeopathic approach & national program in chapter *Mental Health*.
- Use of statistical method in planning, collections, compilation, analysis & interpretation of data in the field of medicine has been detailed in *Biostatistics*.
- Health plan formulation, execution and evaluation with various National Policies and Five Year Plans have been dealt in *Health Planning, Management and Economics*.
- *Health Education* is concerned with objectives, goals, methods, principles & practice of health education along with functions of health communication.
- This book also gives a detailed knowledge about different levels of *Health Care in Community* with their principles & functions.
- Various biomedical wastes creating hazards for the human beings as well as their management has been dealt in *Biomedical Waste Management*.
- People are coming across disasters very frequently and thus is the present need of its management which has been dealt in *Disaster Management* chapter.
- For the sake of revision & mental exercise *Sample Question Papers* have been included at the end of the book.

We hope "Textbook of Community Medicine" will fill the long-felt need for a book which specifically covers the syllabus prescribed by Central Council of Homoeopathy for students of homoeopathy.

Kuldeep Jain
MD, B. Jain Publishers

CONTENTS

		Page
Chapter-1	: Health, Illness and Medicine : History & Evolution	1
Chapter-2	: Concepts of Health and Diseases	11
Chapter-3	: Principles of Epidemiology and Epidemiologic Methods	35
Chapter-4	: Respiratory Infections	71
Chapter-5	: Intestinal Infections	113
Chapter-6	: Arthropod Borne Diseases	123
Chapter-7	: Contact Infections	149
Chapter-8	: Epidemiology of Non-communicable Diseases	155
Chapter-9	: Demography & Family Planning	163
Chapter-10	: Maternal & Child Health	203
Chapter-11	: Nutrition and Health	235
Chapter-12	: Environment and Health	267
Chapter-13	: Occupational Health	301
Chapter-14	: Genetics and Health	323
Chapter-15	: Social Science and Medicine	329
Chapter-16	: Mental Health	333
Chapter-17	: Biostatistics	345

Chapter-18	: Health Planning, Management and Economics	371
Chapter-19	: Health Education	423
Chapter-20	: Health Care of Community	429
Chapter-21	: Biomedical Waste Management	451
Chapter-22	: Disaster Management	459
Sample Question Papers		467
Final Question Papers		473
Bibliography		483

CHAPTER-1

HEALTH, ILLNESS AND MEDICINE : HISTORY & EVOLUTION

Disease and humanity go hand in hand from time immemorial. Since ages one of the most cherished dreams of the human beings to control diseases, mankind has tread a long path in this regard. Some diseases have been eradicated while others are on the verge of being eradicating. We have an extensive knowledge of various diseases, their treatment and control measures. But still we are facing new challenges every day!

In a process of learning the growth and development of human medicine we must look at its history first.

THE BEGINNING

The healing process of art originated out of constraint need, self-protection and urge to provide relief during the time of sickness and suffering.

Then onwards there was no looking back. The knowledge of medicine started increasing gradually and the persons practising the newly evolved methods of healing became 'Physicians'. Then various systems of medicine evolved at various places.

The various ancient systems of medicine are :

The Greek Medicine

The Greek civilization is considered to be one of the most influential civilizations of all times. The Greeks were the first to separate medicine from religion and placed disease on a far more rational basis than ever before by more extrapolation and rationalisation of the observation. The Greeks were the first to note that diseases are natural. The most important person in early Greek medicine is Hippocrates "the father of Medicine" who wrote some seventy books known as the Hippocratic Corpus. During the Greek era medicine became a science and the profession had to be underpinned with theory. The body was thought to consist of four principle humors – **yellow bile, blood, phlegm and black bile** characterised by the same properties – dry, hot, wet and cold as the four elements – fire, air, earth and water.

The four humors, elements and their characteristics according to Hippocrates are :

Humor	–	Yellow bile	Blood	Phlegm	Black bile
Element	–	Fire	Air	Water	Earth
Characteristic	–	Dry hot	Hot wet	Wet cold	Cold dry

One generalised theory was that disease was due to an imbalance in the fluid portion of the body. Hippocratic physicians, studied anatomy, physiology as well as evident, immediate and obscure cause of disease.

Hippocrate was also an epidemiologist, always trying to seek out the causation of the disease. He considered factors like air, water, climate in causation of disease.

In addition to the Hippocratic medicine many other smaller schools with cult or sect characteristic existed. The most renowned university/medical centre built by Greeks was Alexandria.

Roman Medicine

Roman empire was a complex and rigorous combination of Greek and Roman cultural elements forged through centuries of war. Medicine had magic and folklore elements as well as empirical and rational elements. Aulus Cornelians Celsus wrote an encyclopedic work on medicine and Pedanius Dioscorides one of the first herbalist wrote the Materia Medica. According to Celsus the art of medicine could be divided into 3 parts :

(a) cure by diets or life-style.
(b) cure by medication.
(c) cure by surgery.

He rejected the Greek concept of the physician as necessary guide to health and considered it essential for every individual to acquire and understand the relationship between disease and stage of life. The most important medical school in the Roman era is represented by the work of Galen. No other person in the history of medicine has influenced concepts of anatomy, physiology, therapeutics and philosophy as much as Galen. He expanded, commented and supplemented the Hippocratic

Corpus with detailed formulations on the quality and body fluids pathology including their physiology. He increased his anatomical knowledge by animal dissections. The essential features of Galen's system were a view of nature as purposeful and the principle of balance among the four qualities and the four humors as already described by Hippocrates. Although Galen studied anatomy and physiology on a rational basis, he included spiritual elements as well, like in his pneuma theory [pneuma psychikon = Semi pneuma (spiritus anlmalis) and pneuma Zootikon = life pneuma (spiritus-vitalis)]. Hippocrates had nature let heal whereas Galen was willing to interfere with healing process. His most utilised therapy was bleeding, which he used for almost every disorder.

Indian Medicine

The classical system of Indian medicine is called "the knowledge for longevity" or in Sanskrit, Ayurveda. The theoretical doctrine is based on the three body humors – wind, bile and phlegm and its therapies are herbal, massage, ointments, enemas, douches or surgery.

The earliest surviving text books of ayurveda, written in Sanskrit, date from the first centuries A.D. The two most important texts are the Chark Samhita and the Susruta Samhita which form the corner stone of Ayurveda. Both texts emanate from a single medical tradition and contain philosophical passages as well as descriptions of sophisticated surgery. Later new important texts were implemented like the Astangahrdaya Sanhita (700 A.D.) or the Sarngadhara Sanhita (1400 A.D.).

The basic theories of ayurvedic medicine are related to the Sankhya philosophy which postulates that there was no universe before creation occured and all that exists is "pure reality". The cosmos and "pure reality" can not be separated because "pure reality" is the cause and cosmos is the effect. Regarding body and mind this means that body evolves from mind, and the body is thought to consist of the same five elements of which the universe is made up of-earth (hardness), water (moisture), fire (heat), air (vital breath) and space (the interstices and the self by in – dwelling spirit). Combinations of the five elements condense into the three doshas : *vata* (air and space) *pitta* (fire and water) and *kapha* (water and earth). A *dosha* is any fault, error or any transgression against the rhythm of life which promotes chaos. The different doshas are in charge of different functions in the body : *vata* for all motion in the body and mind, *pitta* for all transformation and *kapha* is the stabilising factor.

Life is inconceivable without these three activities and any imbalance causes disease.

The Ayurvedic perspective holds that one should take care of the body for in the absence of the body there is a total extinction of all those characteristics which embodied beings. Diseases, which can affect mind and/or body, are divided into two types – those arising front within, and those arising from without. Both mental and bodily diseases can be transformed into and expressed by each other and intensive emotions are assumed to be of great influence on the onset of disease. Ayurvedic diagnosis concentrates on the relationships between the body and mind of the individual in the "row" and the direction one is changing to. From the side of the physician curative energy towards the patient is demanded since reinforcement of faith and hope during the diagnostic process can initiate the healing process. The applied therapy first has to be rightly timed and is essentially of two kinds purification and palliation. Palliative drugs should protect the tissues from the attack of the doshas.

Although India has been occupied by the British, which suppressed Ayurvedic practises and introduced western medicine, after liberation Ayurvedic medicine still regained an important part of the Indian health care system with its own universities and journals.

Chinese Medicine

The traditional Chinese medical theories are based on the Taoist concept of body functions and its ideas about the internal world of the human body. The body is viewed as a small world, country or model of the universe, where the landscape is governed by a ruler and its assisting officials and ministers. Only the harmony and the co-operation between the members of the government results in health. In addition the body is inhabited by spirits, which live in the body's important areas and take care of its different functions. Inside and outside the body there is a moving thing called *Qi* which has its natural rhythm and direction, is omnipresent and when acted contrary to, is liable to contact diseases because it is blocked somewhere in its circulation. Qi is the representation of movement and change, which is essential as per the Chinese philosophy. Change is created by the interplay of two forces, yin and yang.

The basic cause of disease according to Taoist medicine is the lack of "rest" and so the mind should remain quiet, which can be achieved by exercises. Diseases and their cure are understood in the yin-yang terminology and can be caused by external and internal factors. Diagnosis is based on the four elements :

- looking.
- listening, smelling and tasting.
- interrogation.
- touching.

The therapy of the yin-yang principle is that the opposite of what is causing the disease will cure it (cold versus heat, but heat versus heat when the heat is caused by cold like fever is caused by cold). There are eight methods of therapy that form the basis of any technique of therapy (acupuncture, massage, drugs etc.) namely **sweating, vomiting, lowering, harmonising, warming, purifying, dispelling and supplying**. The best known chinese therapeutic technique is acupuncture which is a method of influencing body functions by inserting needles in the xne or acupuncture points. Acupuncture is often combined with moxibustion or burning of the herb moxa placed on the body. Another therapeutic technique is massage, of different systems of the body. Chinese pharmacology uses herbals, minerals and animal components according to their medical nature and taste. Only when these above mentioned therapeutic techniques fail then the traditional Chinese physician uses surgery.

Chinese medicine is much more diverse than the other Asian medical traditions and sharing of traditions, theories and therapies, for medicine as well as for religion is common among the Chinese people. The mix of traditional Chinese and Western therapies used now-a-days by Chinese physicians, is completely accepted, however it creates paradoxical ways of explaining and curing diseases and is more disconnected from the roots.

THE MIDDLE AGE

During the following period, no important insights in medicine developed. The Roman Empire became divided and most of the ancient medical texts were collected, summarised and newly categorised into compendia, so called the **"Dark ages of medicine"**. This period saw the rise of Arab medicine. During this period Europe was passing through the Dark ages where ignorance and superstitions prevailed.

In the early period of the Arabian middle age, many Greek and Roman medical texts were translated into Arabic. Another significant achievement was the development of hospitals and hospital based clinical training of medical practitioners, which were financially supported by the religious law of charitable endowments. Despite the honours accorded to scholar-physicians, scepticism about medical practise remained strong and Islamic traditionalists warned that the medical art was foreign to Arab culture.

One of the most scientific minded physicians of the Arabic world was Rhazes (850-923 A.D.). He wrote the Continens (comprehensive book of medicine) which was translated into Latin. To Rhazes, the physician patient relation was of great importance, both having an ethical obligation, duty and trust on each other. He established the concept of specific disease (small pox and measles) instead of defining them in terms of symptoms (fever, diarrhoea etc.). The first scholar to create a complete philosopical system in the Arabic language was Avicenna (980-1037 AD). He wrote the *Canon of Medicine* for general practitioners and described the philosophical principles of medicine and the relationship between the mind and the body demonstrating how physiological phenomenon an betrary the hidden thoughts.

Although most of the Arabian medicine comprised the preservation of the ancient Greek wisdom, one important original contribution to medicine was done by the Arab Ibnan-Nafis (Ca 1200 AD), who described the pulmonary circulation correctly.

RENAISSANCE

The Renaissance period in Europe can be described as the age of exploration of the world, the mind and the human body. The Greco-Roman-Islamic traditions were replaced by "modern" science, by the work of the medical humanists. Both artists (Like Leonardo da Vinci 1452-1519) and physicians (like Andreas Vesalius 1514-1564) sought accurate anatomical knowledge of the human body because it is beautiful and worthy to study. During this period, differences between the writings of Galen and own anatomical observations were made, but it was hard to reject the authority of Galen's work. The anatomical knowledge increased greatly during the renaissance, whereas physiology stayed on the level of Galen.

The renaissance was not only a period of rational medical science but also an age of superstition and occult science. Medicine remained entangled with astrology, alchemy and mysticism. Astrology incorporated the motions of the heavenly bodies in diagnosis and therapy. And alchemist tried to develop drugs and thought that the vital functions of the body depended on a mysterious force called the archaevs (internal alchemist). In opposition to the concept of humoral pathology and the doctrine of Galen, the alchemist Paracelsus attempted to substitute the doctrine by the principle that the body is essentially a chemical laboratory. Disease is therefore, the result of derangements in the chemical functions of the body and should be cured by specific chemical substances.

REVOLUTION (SEVENTEENTH CENTURY)

During the sixteenth and seventeenth centuries a great transformation of the physical sciences occured by the works of Copernicus, Galilei and Newton. Revolutions in medical sciences were given by William Harvey, who discovered the minor and major blood heart-lung-circulation and Antony van Leeuvenhoeck who invented the microscope. The increased insight in nature and physics demanded theories in medicine. Two main streams in health and disease concepts developed, namely :

- Paracelsic iatrochemistry
- Iatrophysic, iatromechanics and iatromathematics.

THE AGE OF ENLIGHTENMENT

During the earlier period, thinking, and handling were strongly dominated by the doctrines and religion. This changed in the 18th century as the thinking and reasoning became independent from the church and state. The scientific motive changed to empirism and rationalism, with systematic observations and planned experiments. Different old health and disease concepts were renewed or replaced by new ones. It was during this time Dr. Christian Friedrich Samuel Hahnemann made the induction of the diseases so cured by the medicines were cured by the virtue of the same power in the medicines which produced symptoms like those they cured. He then converted the induction to deduction and said "Let likes be treated by likes", Similia

Simililbus Curentur. Thus homoeopathy was born when Hahnemann published an article in Hufeland's Journal under the title "Essay on a New Principle for Ascertaining the Curative Powers of Drugs," 1796. The 18th century was also the age of the establishment of modern hospitals with inner medicine surgery and pharmacology.

THE NINETEENTH CENTURY

The nineteenth century was the century of the industrial revolution and early capitalism. It was also the century of the origin of the modern empirical to experimental science and medicine, the development of pharmacology, cell pathology and bacteriology (Pasteur). New instruments allowed new scientific investigations, diagnosis and a rationalisation of therapies. During this period, the psychical and physical body were further separated and medicine became more and more the science of "material body". With the evolving knowledge of the different body organs, physicians started to specialise in different disciplines according to the corresponding body organs or functions. Medical treatment became available to almost the whole population. Medical health and accident insurance institutions were established.

The successes booked in physics and chemistry more and more influenced and determined the medical science, methods and therapies. However it did not hinder the appearance of different theoretical schools, such as :

- The natural philosophical physiology with the vegetative (growth, nourishment and reproductive forces) animistic (irritability of the organs, muscles and sensitive sensory nerves and soul) dimension.
- The natural scientific physiology which was completely based on the scientific investigations of the body functions.
- The cell-pathological theory of Virchow (1821-1902); who declared that all diseases resulted out of changes in the cells and that the cell was the true organic unity of the body and the part of departure for all life. His theories were transmitted to society and resulted in the development of bio-socialism.

The development of bacteriology by Louis Pasteur (1822-1885) and Robert Koch (1843-1910) for the first time proved the ill making potency of micro-organisms which initiated the science of microbiology, modern vaccination and the development of disinfecting agents to be used during surgery.

The separation between body and the psychic illness proceeded during this century and the brain became more and more the object of investigation for psychic illness and abnormalities (pathological and somatic psychiatry). As for body medicine, alternatives to the scientific views were established like the psycho-analysis of S. Freud (1856-1939).

Not all physicians accepted the scientific developments in medicine and out of vitalistic and life force theories of the 18th century, alternatives arose like the homoeopathy of C.F.S. Hahnemann (1755-1843). According to Hahnemann disease is an affection of the life by pathogenic disturbers and has to be observed as a holistic phenomenon. Instead of supporting the body's resistance, a homoeopathic physician applies low or lowest doses of substances which evoke the same symptoms as caused by the disease itself. The so provoked artificial disease stimulates the life force to increase resistance, against disease causing force and protect the person.

THE TWENTIETH CENTURY

The last 90-100 years have been years of immense technical improvement in medicine. Newly developed diagnostic (X-ray, nuclear magnetic resonance, bio-chemistry, genetic and molecular methods) as well as therapeutic (antibiotics, chemo and radiation therapy, micro-surgery, gene manipulation etc.) methods have brought great advancements and possibilities to cure diseases which were untreatable up till then. In addition, the work of the early alchemists evolves in modern pharmacology and the research and production of medication is industrialised and commercialised. Medicine and pharmacology become political issues. For example the development of organics during the first and second world was as well as commercial issues such as health care insurance companies. Medical research is no longer determined by exclusively and purely curiosity but is controlled by ethical as well as financial and commercial elements.

One of the highlights of the medical science is the discovery of deoxyribonucleic acid (DNA) by G. Watson and Crick and the gene is the information carrier of all the bio-chemical substances of the organism. Many diseases have now become reduced to gene mutations. The discovery of DNA on the one side reinforced the materialisation of medicine, on the other side lead to the development of Darwinian medicine (the egoistic gene, why do mutated genes survive?).

Because of the enormous technical progress in medicine, the life expectancy increased rapidly, however many people loose their belief in the technical materialistic medicine as they threaten to become a "body without soul" in a factory called health care or hospital. When the advanced techniques fail to cure and the side effects of a therapy are worse than the disease itself, alternatives are searched in old traditional medicine such as Indian or Chinese medicine as well as in new (for example – anthroposophic), partially sect (for example – esoteric, spiritual, aura healers, etc.) or gentle healing methods. Thus medical methods find even more confirmation when it becomes clear that many disease causing micro-organisms and viruses mutate and become resistant to medication like antibiotics faster than new medication which can be designed against them.

In spite of the fact that modern medicine has improved health in western cultures to a standard never seen elsewhere on earth, its achievements stay below its promises. The loss of confidence in modern medicine seems to take place parallel to the loss of confidence in the authority of the Christian church in western countries and stimulates the search for a new life sense, including a new sense of health and disease. On the newest interest is the role of brain in consciousness, mind and soul, and the influence of these non material elements on health and disease. In addition to technical bio-medicine, the call for more holistic, body and soul integrating medicine has become loud.

CHAPTER-2

CONCEPTS OF HEALTH AND DISEASES

CONCEPT OF HEALTH

'Health' is a multidimensional feature of human life. It has various dimensions, concepts, etc. associated with it. Before learning about the dimension or concept one must first try to learn what actually health is.

According to WHO, Health is a state of complete physical, mental and social well being and not merely an absence or disease of infirmity and an ability to lead a socially and economically productive life.

As per **homoeopathic** concept, Hahnemann writes about health in aphorism 9 of Organon of Medicine that, "In the healthy condition of man, the spiritual vital force (autocracy), the dynamics that animates the material body (organism) rules with unbounded sway, and retains all the part of the organism in admirable harmonious, vital operation, as regards both sensations and functions, so that our indwelling, reason-gifted mind can freely employ this living, healthy instrument for the higher purposes of our existence."

He further writes in aphorism 10, "the meterial organism, without the vital force, is capable of no sensation, no function, no self-preservation. It derives all sensations and performs all the functions of life solely by means of the immaterial being (the vital force) which animates the material organism in health and in disease."

DIMENSIONS OF HEALTH

As already stated health is multi-dimensional. As per WHO only 3 dimensions of health are mentioned viz. physical, mental and social, but we have several other dimensions like emotional, spiritual, occupational, etc.

Physical Dimension

It describes the 'functionioning' of human body which includes each and every cell, tissue, organ, system working to their fullest potential and with proper coordination.

Most of the time this is the only dimension people relate to as most diseases result in predominant physically manifested signs and symptoms. So, it becomes important from physician's point of view to understand properly this aspect of 'Human Health'. Some indicators of normal physical health are :
- Normal vitals like weight, height, pulse rate, B.P., etc.
- Normal bowel and bladder function.
- Normal body functions like vision, hearing, muscle coordination, etc.

Mental Dimension

Mental health has been defined (as per WHO) as a state of balance between individual and the surroundings. Its a state of harmony between oneself and others, a coexistence between the realities of the self and that of other people and that of environment. With the evolution of newer diseases, we are realizing the importance of mental health. And with modernisation, mental illnesses have taken a very important more in leading killers of our times.

Intellectual Dimension

It is a cognitive process whereby an individual develops and experiences unique approaches to existing issues and problems, the use of educational and human resources to enhance one's skills and knowledge, decision making, life planning, access and use of knowledge as well as learning disabilities.

Emotional Dimension

It deals with knowledge and acceptance of one's feelings, stress management and psychological awareness.

Social Dimension

It includes acceptance and celebration of diverse populations and their ideas, fostering a positive self image and improving inter personal social skills, building healthy relationships.

Spiritual Dimension

It revolves around finding purpose and meaning of human existence, conscious awareness of the depth and expense of life. A humble appreciation of nature.

Occupational Dimension

It implies goal setting, meaning and purpose in work, work satisfaction.

Environmental Dimension

It is related to injury prevention, safety precautions, establishing a positive respect for ones surroundings.

Some other dimensions are :
- Educational dimension;
- Nutritional dimension;
- Cultural dimension;
- Preventive dimension;
- Curative dimension;
- Economic dimension.

POSITIVE HEALTH

Positive health is a term used to describe the perfect functioning of body and it takes into consideration physical, mental and social dimensions of health.

Positive health is achieved when :
- all the cells, tissues, organs are working to their optimal potential and in perfect harmony.
- the person is mentally compatible, has a sense of normality and is able to have perfect coordination between himself and his environment.
- he is able to fulfill his social obligations to the fullest extent.

But we know that it is impossible to acquire perfect positive health state. The spectrum of factors affecting health is so complex and continuously changing that it is nearly impossible to modify all to achieve the positive health as dreamed.

CONCEPT OF WELL BEING

We are introduced to the term 'Well being' in the WHO's definition of health.

Well being can be defined by studying its objective and subjective components.

- Objective → Standard of living.
- Subjective → Quality of life.

Standard of Living

It takes into account day to day expenses, educational status, income, occupation, nutrition, sanitation, etc. By properly working out these, standard of living can be adjudged for. For simple comparison of the standard of living in different countries we can utilize the per capita GROSS NATIONAL PRODUCT (GNP).

Another term that can be used as an alternative is "LEVEL OF LIVING". It also takes into the account similar factors like housing, occupation, etc.

Quality of Life

It is the subjective component of well being. It is defined by WHO as "the condition of life resulting from the combination of the effects of the complete range of factors such as those determining health, happiness (including comfort in the physical environment and a satisfying occupation), education, social and intellectual attainments, freedom of action, justice and freedom of expression."

Unlike standard of living which is an objective criteria of well being, it takes into account the subjective evaluation of the factors affecting 'WELL BEING' of a person.

There are a many indicators used for measuring the quality of life and standard of living. Some of the important ones are discussed below :

Physical Quality of Life Index

One of the indices used for measuring quality of life. It takes into account three indicators which are :

(a) INFANT MORTALITY RATE
(b) LITERACY RATE
(c) LIFE EXPECTANCY

The index is calculated by taking the average of all three indicators. Then the results are displayed on a scale of 0 to 100.

Concepts of Health and Diseases

After that, using the PQLI various countries can be compared with each other.

Human Development Index

Like PQLI, it is a composite index. It's value is between 0 and 1.

Indicators used in the Estimation of HDI

The provincial HDI is constructed using the average of three development outcomes of each country. These include :

1. Health as measured by life expectancy.
2. Level of knowledge and skills as measured by the weighted average of functional literacy and combined elementary and secondary net enrolment rate; and
3. Access to resources as measured by the level of real per capita income.

Computation of the Human Development Index

The steps performed in the estimation of HDI are as follows :

Step 1 : Generate an index for each component of HDI, i.e. health (H), education (E) and per capita income (Y)

(a) Index for H : $I_1 = \dfrac{H - H^{min}}{H^{max} - H^{min}}$

where H is the life expectancy at birth (in years) by province

H^{max} = 85 years.

H^{min} = 25 years.

The minimum and maximum values adopted for life expectancy at birth are based on the values being used by UNDP and HDN.

(b) Index for E : $I_2 = \tfrac{2}{3}(E_1) + \tfrac{1}{3}(E_2)$

where $E_1 = \dfrac{(Lit - Lit^{min})}{(Lit^{max} - Lit^{min})}$

$E_2 = \dfrac{(Enrol - Enrol^{min})}{(Enrol^{max} - Enrol^{min})}$

E_1 = Index for functional literacy by province

Lit^{max} = 100

Lit^{min} = 0

E_2 = Index for combined elementary and secondary net enrolment rate by province

$Enrol^{max} = 100$

$Enrol^{min} = 0$

(c) Index for Y : $I_3 = \dfrac{(Y - Y^{min})}{(Y^{max} - Y^{min})}$

where Y is the real income per capita by province

e.g. – for 1994
$$Y^{max} = Ph\ P37,070$$
$$Y^{min} - Ph\ P6,533$$
for 1994
$$Y^{max} = Ph\ P48,930$$
$$Y^{min} - Ph\ P8,181$$

The maximum and minimum values set for the income indicator are the highest and lowest values of real income per capita actually attained by the provinces for a particular reference year. As suggested by the HDN, the National Capital Region was treated as one of the provinces in determining the maxima and minima. Hence, the NCR real income figures were adopted as the maximum values in the computation of the HDI for all provinces for the two reference years.

Step 2 : Take the simple average of all three indices.

$$HDI = \tfrac{1}{3}(I_1 + I_2 + I_3)$$

DETERMINANTS OF HEALTH

Health is a multifactorial phenomenon. A number of factors decide the state of health.

The most important determinants of health are :

- *Biological or physiological,*
- *Life-style or behavioural and*
- *Environmental*

The interaction of all these factors can result in health or disease.

Some other determinants are :

Income and Social Status

People's health is affected by the difference in income distribution between the richest and poorest members of society.

When these differences are big, people with lower income and social status have less control and fewer choices in their lives.

Social Support Networks

People need support to handle difficult situations and to feel that they have some control over their lives. These networks can include their family, friends and community.

Education

Education gives people the knowledge and skills they need to make healthy choices to have a better income and more job security, and to participate in their community.

Employment and Working Conditions

People are healthiest when they have control over their work and their working conditions. Their health also benefits when they feel that the work they do is important, their job is secure, and their work place is safe and healthy.

Indoor and Outdoor Environments

Clean air and water, safe houses, communities, work places and roads, all contribute towards the good health.

Genetics

Our genetic make up plays a part in deciding how long we live, how healthy we will be and how likely we are to get certain illnesses.

Personal Health Practices and Coping Skills

Personal practices include whether a person eats well and is physically active, and whether they smoke or drink. Coping skills refer to the way in which we relate to the people around us and handle life's challenges and stresses.

Health Services

People's health throughout their lifeline is affected by prenatal care, and by the kinds of care and experiences they have in early childhood.

Gender

Men and women get different kinds of diseases and conditions at different ages. They also tend to have different income levels, and to work at different kinds of jobs. Many of these realities results from the differences in the way society treats men and women.

Culture

People's customs and traditions and the beliefs of their family and community all affect their health because these factors will influence what they think, feel, do and believe to be important.

Importance

If we are interested in a system that generates health, we need to work beyond medical care system and life-style factors. We need to learn to work across various sectors and systems.

INDICATORS OF HEALTH

Indicators are used to give an idea of the health status of the community. They are very useful in planning, execution and evaluation of health programmes and services.

Some properties of indicators are :
- should be accurate;
- should be valid;
- should be reliable;
- should be sensitive;
- should be specific and
- should be feasible.

But most of the indicators fail to obey these characteristics.

The indicators are as follows :

(1) Morbidity indicators;
(2) Mortality indicators;
(3) Environmental indicators;
(4) Socio-economic indicators;
(5) Mental health indicators;
(6) Nutritional indicators;
(7) Utilization indicators;
(8) Disability indicators;
(9) Quality of life indicators.

Morbidity Indicators

They are used to describe the disease trends in the population. It is one of the most important indicators for studying the

epidemiology of communicable diseases and also for developing efficient disease control programmes e.g. RNTCP, NAMP, etc.
- Number of persons who fell ill.
- The illness experienced.
- Duration of their illness.

These aspects of morbidity are commonly measured by morbidity rates & ratios as frequency, duration & severity.

Incidence – The no. of new cases occurring in a defined population in a defined period of time.

$$\text{Incidence (I)} = \frac{\text{No. of new cases during specified period}}{\text{Population at risk during that period}} \times 100$$

Prevalence – It is the total no. of all individuals who have an attribute or disease at a particular time divided by population at risk of having the attribute or disease at this point in time or midway in that period.

$$\text{Point Prevalence} = \frac{\text{Number of all current cases of specific disease at a given time}}{\text{Estimated population at the same time}} \times 100$$

Stable disease – If the incidence & duration of a disease are constant then the prevalence is also constant i.e. disease is stable.

$$\therefore P = I \times D$$

Other morbidity indicators are :
- Hospital admission, discharge rates.
- Sickness absenteeism.
- Duration of illness, stay in hospital.

Mortality Rates

(a) Crude death rate – Crude death rate is defined as the number of death per 1000 estimated mid-year population in one year, in a given place.

$$\frac{\text{Number of deaths during the year}}{\text{Mid-year population}} \times 1000$$

Though it is not a very good indicator but still useful in rough estimate of overall health situation.

(b) **Life expectancy at birth** – It is defined as the number of years a new born is expected to live, taken into account current age specific mortality rates. It is a very good indicator of health situation of a country. It is a global indicator used as one of the goals of health for all which has given as an universal minimum life expectancy of 60 years at birth.

(c) **Age specific mortality rate** – It is the no. of deaths per 1000 estimated mid-year population of a specific age group.

$$\frac{\text{Number of deaths in a particular age group}}{\text{Mid-year population}} \times 1000$$

Other morbidity indicators are :
- Infant mortality rate;
- Maternal mortality rate;
- Disease specific mortality rate and
- Proportional mortality rate.

Environmental Indicators

They describe the state of environment, like pollution, sanitation etc. Indicators used are – Pollution indices, sanitary facilities available, availability of safe water, housing facilities, etc.

Socio Economic Indicators

They are used to describe the financial and social status which affect the health. These are :

(a) Per capita GNP;
(b) Literacy rates;
(c) Unemployment levels;
(d) Family size and
(e) Housing facilities.

Various scales are used for socio economic clarification like Gupta - Mahajan scale, Kuppu Swami classification, etc.

CONCEPTS OF DISEASE

As per dictionary, we have a number of definitions of disease, some of them are :

- "A condition in which body health is impaired or a departure from state of health, an alteration of the human body interrupting the performance of vital functions" (Webster).

- "A condition of the body or some part or organ of the body in which its functions are disrupted or deranged" (Oxford).

Hahnemann writes about disease. "when a person falls ill, it is only this spiritual, self-acting (automatic) vital force, everywhere present in his organism, that is primarily deranged by the dynamic influence upon it of a morbific agent inimical to life; it is only the vital force, deranged to such an abnormal state that can furnish the organism with its disagreeable sensations, and incline it to the irregular process which we call disease; ..... only recognizable ... by morbid symptoms ..." (Aphorism 11, Organon of medicine).

He writes in §19, "... diseases are ... alternations in the state of health of the healthy individual ..." Simply, any state which does not follow the definition of health is disease.

We have a no. of disease, which can be classified on the basis of :
- Infecting organism,
- Clinical signs and symptoms,
- Pathological effect, etc.

INTERNATIONAL CLASSIFICATION OF DISEASE

It has 21 major chapters, last revised on January 1, 1993 :

I.	Certain infectious and parasitic diseases (A00 - B99)
II.	Neoplasms (C00 - D48)
III.	Diseases of the blood and blood forming organs and certain disorders involving the immune mechanism (D50 - D89)
IV.	Endocrine, nutritional and metabolic diseases (E00 - E90)
V.	Mental and behavioural disorders (F00 - F99)
VI.	Diseases of the nervous system (G00 - G99)
VII.	Diseases of the eye and adnexa (H00 - H59)
VIII.	Diseases of the ear and mastoid process (H60 - H95)
IX.	Diseases of the circulatory system (I00 - I99)
X.	Diseases of the respiratory system (J00 - J99)
XI.	Diseases of the digestive system (K00 - K93)
XII.	Diseases of the skin and subcutaneous tissue (L00 - L99)
XIII.	Diseases of the musculoskeletal system and connective tissue (M00 - M99)
XIV.	Diseases of the genitourinary system (N00 - N99)
XV.	Pregnancy, child birth and puerperium (O00 - O99)
XVI.	Certain conditions originating in prenatal period (P00 - P96)

XVII. Congenital malformations, deformations and chromosomal abnormalities (Q00 - Q99)
XVIII. Symptoms, signs and abnormal clinical and laboratory findings, not elsewhere classified (R00 - R99)
XIX. Injury, poisoning and certain other consequences of external causes (S00 - T98)
XX. External causes of morbidity and mortality (V01 - Y98)
XXI. Factors influencing health status and contact with health services (Z00 - Z99).

CLASSIFICATION OF DYNAMIC DISEASES UNDER HOMOEOPATHY

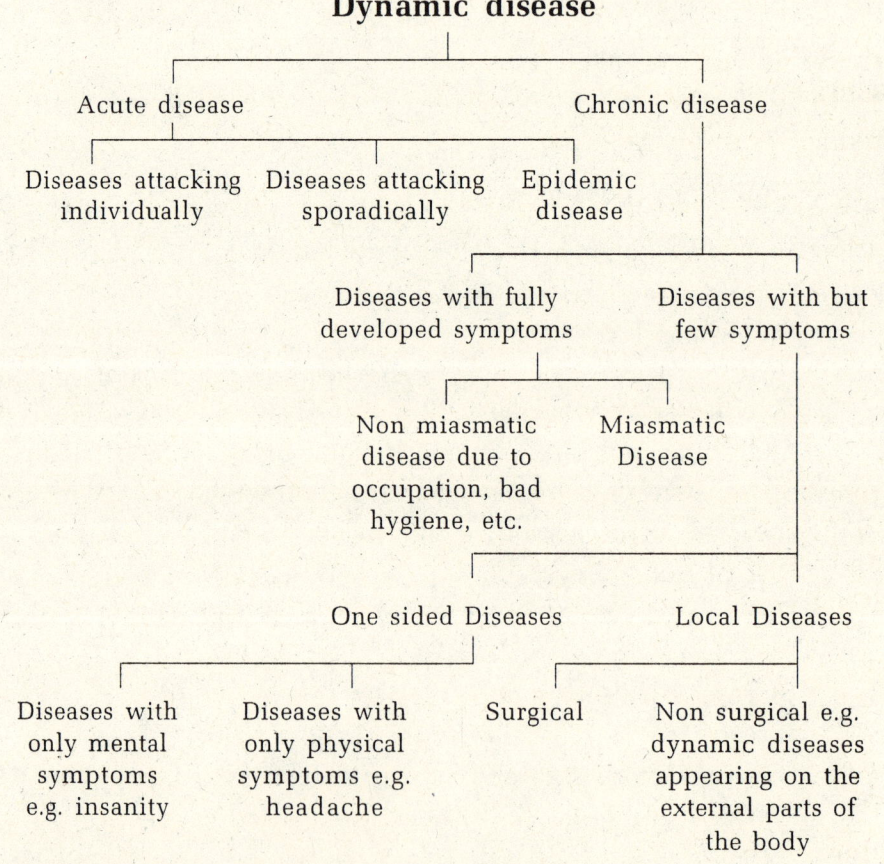

CONCEPTS OF DISEASE CAUSATION

Earlier we learned about various theories prevalent in ancient times, in old civilization like super natural theory of disease; the 4 humors

Concepts of Health and Diseases

theory (Greek), miasmatic theory of disease, etc. But a new revolution occurred with the advent of microbiology.

Germ Theory

It is based on the observation that most of the disease are caused by microorganisms like bacteria, viruses, etc. Koch's postulates form the back bone of this theory.

Koch's Postulates for infectious diseases are :

1. The microorganism must be observed in every case of the disease.
2. The micro organism must be isolated and grown in pure culture.
3. The micro organism grown in pure culture must produce the disease when inoculated into a susceptible host.
4. The micro organism must be observed in and recovered from the experimentally diseased host.

Miasmatic Theory

Hahnemann evolved the miasmatic theory as causes behind the disease after long years of research in this direction. According to him psora, sycosis and syphilis are the fundamental causes behind all cronic diseases and acute diseases are caused by acute miasm or half acute miasm.

Classification

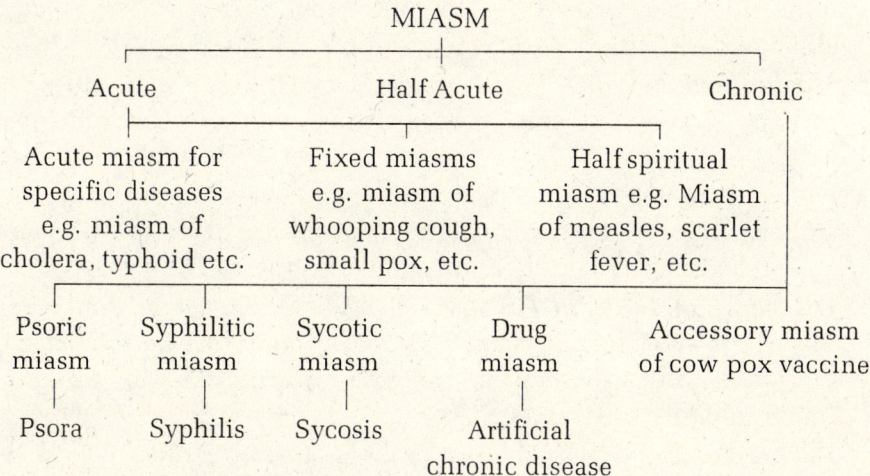

Epidemiological Triad Model

Modern medicine evolved using the germ theory of disease to explain the concept of aetiology. But the germ theory of diseases is having a no. of limitations. Each and every disease cannot be explained on the basis of it, e.g. diabetes, cancers etc. So, we use a more advanced and broad model for explaining disease. It is called the EPIDEMIOLOGICAL TRIAD having AGENT, HOST AND ENVIRONMENT. It states that mere presence of these three factors is not responsible for producing the disease but a proper **interaction** is required.

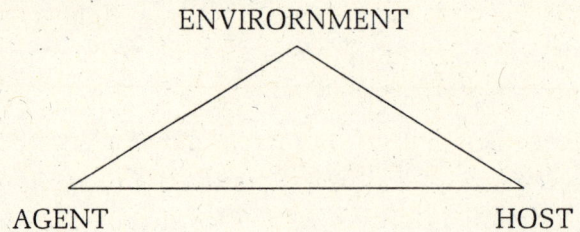

Now, we have three factors as AGENT FACTORS, HOST FACTORS and ENVIRONMENTAL FACTORS

Agent Factors

An agent is the living or non living substance or a force which may initiate a disease in a susceptible host.

- ***Biological Agents*** – e.g. bacteria, viruses, protozoa, rickettsiae etc.
- ***Physical agents*** – e.g. heat, cold, humidity, pressure, etc.
- ***Chemical Agents*** – Either endogenous like ketone bodies, bilirubin etc. or exogenous like allergies, poisons, gases, acids, alkalies, etc.
- ***Mechanical Agents*** – Forces which damage the tissues and parts of body e.g. bones, skin, etc. resulting in fractures, abrasions, lacerations, etc.
- ***Nutrient Factors*** – It includes proteins, fats, vitamins, minerals, carbohydrates and water. Deficiency or excess of these can result in diseases like malnutrition, night blindness, etc.
- ***Disorders of Internal Factors*** – It includes excess or deficiency of various substance normally formed in body like hormones and enzymes, body structure defects, chromosomal defects, immunological factors, etc.
- ***Social Factors*** – It includes smoking, unemployment, poverty, alcohol, sanitation etc.

Environmental Factors

It is the one which contains, both agent and the host, and is in close interaction with both. It has 3 parts :

Concepts of Health and Diseases

- *Physical environment* – Air, water, soil, etc.
- *Biological environment* – Living organisms and
- *Psycho-social environment* – It include social customs, traditions, religion, education, beliefs, habits, behaviour, etc.

Host Factors

They vary from person to person. They are :
- *Age*
- *Sex*
- *Race*
- *Genetic make-up* – Haemophilia, down's syndrome, etc.
- *Blood groups*
- *Immunological responses*
- *Biochemical factors* – Blood, enzymes, CSF, etc.
- *Organ systems* – Respiration, etc.
- *Life Style* – Habits, alcohols, drugs, etc.
- *Social and economical factors* – Education, occupation, marital status, etc.

There are also diseases where it is difficult to identify the 'agent' completely. In that situation aetiology is discussed in terms of "Risk Factors" but they are not the absolute proof of causation. Mere presence of a risk factor doesn't mean that the disease would be occurring. e.g. – smoking, hypertension.

Multifactorial Causation

Many a times we find that it is impossible to explain the aetiology of the disease using only a single factor, at such occasions multifactorial causation theory proves quite useful. It can explain modern diseases like mental illnesses, cancers, diabetes, etc.

Sir Bradford Hills in 1965 gave 8 postulates for multifactorial causation.

Bradford Hills postulates for multi-causal diseases :
1. Strength of association : The stronger the association, the greater the chances are of a causal relationship.
2. Consistency upon repetition : The association between exposure and outcome should be similar in different persons, places and times and among different study designs. The more the supporting studies the stronger the evidence.

3. Specificity : As with Koch's postulates – one exposure, one disease. However, a given disease may have multiple causes, and a given exposure may influence many disease states. When a specific exposure is associated with a specific disease, there is strong evidence of causality with multi-causal diseases, lack of specificity does not weaken the possibility of a causal relationship.
4. Time sequence : The temporal relationship should be such that the exposure precedes the outcome.
5. Biologic gradient – If there is the presence of a dose response curve suggesting that larger or longer exposure increases the risk of outcome, the results are more reliable. However, there may be thresholds below which no disease occurs, and greater exposure may not necessarily cause more disease (*ceiling effect*).
6. Plausibility : If there is some biologically plausible explanation for the observed association, the causality is more plausible. However, this depends on the state of knowledge at the time of the study.
7. Coherence of explanations : The observed association should be in agreement with the previous knowledge about the natural history and the biology of the disease and the known biological effects of the exposure.
8. Evidence from experimentation : There may be evidence from true experiments or natural experiments. Presence of experimental evidence strengthens the possibility of causality, however, it may be impossible to gather experimental evidence in many situations because of ethnical considerations, or the rareness of the outcome.

NATURAL HISTORY OF DISEASE

Natural history of disease looks into the evolution of disease from its earliest phase, termed as 'Pre-pathogenesis phase' to the terminal phase which may result in recovery, disability or death; termed as 'Pathogenesis phase'

Pre Pathogenesis Phase

It describes the time span that occurs before the onset of disease.

All three factors i.e. agent, host and environment are ready to interact and the moment the interaction is established the 'Pathogenesis Phase' begins.

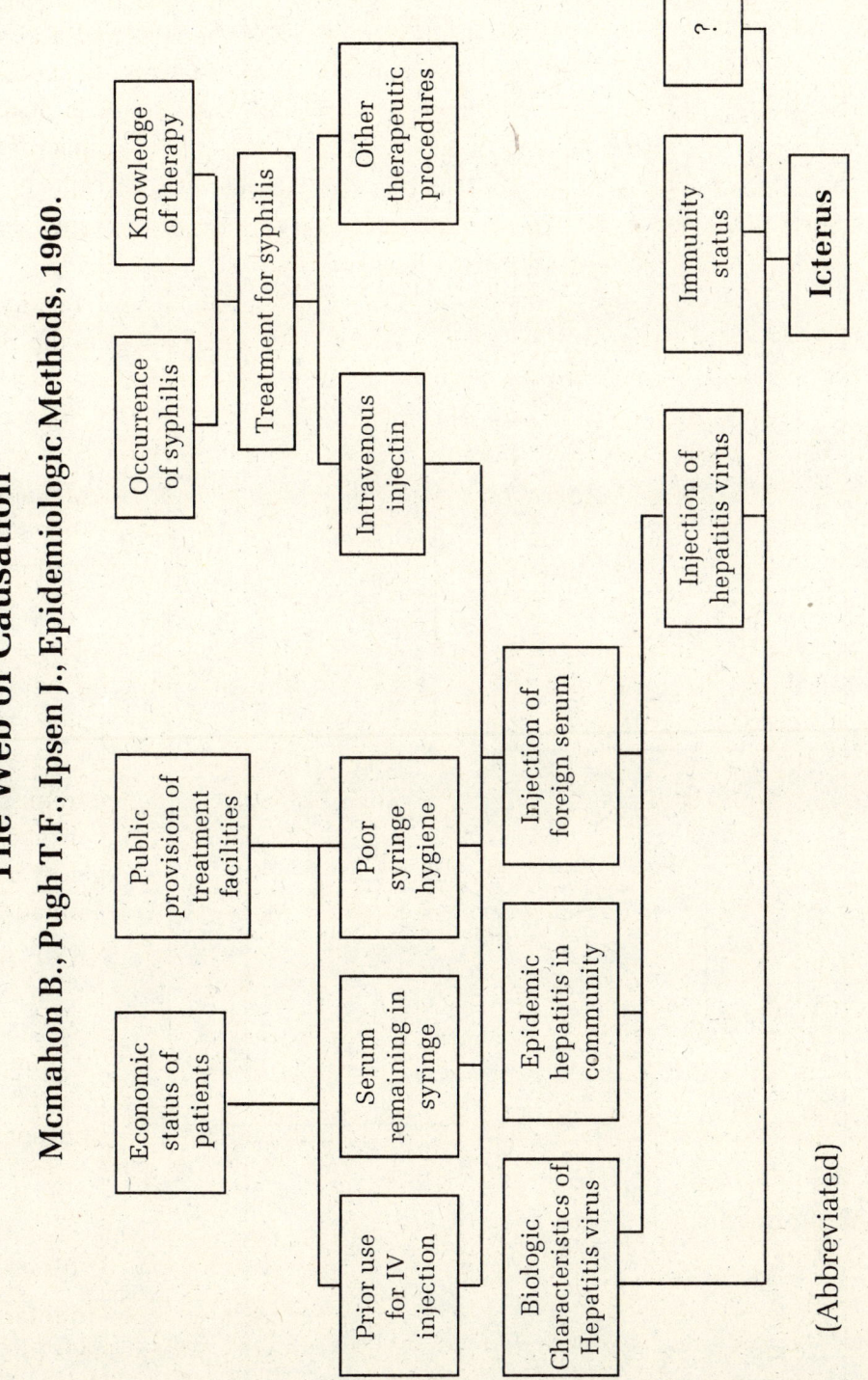

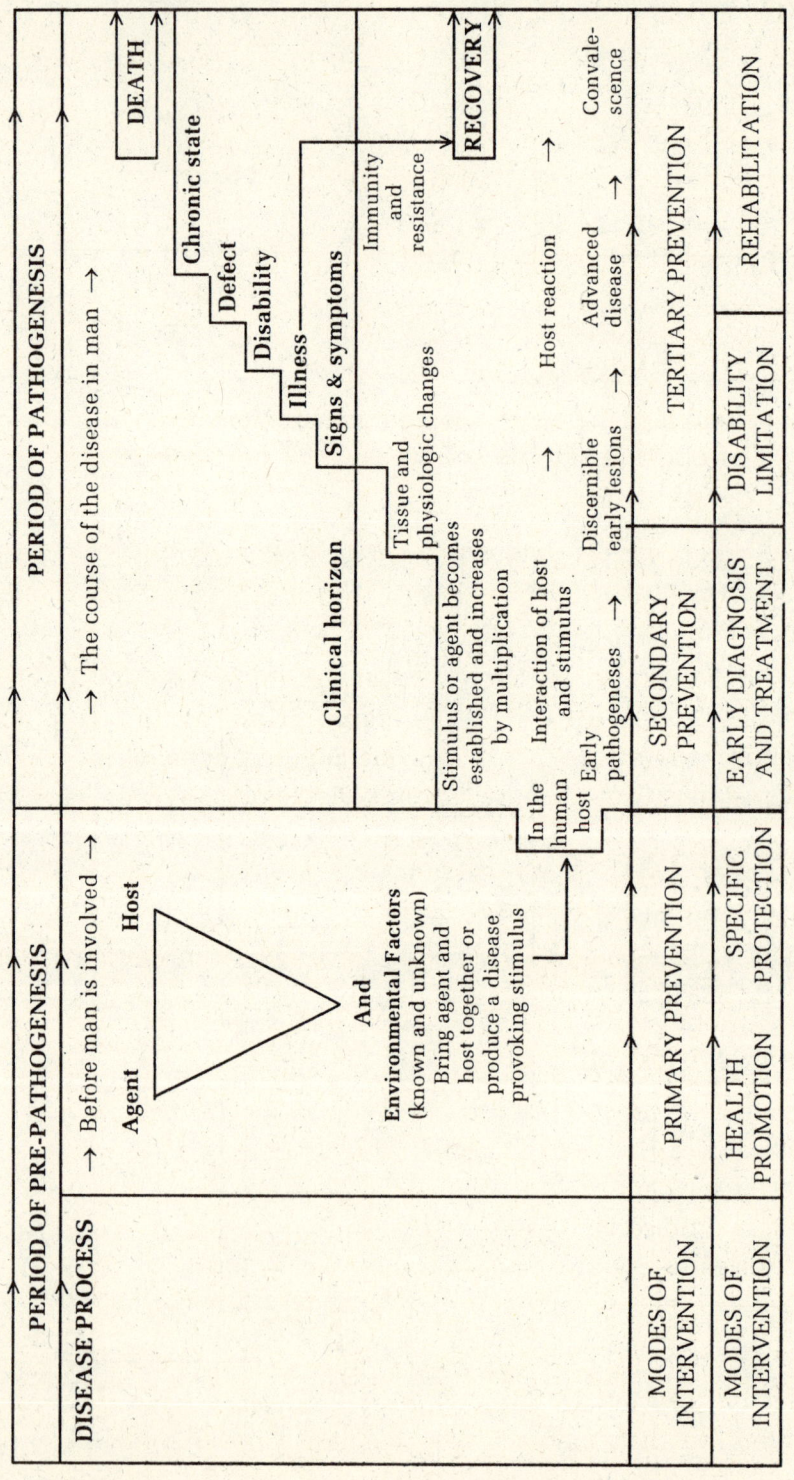

Natural History of Disease

(From Preventive Medicine for the Doctor in his Community by Leavell & Clark with permission of McGraw-Hill Book Co.)

Pathogenesis Phase

The phase takes its course with the onset of disease. Then many changes then take place resulting in clinical symptoms and signs. The disease from there can take a no. of courses available such as recovery, chronic state, disability or death.

Most of the medical intervention are found in this phase like chemo therapy, surgery, etc. But this general course of disease differs for different diseases.

Homoeopathic Concept

Hahnemann noticed "Three different important moments" with respect to the origin of acute infectious diseases, which are as follows :

1. The moment of infection;
2. The period of time during which the whole organism is being penetrated by the disease infused, until it has developed within; ('incubation period' in modern terminology) and
3. The breaking out of the external ailment, whereby nature externally demonstrates the completion of the internal development of the miasmatic malady throughout the whole organise (vide Hahnemann's Chronic Diseases pp. 33, 2nd edition).

CONCEPTS OF PREVENTION

It is often said 'prevention is better then cure'. Prevention is one of the best approach in combating disease. Many times prevention is the only cure e.g. HIV.

Hahnemann's View on Concept of Prevention

The concept of prevention also exists in homoeopathic system of therapeutics. Infact Hahnemann dreamt about the scope of prevention long before the modern medical science, and expressed in aphorism 4. "He is likewise a preserver of health if he knows the things that derange health and cause disease, and how to remove them from persons in health."

Hahnemann's essay "Friend of Health" 1792 and 1795 give an elaborate discussion about prevention and prophylaxis.

For effective prevention nature history of disease must be known and depending on that, methods of prevention can be derived.

Levels of Prevention

There are four levels of prevention :
- Primordial prevention;
- Primary prevention;
- Secondary prevention and
- Tertiary prevention.

Primordial Prevention

It is based on prevention of the emergence or development of risk factors e.g. primordial prevention of lung cancer by health giving education to small children about the harmful effects of smoking.

Primary Prevention

It is based on intervention before the onset of the disease i.e. action taken for the prevention of the disease in 'Pre-pathogenesis phase'.

The mode of intervention at this level of prevention are :
- Health promotion.
- Specific protection.

For primary prevention of chronic diseases WHO recommends following strategies :

(a) Population (Mass) Strategy : Whole population is aimed at for intervention in the form of health education, environmental modifications, life-style and behavioural changes.

(b) High Risk Strategy : It is aimed at persons who are at risk of getting a particular disease when the risk factors are already present.

Secondary Prevention

It can be defined as action which aims to the disease at its incipient stage and prevent the future outcome and complications. The modes of intervention at this level of prevention are 'early diagnosis and treatment'.

Tertiary Prevention

Here the disease has already done the damage, so, the aim is to reduce the impairments, disabilities, sufferings and help patient return to normal social life.

The modes of interventions at this level are :
- Disability limitation and
- Rehabilitation.

Impairment : Loss/abnormality of physical/psychological/anatomical structure or function e.g. loss of foot, mental retardation, etc..

Disability

The impaired person is unable to carry out certain activities normal for his age & sex. This is disability. It is the restriction or loss of ability to perform an activity in the normal manner.

Handicap : A disadvantage for a given individual, resulting from disability or impairment due to which his normal functions in the society are hampered.

Rehabilitation

Combined & coordinated use of medical, social, educational & vocational measures for training & retraining the individuals to the highest possible level of functional ability (WHO).
- It is not centered around the community.
- Preventable & curative measures not included.

Objectives

- To help individual adapt to his surrounding.
- To reduce the impact of inabilities due to disability/handicapping.
- Social integration of individual.

    Impairment → Disability → Handicap.
- Serial & enviornmental factors can increase/decrease the condition of handicapping.

    Rehabilitation should be aimed at integrating the individual & his/her environment.

Special problems with disabled/handicapped

1. Decreased/complete loss of bodily/mental incapabilities.
2. Treated with suffer ignorance, prejudices, revulsion,
3. Economic, social, eduucational, legal etc. barriers hamper achievement of fulfilled life.
4. Frequently suffer humiliation.

5. Fidelity excluded from school, play, marriage & employment.
6. Lack of facilities for treatment, education & rehabilitation except big urban centres.

Principles of Rehabilitation

(1) Detailed house to house survey at the onset.
- It include those persons who are actually considered disabled by the community without superimposing medical/cultural preoccupied definition.

(2) Community based rehabilitation.
- Mass IEC campaign.
- Resource generation.
- Manpower (voluntary disabled workers) development.

(3) Most rehabilitation & treatment should take at the home or in the community with loving support of family, neighbours & friends.

(4) Therapy

Physiologist : Art of improving position, movement, strength, balance & control of the body.

Occupational treatment : The art of helping a disabled person to learn the useful/enjoyable activities.

(5) Detailed examination of each disabled person by specialists/trained persons.

(6) Aids & appliances using local materials & skill.

(7) Promoting self help groups.

(8) Ensure access to educational facilities.

(9) Promoting special schools having the facilities of different learning aids for disabled persons.

(10) Vocational rehabilitation : Ultimate mission of entire rehabilitation process.
- Vocational guidance.
- Training.
- Selective placement.

(11) Promoting accessibility to recreational facilities.

E.g. visually impaired child/person :
- Treatment if possible to decrease impairment.

- Blind school : **Braille**, etc.
- Recreational facilities.
- Vocational guidance.

Resources for Disabled

Education & Training :

(1) Scholarship :

  (a) *Ministry of Welfare* → For general education from Class IX onwards.

    Reader's allowance → For the blinds.

  (b) Deptt. of Social Welfare State Govt. : To pursue education from Class 1 to 8.

(2) Programme of Integrated Education :

- Ministry of HRD & Deptt. of Education : Central Govt. bears 100% expenditure.
- UGC provides a special grant to cover the appointment of reader.

Employment

- Special employment exchange (Ministry of Labour & State Govt.).
- Vocational rehabilitation centres : Madras, Ludhiana, Bombay, Calcutta & Kanpur.
- DRC (Distt. Rehabilitation Centres) : Ministry of Welfare.
- National awards (Ministry of Welfare)
  - outstanding physically handicapped employee.
  - efficient handicapped employee.
  - outstanding placement officer.
- Economic assistance for self employment.
- 1% vacancies resumed for each of blind, deaf & handicapped in group C&D in central services.
- Concessions/relaxation of age.

Other facilities

By railways : 75% concession for blind & the escort.

Roadways : Full to 50% concession in state bus.

Air : 50% concession for blinds.

Legislation

(1) Rehabilitation council of India act 1992
- Regulates training of rehabilitated professionals & maintenance of Central Rehabilitation Register.

(2) Persons & Disability Act 1996.
- Previous & early detection of disables.
- Education.
- Employment.
- Affirmative axes.
- Non-discrimination.
- Mass IEC campaign.

CHAPTER-3

PRINCIPLES OF EPIDEMIOLOGY AND EPIDEMIOLOGIC METHODS

BRIEF HISTORY OF EPIDEMIOLOGY

In the 5th century BC, Hippocrates described the importance of the environment in disease development.

Classical Epidemiology : Study of infectious disease epidemics.

Edward Jenner (1749 – 1823)

In 1978, Jenner observed that the "person who has been thus affected is for ever after secure from the infection of the small pox".

Inoculation against small pox up to that time had been with small pox effluence – the inoculation caused a milder from of the disease. Jenner performed an experiment with only one subject : a boy was inoculated with cox-pox effluence; several months later he was inoculated with Small pox effluence and did not become ill. Following this experiment, use of cox-pox effluence to prevent small pox became norm. The orthopox virus was not identified until 1958.

John Snow (1813 – 1858)

Snow postulated that cholera was transmitted by contaminated water, although the mechanism was not known. Snow observed that death rates for cholera were high among those receiving water from the Lambeth company and the South wark & Vauxhall company Both the companies took their water from a heavily polluted point in the Thames River. The Lambeth company changed its source to an area with less pollution, and cholera death rates declined in areas of the city supplied from this new source. Snow charted the occurence and distribution of cholera among houses supplied by both water companies and was able to show convincingly that the South wark and Vauxhall company was responsible for the outbreak of cholera in London in 1849. Vibrio cholera was discovered as the causal agent in cholera 44 years later in 1893.

James Lind (1716 – 1794)

Classical Epidemiology : Study of nutritional deficiencies.

In 1753, Lind described the occurrence of scurvy in relation to environmental conditions and dietary habits on board the ship, Salisbury. Based on observations, he conducted an experiment where he treated men with scurvy with a variety of nutritional supplements, including vinegar and citrus fruits. The results showed that scurvy could be prevented and successfully treated with the addition of oranges, lemons and limes to the diet of the sailors. In 1928, ascorbic acid was identified as the vitamin which prevents scurvy.

Joseph Goldberger (1874 – 1927)

Pellagra was originally considered an infectious disease until Goldberger recognized that there seemed to be no transmission from sick patients to the healthy nurses. He observed that the diets of those affected with pellagra had very little meat or other animal protein food, and substantially more vegetable foods, especially corn. He then investigated whether it was a lack of meat or milk that lead to the disease, by examining households with low milk intake by the amount of milk consumed, and by examining households with low milk intake by the amount of meat consumed. Both meat and milk were independent contributors to the development of pellagra. An experiment began is 1914 in which he increased the dietary offerings of meat, milk and eggs, and replaced grits with oat meal in several institutions, following institution of the new diet, pellagra essentially disappeared. Niacin, the specific food factor associated with development of pellagra, was identified in 1924.

MODERN EPIDEMIOLOGY

Some very important studies conducted during the phase of epidemiology of chronic diseases were :

- **Case-control study** design of Doll & Hill for relation of smoking and lung cercinoma.
- **Cohort design** (Framinghem 1948). The most important contribution of this study was coining of the term "Risk factor".

Various risk factors associated with development of heart diseases were identified.

- **Randomized Clinical Trial (RCT)** : Hypertension detection and follow up program cooperative group. For testing two treatment modalities used for treating hypertension.

DEFINITION OF EPIDEMIOLOGY

Epidemiology is a quantitative science and practice concerned with the occurrence and determinants of states of health and disease in populations.

Epidemiology is defined by Last as the study of the distribution and determinants of health – related states or events in specified population, and the application of this study to control health problems. Elements of this definition includes :

Study : Surveillance, observation, hypothesis testing, analytic research and experiments.

Distribution : Analysis by time, place and person.

Determinants : Physical, biological, social, cultural and behavioral factors that influence health.

Health – related states or events : Disease, causes of death, behaviour, reactions to preventive regimens, and provision & use of health services.

Specified populations : Groups of people with identifiable characteristics.

Application to control : It refers to the goal of epidemiology, that is to assess the public health importance of diseases, identify the population at risk, identify the causes of disease, describe the natural history of disease, and evaluate the prevention & control of disease.

Epidemiology is based on the scientific method; a systematic approach that incorporates observation, experimentation, measurement, hypothesis testing and refinement of theory.

In the epidemiologic process, researchers :

(a) Ask a well focused question;

(b) Test the hypothesis;

(c) Interpret the results;

(d) Assess causality.

Epidemiologic methods are used in clinical medicine for disease surveillance, disease causality, diagnostic testing, describing the natural history of diseases, screening for prognostic factors and testing new treatments.

Aims

To describe the health status of populations :
- Enumerating the occurrence of diseases.
- Obtaining relative frequencies within groups.
- Discovering important trends.

To explain the etiology of diseases :
- Discovering causal factors.
- Discovering modes of transmission.

To predict the occurrence of disease :
- Actual numbers of cases.
- Distributions within populations.

To control the distribution of disease :
- Prevention of new occurrences.
- Identification and timely treatment of existing cases.
- Reduction of sequela of disease.
- Prolongation of life for those suffering with the disease.

Frequency Measurements

The occurrence of disease or outcome or other factors of interest are described using two primary measurements of frequency : prevalence and incidence.

Measures of disease frequency can be ratios, proportions or rates. Number alone are less helpful because they lack denominator data. So, there is no sense of the relative importance of the frequency.

Frequencies can be measured as :
1. **Ratio** : Value obtained by dividing one quantity by another.
2. **Proportion** : A ratio where the numerator is always part of denominator and often expressed as a percentage.
3. **Rate** : The rapidity with which newly diagnosed diseases develop; a change in one quantity per unit change in another, the denominator is usually person-time. In a cohort study, 50 participants were followed over 5 years to determine if they

developed lung cancer. The rate of developing lung cancer in this study was 17/50 persons 5 years or cases of lung cancer per person — year.

MEASUREMENTS IS EPIDEMIOLOGY

(a) Measurement of morbidity.
(b) Measurement of mortality.
(c) Measurement of disability.
(d) Measurement of fertility (natality).
(e) Measurement of health care facilities, utilization, of health care services and other related events.
(f) Measurement of the pressure, absence or distribution of the environmental, socio-economic factors suspected of causing the disease.
(g) Measurement of nutritional status.
(h) Measurements of demographic variables.
(i) Measurements of the pressure, absence or distribution of the characteristic or attributes of the disease.

Measurement of Morbidity

1. Prevalence (a proportion):

The number of existing cases in the population to the proportion of the population at a given time that have the factor of interest. We can describe the prevalence of an exposure or we can describe the prevalence of outcome. The numerator includes all these with the attribute at a particular time; the denominator includes all the population at risk of having the attribute during that same period.

$$p = \frac{\text{Number of current prevailing cases (old and new)}}{\text{Estimated population at the same point of time}} \times 100$$

There are two general type of prevalence used in epidemiology, point prevalence and period prevalence.

(a) Point Prevalence

The probability of an individual in the population having the disease at a specific point in time. The point in time is the point of actual physical examination or data collection.

$$p = \frac{\text{Number of prevailing cases at a point in time}}{\text{Number in the population at the same point of time}} \times 100$$

(b) Period Prevalence

The probability of an individual in the population for the disease during a specific period of time.

$$p = \frac{\text{Number of prevailing cases at the start} + \text{New cases during follow up}}{\text{Number in population at start}} \times 100$$

2. Incidence :

The probability (risk) of an individual developing the disease during a specific period of time.

$$p = \frac{\text{Number of new cases of disease over a study period}}{\text{Population at risk at the start of the study}} \times 100$$

There are two types of incidence measured in epidemiology; cumulative and incidence density.

(a) Cumulative Incidence : A proportion or a risk. Risk is a measure of the occurrence of new cases in a population. Risks are most useful to the individual; risks describe the probability that this patient will develop disease over a specified time period.

$$I_{c1} = \frac{\text{Number of new cases developing among disease free during a defined time period}}{\text{Number in the population at risk for developing the disease}}$$

(b) Incidence Density : A rate. The rate which describes the rapidity with which new cases develop.

$$I_{density} = \frac{\text{Number cases of disease during a time period}}{\text{Total person - Time of experience}}$$

Measurement of Mortality

Various types of mortality rates and ratios are there to express mortality data.

Mortality Rate (cumulative mortality)

Denominator : Population group exposed to the risk of death.
Numerator : Number of death in a specified population.
Time period : Year in which death occurred.

Crude Mortality Rate

Crude measures are often calculated with mid-year population as the denominator.

Expressed per 1,000 or 10,000 and with reference to year and place.

$$\text{Crude Mortality Rate} = \frac{\text{Number of deaths from a disease or all causes}}{\text{Estimated mid-year population}}$$

More specific mortality measures can be calculated by restricting the numerator to a certain group, such as cause of death, age, gender or ethnicity or a combination of any of these factors.

Cause Specific Mortality Rate

$$\text{Cause specific mortality rate} = \frac{\text{Deaths from a specific cause}}{\text{Estimated mid-year population}}$$

Age Specific Mortality Rate

$$\text{Age specific mortality rate} = \frac{\text{Number of deaths in a specific age group}}{\text{Number of person of that age in mid-year population}}$$

Sex Specific Mortality Rate

$$\text{Age specific mortality rate} = \frac{\text{Number of deaths in a specific sex group}}{\text{Number of persons of that sex in the mid-year population}}$$

Infant Mortality (a ratio)

$$\text{Infant mortality rate} = \frac{\text{Number of deaths in a year among infants less than 1 year of age}}{\text{Number of live births in the same year}}$$

Usually presented per 1000 live births per year.

Neonatal Mortality (a ratio)

$$\text{Neonatal mortality rate} = \frac{\text{Number of deaths in a year among infants less than 28 days of age}}{\text{Number of live births in the same year}}$$

Parinatal Mortality (a ratio)

$$\text{Perinatal mortality rate} = \frac{\text{Fetal death } (\geq 28 \text{ weeks of gestation}) + \text{perinatal death } (<7 \text{ days of life})}{\text{Fetal death + live births in the same year}}$$

Case Fatality Rate (a proportion)

$$\text{Case Fatality Rate} = \frac{\text{No. of deaths after onset of specific disease}}{\text{Number diagnosed with disease}}$$

METHODS OF EPIDEMIOLOGY

The steps in the epidemiological approach to study disease etiology are :

(1) Initial observation of the event, disease, etc. in population.
(2) Definition of the disease or process by
   (a) Clinical presentation (signs and symptoms).
   (b) Specific etiological agent.
(3) Descriptive epidemiology : identifying associations of disease in relation to :
   (a) time,
   (b) place and
   (c) person
(4) Analytical Epidemiology :
   (a) Identification of associations of disease with possible etiological factors like genetic, environmental etc.
   (b) Refining and testing of hypotheses.
(5) Experimental Epidemiology : For evaluation of the effectiveness of interventions and of preventive and therapeutic programs.

   It involves various study trials like :
   (a) Randomized controlled trials or clinical trials.
   (b) Field trials.
   (c) Community trials.

Analytical Epidemiology

The main utility of Analytical studies is not formulation of hypotheses but testing them with various study designs unlike descriptive

epidemiology which takes into account the whole population, in analytical studies individuals or groups of individuals are taken up for study. 3 types of analytical studies are used etc. :
- (a) Cross sectional studies.
- (b) Case control studies.
- (c) Cohort study.

Cross Sectionmal Studies

A observational study also called as disease frequency survey or prevalence Study. They are more useful for recording disease prevalence rather than incidence. Here a cross section of population is examined at a point of time and the results are projected on the whole population. They are useful for presence of association rather than hypothesis testing. These studies are unable to determine temporality or draw casual inferences. It can possibly help in formation of casual hypothesis from study of distribution patterns and can be considered cross sectional study is exposure is unalterable over a period of time.

It provides very little information regarding incidence and "natural history of disease" e.g. a cross sectional study of pap smear in sex workers (no. = 10,000)

Trait	Number	% of Sample
(i) Ever had Pap smear?		
No	3000	30%
Yes	7000	70%
(ii) Number of Pap Smears (at 3 years interval)		
One	2500	
Two	2000	
Three	1200	
Four	800	
Five or more	500	

Longitudinal Studies :

They are also called as **incidence studies**. They are based on repeated observations in the same population over a period of time by means of follow up examinations. This way new cases appearing are picked up and thus helps in calculation of incidence rates of that disease. Unlike cross sectional studies they give information about the natural history of disease and its future course. As they require follow up attrition problems arise and are costly too.

Case Control Studies

It is also known as "Retrospective Studies". They are 1st approach to test causal hypothesis. It is a study that starts with the identification of persons with the disease of interest and a suitable control group of persons without disease. The relationship of an attribute to the disease is examined by comparing the diseased and non diseased with regard to how frequently the attribute is present or if quantitative, the levels of the attribute in each of the groups.

Some important features of this type of study are :

(a) Both exposure and disease have occurred before the study starts.

(b) Starts after the onset of disease and proceeds to postulated cause i.e. it proceeds backwards from effect to cause.

(c) Preferred study if :

    (i) The disease to be studied is relatively rare and only a little information is available about the disease.

    (ii) Several exposures may be associated with the disease of interest.

'Cases' and 'Controls' are used for this type of study. For explaining 'case' and 'control', we have take a simple design or a case control study.

The hypothesis selected for our example is "high fat diet causes coronary artery disease". First for 'cases' we take patients with the disease and for 'controls' persons free of the disease. Further the 'cases' and 'controls' are divided on the basis of presence or absence of suspected etiological factor i.e. high fat diet.

Risk factor	Cases (Disease present)	Controls (Disease absent)
Present	a	b
Absent	$\dfrac{c}{(a+b)}$	$\dfrac{d}{(c+d)}$

Procedure

(1) Selection of cases.

(2) Selection of controls.

(3) Comparison of demographic information.

(4) Measurement of exposure.

(5) Analysis and interpretation.

Selection of Cases

It is very important first to make sure that the case selected is representative of the disease. There is a diagnostic and eligibility criteria for the selection of the case. Same diagnostic method must be used for all cases. The various sources for obtaining cases are — hospitals, general population etc.

Selection of Controls

Controls are the ones who are free of disease. They must be selected along with cases. They can be obtained from hospitals, neighbourhood controls, relatives, etc.

The selection of both cases and controls is very important because they form the basis of the study. 'Selection bias' must be avoided at this stage.

Comparison and Matching

Matching is defined as a process by which controls are selected in such a manner that they are similar to cases with regard to certain selected variables which are known to influence the out come of the disease and if not properly matched can 'confound' the results. A confounding factor is associated to both exposure and disease and distributed unequally in cases and controls.

Confounding

It is mixing of effects between the exposure and the disease by other factors associated with both the exposure and the disease such that the effects of the two processes are not separated e.g. in a study of effect of exercise on the occurrence of coronary artery disease, age could be a confounding agent. Confounding may be adjusted in the study design or in the final analysis of the data collected by —

- Randomization : Assures equal distribution of confounders between study and control groups.
- Restriction : Subjects are restricted by the levels of a known confounder.
- Matching : Potential confounding factors are equally distributed between the study groups.
- Stratification in the analysis : Risk estimates are computed for the various levels of potential confounders.
- Can control for confounding in the analysis of the data.

While matching it should be kept in mind **not to match the suspected etiological factors** we want to measure. The matching can be done by group matching or pair matching.

Measurement of Exposure

It can be done by obtaining data from hospital records, medical records, death certificates, registries, questionnaires, surveys etc.

Analysis and Interpretation

Two types rates ratio are used to express the results. Exposure and Odds ratio :

(a) Exposure Rates :

Here the frequency of exposure is calculated in both case and control groups.

For cases exposure rate is = $\dfrac{a}{a+c}$

For controls exposure rate is = $\dfrac{b}{b+d}$

(b) Relative Risk :

It is used for estimation of the risk associated with exposure. It is also called 'risk ratio'.

$$\text{Relative risk} = \dfrac{\text{Incidence rate of exposed group}}{\text{Incidence rate of non exposed group}} \times 100$$

$$= \dfrac{a}{(a+b)} \Big/ \dfrac{c}{(c+d)}$$

(c) Odds Ratio :

It describes the strength of association of between the risk factor and disease.

Odds Ratio = a d/b c

Bias in Case Control Studies

Bias – 'Systematic' errors in 'collecting' or interpreting data such that there is deviation of results or inferences from the truth. Bias results from the systematic faults in study design, data collection, the analysis or interpretation of results.

There are various kinds of bias like confounding bias (discussed earlier), selection bias, information bias, Berkesonion bias (based on problem of difference in admission rates in hospital), etc.

1. Selection Bias : Non-comparable criteria used to enroll participants. Theoretically, the controls and the cases must have had same opportunity to be exposed to the factors of interest.

2. Information Bias : Non-comparable information is obtained from the study group, due to interviewer bias, or due to recall bias.

Example of case control studies

(Doll & Hill, Smoking and carcinoma of the lung : Preliminary report. British Medical Journal 2:739, 1950) Information was obtained from over 700 men and women with lung cancer and a similar number of patients hospitalized for nonmalignant conditions. Cigarette smoking was associated with lung cancer but not with the other nonmalignant conditions.

Cohort Study

It is another type of analytical study also known as prospective study, longitudinal study, incidence study. It is just opposite to case control study as it proceeds forward from cause to effect i.e. the cohorts are selected prior to occurrence of disease and are then observed over a period of time to estimate the disease frequency among them. Most of the times done it is only after supplementation from other studies:

- Cohort is a group of individuals sharing a common trait or a experience among them e.g. age, exposure, occupation, etc.

Cohort studies are useful when :

- There is evidence supporting that a relationship exists between the risk factor and the disease.
- The incidence of disease is higher among the exposed ones even though the exposure is rare.
- Follow up is possible i.e. nutrition problem, lack of funds, etc. can be minimised.

The cohorts are free of disease at the time of commencement of the disease. Both the exposed ones and non exposed ones are equally susceptible to the disease under study and are comparable to each other in respect to all the possible variable.

Types of Cohort Studies

(a) Prospective Cohort Studies :

Here the disease has not yet occurred among the cohorts, exposure level is measured at the base line and then cohorts are followed for occurrence of disease.

(b) Retrospective Cohort Studies

Disease has already occurred before the start of the study. The researcher uses the historical data to determine exposure level at base line then find out the disease frequency i.e. form cohorts from the data available; then looks for disease frequency among the exposed ones and non exposed ones. Data is obtained from hospital records, employment records, mortality records, etc.

(c) Historical Prospective Cohort Study

Also called 'embispective study', here both type of studies i.e. prospective and retrospective studies are combined.

Procedure

(1) Selection of cohorts
(2) Obtaining exposure data
(3) Selection of comparison groups
(4) Follow up
(5) Analysis.

Attributable Risk Percent

It is the percent of disease/death among exposed, that is attributable to exposure. It is not affected by prevalence of exposure.

$$\frac{\text{Incidence in exposed - Incidence in unexposed}}{\text{Incidence in exposed group}}$$

It is same as :
- Attributable proportion and
- Etiologic fraction (for exposed).

Preventable Fraction

It is the estimation of what might be achieved by a community based public health program.

Prevented Fraction

It is a useful measurement of what has been achieved by a program : $= P_1 (1-RR) (RR + P_1[1-RR])$

P_1 is the proportion of the population that accepts the intervention.

Relative Risk

As discussed earlier relative risk is the ratio of incidence of the disease/death among the exposed and the incidence among non exposed.

e.g.

Smoking	Disease	No disease
Yes	a	b
No	c	d

disease = Lung cancer

So, Relative risk = $\dfrac{a}{(a+b)} \Big/ \dfrac{c}{(c+d)}$

Attributable Risk

It is the difference in the incidence rates of disease/death among the exposed and non exposed group.

$$= \dfrac{\text{Incidence of disease among exposed minus incidence of disease among non exposed}}{\text{Incidence rate among exposed}} \times 100$$

Population Attributable Risk (PAR%)

- Percent of disease/death in the population attributable to an exposure.
- High prevalence, high PAR, and vice versa.
- $\dfrac{\text{(Incidence in entire population - incidence in unexposed)}}{\text{Incidence in entire population}}$

Experimental Epidemiology

It is study of diseases in experimental animals and clinical trials in human.

Clinical Trials

I. **Definition** : A prospective study comparing the effect and value of interventions against a control in human subjects.

II. **Essential features** :
   (a) Subjects are followed forward in time : prospective.
   (b) Employ one or more interventions : may be prophylactic, diagnostic, therapeutic agent, devices, regimens or procedures.
   (c) Must have a control group which must be similar to the intervention group at base line.

   Phase I : Evaluates dose and toxicity.
   Phase II : Assesses drug activity.
   Phase III : Clinical trials – comparative trial.

The control group is selected to be virtually similar to the study group in all respects.

(d) Human subjects :
- Concerns regarding subject safety.
- Issues of research ethics and informed consent.

(e) The ideal clinical trial includes both the randomization of subjects and blinding of subjects and care providers.

1. Randomization makes the equal allocation of potential confounders and effect modifiers between the two study groups. These are the factors which are possibly unknown or unpredictable at the onset of the study.
2. Blinding attempts to eliminate bias, which might be introduced by either the participating subject or care providers :
   - Single blinding
   - Double blinding.

III. Other Characteristics

(a) Need :
   1. Most definitive method of determining whether an intervention has the postulated effect.
   2. Uncertainty regarding diseases, their natural history and therapy and its positive and negative effects.
   3. The consequences of not conducting appropriate clinical trail can be serious and costly in the long run.

   E.g.
   - Use of CPAP in COPD patients.
   - Use of digitalis in congestive heart failure.
   - Uncontrolled use of high concentrations of O_2 in premature neonates.

(b) Timing :
   1. Must be performed before drugs or interventions have become part of routine medical practice.
   2. Early in the development of new therapies, but
   3. Only after sufficient knowledge is available concerning efficacy and safety.
   4. Should not be conducted if therapy will be outdated before or shortly after the trial has conducted.

(c) Ethics :
1. Fundamental ethical principles regarding research are :
   (i) Respect for persons : Individuals should be treated as autonomous. Those with diminished autonomy need protection.
   (ii) Beneficence :
   - Secure the well being of the individual.
   - Benefit for society/class of patients.
   (iii) Justice : treat persons fairly. Equally share the risks and benefits.
2. Ethical Norms dictate that there should be :
   (i) Good research design :
   - Randomization
     * May be a problem if the treatment is known or perceived to be superior to placebo.
     * Trial may be unethical.
   - Placebo control
     * Problems of an acceptable placebo.
     * Deprivation of treatment.
   - Monitoring of the trial
     * How to handle available data as it acrues.
     * Safety monitoring committee.
   (ii) Competent investigators.
   (iii) Favorable balance of harm and benefit :
   - Welfare of the subject/physician's obligation to his patient.
   - Societal good.
   (iv) Informed consent : cannot always be obtained.
   E.g. minor (infants), comatose subjects, mentally incompetent, prisoners, emergency procedures, pregnant woman/foetus.
   (v) Equitable selection of subjects.
   (vi) Compensation for research related injury.

IV. Essential Components

Generally, these criteria may be applied to virtually all clinical investigations.

A. Review of the scientific background for the study.
- Previous animal investigations or laboratory works.

- Preliminary human evidence from case reports or case series.
B. Development of specific written hypothesis to be tested.
    - Random testing for statistical significance is unjustifiable.
    - Specific methods are available if multiple testing is to be used.
C. Study Design :
   1. Basic study design.
      (a) Randomized or controlled trial.
      (b) Non-randomized concurrent controlled study.
      (c) Historical controls : Non-randomized, non-concurrent.
      (d) Cross over designs : Subject serves as own control.
      (e) Withdrawal studies : Assesses response to withdrawal of intervention or a reduction of dosage.
      (f) Factorial design : Assesses the response to more than one intervention.
   2. Study population.
      (a) Specific inclusion and exclusion criteria are necessary.
      (b) Calculation of sample size – Power calculations or curve.
   3. Planned statistical analysis/data needs.
      (a) What is/are the dependent and independent variables? How will these be measured or evaluated?
      (b) How will the bias be controlled?
      (c) Are there specific effect modifiers and or confounders which need to be considered in the planning of the study and analysis of the data?
      (d) What measurements are needed and how is the validity and accuracy of the measure to be confirmed?
      (e) What are the preliminary plans for statistical analysis?
      (f) On the basis of sample size calculations can the study be completed?
         - Alpha error, beta error, effect size and estimation of variance.
         - What about the loss of subjects and how will this be considered in the final analysis?

- If a significant difference exists between groups, can it in fact be demonstrated : does the study have adequate power?
- (g) How will attrition or loss to follow up be handled?
- (h) Did the investigators employ the services of a bio statistician or epidemiologist : check authors and acknowledgments?
4. Enrollments of subjects.
   - (a) Informed consent.
   - (b) Assessment of eligibility.
   - (c) Base line studies/examinations.
   - (d) Allocation to study group :
     - Random allocation involves more than alternate assignment.
     - Use of randomization scheme.
     - Blocked randomization schemes are sometimes used to assure equal distribution of study subjects between groups.
5. Intervention.
   - (a) Description and schedule.
   - (b) Measures of compliance.
   - (c) Measures of the reliability of tools used.
   - (d) Criteria for termination of intervention.
   - (e) Criteria for withdrawal or loss of subject.
6. Follow-up of subjects.
7. Ascertainment of response variables.
   - (a) Training.
   - (b) Data collection.
   - (c) Data monitoring and quality control.
   - (d) Data analysis.
   - (e) Are there criteria to determine when the study should be terminated?

D. Organisation :
   1. Participating investigators.
   2. Study administration.
   3. Data monitoring committee.
   4. Human subjects review.

COMMUNICABLE OR TRANSMISSION DISEASE

Agent : A factor that must be present for a disease to occur in a susceptible host. Environmental health professionals are normally concerned with physical, chemical or biological agents. However, psychological and sociological agents are also included.

e.g. – pathogenic microbes, parasitic worms and chemical poisons.

Infection : Growth of a pathogenic microbe in a host (with or without evidence of disease).

Pathogenicity : Capability of producing disease by the infecting organism.

Virulence : Harmfulness of a disease. The most commonly used measure for virulence is, case fatality rate.

Reservoir : Any place where an infectious agent depends primarily for survival in animate objects, but may also include humans.

Host : Any animal (especially human) infected by an agent. Host may be diseased or may be an intermediate host.

Incubation Period : It is the time interval between invasion by infective agent & the appearance of clinical features i.e. signs and symptoms of the disease. During the period the infectious agent multiplies in the host.

Carrier : A person or animal that harbors an organism of disease without showing symptoms.

A Symptomatic Carrier : A carrier that never shows symptoms. Process is also called as 'inapparent infection'.

Transmission : Any mechanism by which a susceptible human host is exposed to an infectious agent.

Fomites : Inanimate objects which harbor or transmit infectious organisms.

Vector : Insect or other animal that may transfer pathogens to humans.

Serial Interval : The period between 1° & 2° cases is called **serial interval**. It is in the pathogenesis phase of the natural history of disease.

Attack Rate : It is the incidence rate used only when the population is exposed to risk of a disease only for a limited period of time, as in epidemics.

LD-50 or LD_{50} : Lethal dose for 50% of the exposed subjects. A low LD_{50} indicates a very toxic substance, because it says that a small dose is capable of killing half the population. A different measure is LD_{50} which is the lethal concentration for 50% of the population. Concentration refers to measured amounts in the environment, whereas dose refers to measured amounts in the body.

Epidemic : In a community occurrence of an illness of similar nature in excess of normal expected frequency & derived from a common source or propagated source. It consists of acute as well as chronic cases.

Endemic : Continuous occurrence of a disease in a specific geographical area.

Pandemic : When a disease spreads from one country to another (or across continents) in a short time or at the same time in different countries.

Trend : The general pattern or time distribution of a disease is known as a trend. It may be described by the time of its occurrence.

Types :

1) Short term fluctuations : Occurrence of a disease as an epidemic.
2) Mid-term fluctuations : Seen in communicable diseases.
3) Long-term fluctuations : Secular trends implying changes over time, generally several years/decades.
   e.g. : In diabetes/long term diseases.

Case Fatality Ratio : The ratio of total no. of deaths due to a particular disease & total no. of cases due to that disease expressed as percentage is called case fatality ratio.

$$CFR = \frac{Number\ of\ death\ due\ to\ diseases}{Number\ of\ cases} \times 100$$

Importance : It represents killing power of the disease. It is used only in acute infectious diseases. Its use in chronic diseases is limited as the period of onset to death is variable. It is closely related to virulence of organism.

DISEASE TRANSMISSION

This section looks at how the disease is transmitted and introduces the concepts of standard and additional precautions which are used to control the transmission of disease. Many micro-organisms, important in endoscopy are also covered.

Transmission of Disease

The world is teeming with micro organisms, many of which are harmless to humans. To cause an infection, pathogenic organisms need to gain access to a susceptible human body.

The spread of infection requires three elements :
- Source of infecting micro-organisms.
- Means of transmission for the micro-organism.
- A susceptible host.

To prevent infection, it is necessary to eliminate at least one of these elements.

Source of Infecting Micro-Organisms

Some infections are caused by the micro-organisms that are already present on or in human body, the reservoir of an infection. These are called as **endogenous infections**. Other infections are caused by the micro-organisms from external environment and are called **exogenous infections**.

Organisms that cause exogenous infections usually have a preferred portal of entry such as the gastrointestinal and respiratory tracts. The intact skin and mucous membrane of the respiratory, gastrointestinal and genitourinary tracts provide a protective barrier against these organisms. If this barrier is damaged or penetrated, then the organisms can potentially gain entry into the body. In most endoscopic procedures the endoscope only comes in contact with intact mucous membranes. However, in some procedures, as in a biopsy, the mucous membrane is damaged.

Transmission of Micro-Organisms

To cause an infection, pathogens have to be transferred from a reservoir or source to a susceptible host. Transmission of most micro-organisms usually occurs from person to person, known as **horizontal transmission**. Transmission from mother to foetus across the placenta is called **vertical transmission**. Horizontal spread of organisms can occur by contact transmission, which involves direct or indirect contact with the reservoir or source.

- Direct contact refers to close contact that results in exposure to skin and body secretions. Organisms can be transmitted from one part of a person's body, such as their skin or an infected wound, to another part of their own body or to another individual.
- Indirect contact occurs when organisms from an infected host or other reservoir are transmitted to a susceptible host via an inanimate object or fomite. In the hospital environment, fomites

can become contaminated and act as sources of infection including medical equipment such as endoscopes, clothing, bedding, dressings and sinks. Gastro-intestinal pathogens such as salmonella can be transmitted by this way.

- Droplet transmission : The transmission of infectious agents in droplet from respiratory secretions by coughings, sneezings or talking, is another form of contact transmission. Pathogens that are transmitted in this way are the cold and influenza viruses and the bacteria responsible for tuberculosis.

Infectious agents can also be transmitted over a wide area to many people by a common vehicle such as food, air or water. Legionnaires' disease is typically transmitted in this way. If the bacteria are present in water they can be dispersed in a fine aerosol spray then carried by air currents over a wide area. Transmission of the disease in this manner is referred to as **airborne transmission**.

Susceptible Host

Whether a particular micro organism infects a person or not depends on the balance between the power of the organism to cause disease, and the power of the body to resist it. A variety of circumstances may increase the risk of infection associated with endoscopy. These include :

- Compromised immune status.
- Procedurally induced tissue damage.
- Presence of intrinsic infective foil.
- Endovascular surface integrity.
- Indwelling foreign material.
- Number and type of infectious agents present on or in the endoscope, its water feed system and accessories.

PRINCIPLES OF DISEASE PREVENTION & CONTROL

Based on the epidemiological triad we can have following interventions :

Control the Agent

For example, we can remove agents before their entry into air, water, and soil. If it is a chemical agent, this may involve simple changes in production processes. If it is a microbial agent, it may involve prohibiting consumption of affected foods, or use of bactericides on preparation surfaces.

Control the Environment

For example, we can control vectors, or treat polluted air, water, and soil. We can also prevent access to an area.

Control the Host

For example, we can take steps to protect the young, the old, and the sick, each of whom may be the high risk individuals. This may involve personal hygiene, immunizations, or health education.

IMMUNITY

The word 'immunes' means exempt. The term immunity signifies all those properties of the host which confer resistance to a specific infectious agent. So the immunity is the ability of the body to resist or overcome infection. The state of resistance is indicated either by the failure of the individual to develop the disease upon exposure or in some cases by the demonstration of specific anti-bodies in the blood which are considered effective against the invading organism.

So, the term immunity implies resistance or non susceptibility to a disease or any organisms, naturally or artificially acquired. It may be against the organisms or the toxin liberated by them.

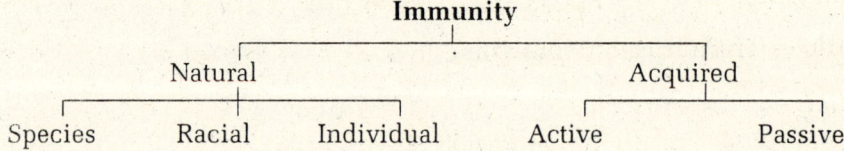

Immunity may be :

(1) Natural or congenital (i.e. from birth).

(2) Acquired (a) Active : By suffering from disease or by vaccination.

        (b) Passive : By serum.

Natural immunity is of following types :

(a) Species : Rats to diphtheria, fowl to tetanus and goat, horse to tuberculosis.

(b) Racial : Negroes to yellow fever, Jews to tuberculosis.

(c) Individual : In smallpox, influenza etc.

Factors Responsible for Immunity

Physical Factors

(a) Integrity of skin and living epithelium of skin and stratified squamous epithelium.

(b) The living epithelium of respiratory and alimentary tract secrete thick tenacious mucus which provides a protective coating, so that bacteria can not penetrate. The ciliated epithelium of respiratory tract by their ciliary movement helps expel out the foreign bodies, bacteria gets entangled due to its stickiness and they are expelled out. This is why, lowering of muco-ciliary resistance of respiratory tract due to any factor will predispose to bacterial infection.

(c) The acid sweat liberated by the skin helps to protect the skin from infection. In other words the sweat acts as outo – sterilising agents.

2. Chemical Factors

(a) Gastric Mechanism : HCL content of stomach has a bactericidal action and it protects against infection of alimentary canal.

(b) Lysozyme : It has bactericidal action and present in all secretion and excretion of the body except urine, sweat and C.S.F. It is present in maximum concentration in lachrymal secretion and cartilages. The conjunctiva is normally kept free from bacterial infection as it is bathed in the lysozyme.

3. Cellulo – Humoral Mechanisms

(a) Cellular Mechanisms : The various phagocytic cells of the system help in the process of phagocytosis of bacteria that lates undergoes intra-cellular lysis. The following are the phagocytic cells :

(i) Cells of circulating blood – Polymorphs and monocytes.

(ii) Cells in the tissue – These are of 2 types –

(I) Fixed cells of particular organs :

(a) Kupffer's cells of liver.

(b) Endothetial cells of bone marrow.

(c) Living cells in the sinus of the lymph gland.

(II) Wandering Cells : Histiocytes and mononuclear cells.

(b) Humoral Mechanisms :

(i) Bactericidal element in blood : There are some bactericidal substances present normally in serum e.g. – L-lysin, Lukin, Plakin, etc.

(ii) Antibodies like : Agglutinin, Bacteriotropin, etc. are produced in the serum which are defensive against infection.

(iii) **Artificial immunity** : It results by the artificial means. It is of 2 types :
   (a) Active
   (b) Passive.

Immunizing Agents

VACCINES

Live attenuated vaccines
- BCG
- Typhoid oral
- Plague ⎫ Bacterial
- Oral polio
- Yellow fever
- Measles
- Rubella ⎬ Viral
- Mumps
- Influenza
- Epi. typhus — Rickettsial

Inactivated or killed vaccines
- Typhoid
- Cholera
- Pertussis
- C.S. Meningitis
- Plague ⎫ Bacterial

- Rabies
- Salk (polio)
- Influenza
- Hepatitis B
- Japanese Encephalitis
- KFD ⎬ Viral

Toxoids
- Diphtheria
- Tetanus ⎫ Bacterial

IMMUNO-GLOBULINS

Human Immuno-globulins
- Hepatitis A
- Measles
- Rabies
- Tetanus
- Mumps ⎬ Human Normal Ig

- Hepatitis B
- Varicella
- Diphtheria ⎬ Human Specific Ig

Non-human (Antisera)
- Diphtheria
- Tetanus
- Gas gangrene
- Botulism ⎫ Bacterial
- Rabies — Viral

Anti Bodies

- Ig G : It is the major serum Immuno-globulin. It may be seen in polymerised form. It is transported across placenta to new born providing natural passive immunity. It acts via :

  (i) Complement fixation.
  (ii) Precipitation.
  (iii) Neutralization of Toxoids etc.
  (iv) Killing target cells coated with Ig G.

- Ig A : It is mostly found in body secretions providing local immunity. It inhibits 'adhesion' of micro organisms to surface of mucosal cells, promotes and intracellular killing of pathogen.

- Ig M : It is a polymer with 5 molecules of Immuno globulin. It is seen in recent infections mostly, as they are short lived. It causes opsonisation of bacteria, immunohemolysis, agglutination, neutralisation of toxins and viruses.

- Ig D : Found mostly intravascularly on surface of B-Lymphocytes (B-cells).

- Ig E – It is an extravascular antibody. It increases in allergic conditions like asthma, hay fever, eczema, etc. It is also responsible for anaphylaxis. It acts via binding to antigen which then leads to degranulation of the mast cell on whose surface it is present. Inflammatory mediators stored in the granules like histamine, serotonin, heparin etc. are released which bring about the inflammatory changes like vasodilatation, increased capillary permeability, migration of other inflammatory cells like neurophils, etc.

Cold Chain Maintenance

Cold Chain : It is a system of storage & transport of vaccines at low temperature from the manufacturer to the actual vaccination site. It is necessary because vaccine failure may occur due to failure to store & transport under strict temperature control.

(1) Polio vaccine : most sensitive to heat.
    : requires storage at $-20°$ C.

(2) Vaccines stored in freezer compartment : OPV & measles.

(3) Vaccines that must be stored in the cold part but never allowed to freeze : DPT, DT, tetanus toxoid, BCG, typhoid vaccine.

(4) At the health centre, most vaccines (except polio) can be stored upto 5 weeks if the refrigerator temperature is strictly kept between 4-8° C.

(5) Opened multi dose vials that have not been fully used should be discarded within 1 hr, if no preservative is present (most live virus vaccines) within 3 hrs., or at the end of a session when a preservative is used.

Cold Chain Equipment :

1. Walk in cold rooms (WIC) : Located at regional level meant to store vaccines upto 3 months and serve 4-5 districts.

2. Deep freezers (300 liters) & ice lined refrigerators (ILRs 300/240 l capacity) : Supplied to all districts & the WIC location to store vaccines. Deep freezers are used for making ice packs & to store OPV & measles vaccines.

3. Small deep freezers & ILR (140 liters) : One set is provided to PHC, Urban Family Planning Centres & Post-partum Centres. Deep freezers are used to prepare frozen ice packs & are used in cold boxes, vaccine carriers for transportation of vaccines & during the sessions. All vaccines at PHC level are stored in the ILR. Vaccines like TT, DPT, DT & diluents are kept in the basket provided in the ILR. A dial thermometer is kept in the ILR & temperature is recorded twice a day. In case of equipment failure or powercut, vaccines should be transferred to ice boxes & then to alternative vaccine storage. Depositing should be done in every 2-3 weeks.

4. Cold Boxes : Supplied to all peripheral centres. These are used mainly for transportation of the vaccines. Before placing the vaccines inside, fully frozen ice packs are placed at the bottom & the sides. The vaccines are first kept in polythene bags. The vials of DPT, DT, TT vaccines & diluents should not be placed in direct contact with frozen ice packs.

5. Vaccine Carriers : For carrying small quantities of vaccines (16-20 vials) for the out-reach sessions & fully frozen ice packs are used for lining the sides. Vials of DPT, DT, TT & diluents should not be placed in direct contact with frozen ice packs.

6. Day Carriers : For 6-8 vials to be carried for a nearby session. Fully frozen packs are to be used. It is used only for few hours period.

7. Ice Packs : They contain water & no salt should be added to it. The water should be fitted upto the level marked on the side. If there is any leakage such ice packs should be discarded.

The risk of cold chain failure is greatest at the sub-centre and village level. Vaccines are not stored at the sub-centre level & must be supplied on the day of use.

8. Portable Vaccine Carrier : Made of polyurethane. Its interior contains 4 recesses to hold ice packs which are plastic containers with screw caps.
9. Reverse Cold Chain : System of storage & transport of vaccines at low temp. from the actual vaccination site to the manufacturer i.e. maintaining cold chain from periphery to the laboratory.

Vaccines

1. **BCG (Bacilli Calmette Guerin) vaccine :**
   - Live attenuated bovine bacilli.
   - Freeze dried preparation – diluent is normal saline (d. H_2O not used – acts as an irritant).
   - Dose 0.1 ml (newborns or < 4 wks – 0.05 ml).
   - Intradermally, just above insertion of deltoid muscle, on left arm.
   - Given at birth in case of institutional deliveries; along with OPV–0 dose or with DPT–1 at 6 wks.
   - Vaccination – Papule in 2-3 wks → Increased diameter to 4-8 mm in about 5 wks. → Subsides & forms a shallow ulcer covered and a crust → Healing occurs in 6-12 wks. → Permanent tiny round scar, typically 4-8 mm in diameter.
   - Contraindication : Patient suffering from generalized eczema, infective dermatitis, hypogamma globulinemia with those & H/O deficient immunity.

2. **DPT (Diphtheria, Pertussis, Tetanus vaccine) :**
   - Mixed vaccine containing diphtheria toxoid, pertussis vaccine (killed) & tetanus toxoid.
   - Dose : 0.5 ml. deep in lateral aspect of thigh or upper outer quadrant of buttocks.
   - Dose : Given at 6 wks. 10 wks., 14 wks. (interval between 2 doses can be 4-6 wks., but not less than 4 wks.).
   - Booster dose given at 16-24 months.
   - Pertussis component not given after 4 years since complications can occur.
   - Complications : Fever, mild local reaction, neurological effects (encephalopathy, prolonged convulsions).
   - Contraindication : Not given in H/O convulsions.
   - OPV is also given with DPT.

3. **OPV (Oral Polio Vaccine – Sabin) vaccine :**
   - Live attenuated Polio virus (Types 1, 2, 3) grown in primary monkey kidney or human diploid cell cultures. Thus, it is a trivalent vaccine.
   - 2 drops given as 1 dose.
   - 6 wks., 10 wks., 14 wks. & DPT.
   - OPV- '0' dose at birth in institutional deliveries.
   - 16-24 months – OPV booster.
   - Also given during pulse polio immunization to all children between 0-5 years of age for polio eradication (herd immunity).
   - Complications : None.
   - Contraindication : Acute infectious diseases, diarrhoea, dysentery, leukemia, malignancy, corticosteroids.
   - Polio vaccine is sensitive to heat → stored at -20°C.
   - Stored in freezer compartment of refrigerator.
   - Vial contains a vaccine vial monitor (V.V.M.) for checking the potency of the vaccine.

4. **Measles vaccine :**
   - Freeze dried live attenuated vaccine – tissue culture vaccine.
   - To be frozen in upper most/freezer compartment.
   - Diluent : H_2O.
   - Dose : 0.6 ml. Subcutaneous in lateral aspect of thigh.
   - Age : 9 months (not given before 9 month – since maternal Antibodies are sufficient to interfere with response).
   - Induces mild illness (fever & rash), so the mother should be informed about this.
   - Contraindication : Acute illness, deficient CMI, immunosuppresive therapy, pregnancy.
   - Strain used : Edmonston – Zagreb strain.

5. **MMR (Mumps, Measles, Rubella) vaccine :**
   - Dose : 0.5 ml. Subcutaneous at 15 months of age (Rubella vaccine is important for female child at 15 months of age) or after 6 months of giving measles vaccine.
   - Reconstituted with sterile H_2O.
   - Contraindication : Same as for measles.
   - Measles (E-Z strain), mumps (L-Zagreb strain), rubella (RA 27/3 strain).

Injection Techniques
Parenteral Administration :

It refers to the administratioin by injection, & the drug is directly take into the tissue fluid or blood w/o having to cross the intestinal mucosa.

Advantages :
1. Action is faster & more sure (valuable in emergencies).
2. Bypass 1st pass metabolism.
3. Employed even in unconscious, uncooperative, vomiting patients.
4. Gastric irritation & vomiting are not provoked.

Disadvantages :
1. Preparation has to be sterilized, along with the instruments.
2. Costly.
3. Invasive & painful.
4. Trained personnel is required.

Commonly used parenteral routes : Subcutaneous, i.m, i.v., i.d.

Other routes : Intraperitoneal, intraosseous, intrathoracic, intra-arterial, intra spinal.

Syringes : 1 ml., 2 ml., 5 ml., 20 ml., 50 ml.
20 ml. and 50 ml. used for suction lavage.
- 1ml. insulin syringe, 1ml. tuberculin syringe.
- All have same length, only the diameter varies.
- Parts : Tip, barrel, plunger.

Needles : Needle length measured in inches – ¼, ½, ¾, 1, 1½ inches.
- Diameter measured in gauge (G) : 14, 16, 20, 21 G – for infusion.
  24, 25, 26 G – for paediatric age group.
  22, 23 G – i.m. injection.
- More the value, less is the diameter of the needle (fixer).
- Parts : Bevel, shaft, heeb.

Different Parenteral Routes
1. Subcutaneous : For injecting insulin, heparin and measles vaccine.
   Site – Anterior abdomen, anterior thigh, dorso gluteal area, scapular area, upper arm, beneath breast.

Technique : Relax the muscle by flexing the limb. Clean the area with spirit. Grasp the muscle in one hand & inject the needle at an angle of 45°. First aspirate to see the blood. If no blood comes, inject the drug slowly. Remove the needle and press the area with a cotton swab. Absorption is faster than intradermal route.

2. Intradermal : It is used for sensitivity testing and BCG vaccination. Absorption is very slow.

   Site : Volar aspect of fore arm, upper back (less hair & appendages & lighter areas of skin for easy measurement of reaction), above deltoid insertion in arm (for BCG).

   Technique : Clean area with spirit. Stretch the skin. Pierce the skin at an angle of 5-15°, raising it such that the needle is seen through the skin. Inject the drug slowly, raising a bleb (1mm diameter or size of a mosquito bite). Remove the needle. Don't massage the area otherwise circulation would improve, leading to greater absorption Mark the area.

   Scarring/multiple puncturing of the epidermis through a drop of the drug (small pox vaccine) can also be done.

3. Intravenous : It is the best method.

   Site : Any superficial vein is chosen.

   Technique : Make vein prominent by stretching the skin. Inject parallel to surface.

   It is useful in an emergency situation & for injecting highly irritant drugs.

4. Intramuscular : Absorption is faster than in intradermal & subcutaneous but slower than in intravenous

   Site : Deltoid, dorsolateral, ventrogluteal, ventro laterals.

   Technique : Relax the muscle by flexing the limb. Clean the area with spirit. Stretch the skin. Pierce quickly at 90° angle. Aspirate to see that no blood is present (blood vessel). Inject the drug slowly. Place cotton swab on needle. Withdraw the needle quietly & massage the area. Here thumb is placed on the stem of syringe & index finger on hub of the needle or all fingers encircle the hub of the needle.

STERILISATION AND DISINFECTION

Sterilisation

It is the process by which an article, surface or medium is made free of all living micro organisms both in vegetative or (resting) spore stock.

Disinfection

It is destruction of all pathogenic organism which are capable of giving rise to infection.

Agents used for Sterilisation are :

A) Physical Agents
    (1) Solar Rays
    (2) Heat   – (i) Dry heat – flaming, incineration
                 (ii) Moist heat – boiling, pasteurisation.
    (3) Filtration.
    (4) Sun drying.
    (5) Radiations.

B) Chemical Agents
    (1) Alcohols   – Ethyl alcohol, isopropyl alcohol.
    (2) Aldehydes   – Formaldehyde, glutard dehyde.
    (3) Halogens   – Iodine, chlorine (eshypochlorites).
    (4) Phenols   – Chlorhexidine, lysol, cresol.
    (5) Gases   – Ethylene oxide, formaldehyde gas.
    (6) Dyes   – Choline and acridine dyes.
    (7) Surface active agents – Cetrimide, benzalkonium Chloride.

Heat

Most effective method. It depends on nature of heat, time duration, level of temperature, bacterial load, characteristic of microbes present, etc.

Dry Heat – It acts by denaturing the bacterial proteins, oxidation and electrolytic damage.

Moist Heat – Acts by denaturing and coagulating the bacterial proteins.

Dry Heat Methods – Flaming, incineration, hot air.

(i) **Incineration** – Used for destruction of contaminated cloth, carcasses and pathological materials.

(ii) **Hot air oven** – Used for sterilisation of glass articles, forceps, scissors, scalpel, syrings (glass), liquid paraffin, dusting powder, etc.

    As hot air is a bad conductor of heat and its penetration is poor, a temperature of 160° C is applied for 1 hr. for sterilising the above mentioned articles.

Moist Heat Methods

Used for pasteurisation for milk. Two methods :

(a) **Holders method** – 63° C temperature for 30 minutes.

(b) **Flash process** – 72° C for 15-20 seconds.

Media like L.J. Medium; Loeffler's serum slope are made sterile by heating at 80-85°C for ½ hr. on 3 successive days in an – Inspissator.

Auto Clave

It is based on the concept of use of steam under pressure. The steam is having a good penetration and it gives up its latent heat when it comes into contact of a cooler surface and condenses into water.

It is used for instruments, dressing, laboratory ware, pharmaceutical products, etc. Aquous solutions can also be sterilised.

Temperature used : 108° C – 147° C.

121° C – 15 minutes, 126° C – 10 min., 134° C – 3 min.

Lab. autoclave – It is made up of stainless steel. It has a lid. On the upper side of, the lid there is a discharge tap for air and steam. A safety valve is also installed on the lid.

Sufficient water is put inside the container and the material to be sterilised is placed on the tray and auto clave is heated. The lid is screwed tight with discharge tap open. The steam air mixture is allowed to escape through the tap which is then closed. The steam pressure rises and when the desired level is achieved safety valve opens for escape of the excess steam. Then heating is done till certain period after which auto clave is turned off, cooled off and pressure is allowed to fall. Then discharge tap is opened.

Filtration

Used for sterilisation of heat labile liquids like serum, sugar solution, antibiotic, etc. Some commonly used filters are :

- Ceramic filters, diatomaceous earth filters like Berkefeld and Meddler filters.
- Asbestos filters : Disposable, single use e.g. Seitz filters.
- Membrane filters : Made up of cellulose esters used for water purification, injectable drug sterilisation, etc.

Chemical Agents

The properties of an ideal antiseptic :

- Wide spectrum of activity and easy availability.

- Speedy action and deepenetrating power.
- Cheap and should not interfere with healing.
- Not toxic if absorbed into circulation.

Mode of action are
1. Disruption of cell membrane resulting in exposure, damage or loss of the contents.
2. Protein coagulation.
3. Removal of free salphydryal (-SH) groups executed for proper activity of enzymes.
4. A compound which has structural similarity to the substrate, competes with the substrate for formation of enzyme substrate complex. It also inhibits the enzyme function thereby :
   - Metabolic reactions are disturbed.
   - Cell death.

INVESTIGATION OF EPIDEMIC
- Epidemic : Frequency more than 2 SD i.e. disease occurrence for more than n frequency in 3 years/5 years (more than 2 standard error)
- Collection of data : Govt. sector and private practitioners.

Management of Epidemic
1. Symptomatic.
2. Break chain of transmission.
   - By removing immediate provocative factor.
     e.g. personal protection, sprays, etc. in case of dengue.

Epidemic
- Signifies significant shift in existing balance between agent, host & environment.
- Call for prompt investigation into cases to find out factors responsible for spread and prevent further occurrence.

Objectives
1. To define the magnitude of the epidemic outbreak in terms of time, place & person.
2. To undermine the particular condition & factors responsible for the occurrence of epidemic.

3. To identify the cause of infection, method of transmission and determine the measures necessary to control the epidemic.
4. To make recommendations so as to prevent occurrence.

Steps
1. Verification of the diagnosis – only sample is needed.
2. Confirmation of occurrence of an epidemic.
   (i) There should be a standard case definition.
   (ii) Investigations.
3. Defining the population at risk.
   (i) Map of area.
   (ii) Counting the population.
4. Rapid search for all cases and their characteristics :
   (i) Medical survey.
   (ii) Epidemiological case sheet – no fired out the migration of people during incubation period of epidemic.
   (iii) Search for more cases.
5. Evaluation of ecological factors.
6. Further investigations of populations at risk.
   (i) Exposure to specific patent vehicle.
   (ii) Whether ill/not.
7. Hypothesis
8. Formulation of hypothesis.
9. Testing of hypothesis.
10. Writing the report.

Final Report
1. Background.
2. Historical datas' investigations.
3. Methodology of investigation.
4. Analysis of data.
5. Control.

CHAPTER-4

RESPIRATORY INFECTIONS

SMALL POX

Smallpox was a serious, contagious and sometimes fatal infectious disease. There was no specific treatment for this disease, the only prevention was vaccination.

The name small pox is derived from the Latin word for "spotted" and refers to the raised bumps that appear on the face and body of an infected person.

There were two clinical forms of smallpox, variola major and variola minor. Variola minor was the severe and most common form of smallpox, with a more extensive rash and high fever. There were further four types of variola major smallpox :

- Ordinary – the most frequent type, counting for 90% or more of cases.
- Modified – mild and occurring in previously vaccinated persons.
- Flat – rare and severe.
- Haemorrhagic – rare and severe.

Historically, variola major had an overall fatality rate of about 30%, however flat and hemorrhagic smallpox usually were fatal. Variola minor was a less common presentation of smallpox, and a much less severe, with death rates 1% or less.

Smallpox outbreaks have occurred from time to time for thousands of years, but the disease is now eradicated after a successful worldwide vaccination program. The last naturally occurring case in the world was in Somalia in 1977. After the disease was eliminated from the world, routine vaccination of people against smallpox was stopped because it was no longer necessary for prevention.

Smallpox was caused by the **Variola virus** that emerged in human population thousands of years ago. Except for laboratory stockpiles, the variola virus has been eliminated. However, in the aftermath of the events of September and October, 2001, there is heightened concern that the variola virus might be used as an agent of bioterrorism. Thus, the US government is taking precautions for dealing with a smallpox outbreak.

Transmission

Generally, direct and fairly prolonged face to face contact was required to spread smallpox from one person to the another person. It also could be spread through direct contact with infected bodily fluids or contaminated objects such as bedding or clothing. Rarely, smallpox had been spread by virus carried in the air in enclosed settings such as buildings, buses and trains. Humans were only natural hosts of variola. Smallpox was not known to be transmitted by insects or animals.

A person with smallpox was sometimes contagious with onset of fever (prodrome phase), but the person becomes most contagious with the onset of rash. At this stage the infected person was usually very sick and not able to move around in the community. The infected person was contagious until the last smallpox scab falls off.

Incubation Period

(Duration – 2 to 4 days)

Exposure to the virus is followed by an incubation period during which people do not have any symptoms and may feel fine. This incubation period averages about 12 to 14 days but can range from 7 to 17 days. During this time, people are not contagious.

Clinical Features

Initial Symptoms (Prodrome)

(Duration – 2 to 4 days)

The first symptoms of smallpox include fever, malaise, headaches, body aches, and sometimes vomiting. The fever is usually high, i.e. 101 to 104 degrees Fahrenheit. People are usually too sick to carry on their normal activities. This is called the prodrome phase and may last for 2 to 4 days.

Early Rash

(Duration – about 4 days)

A rash emerges first as small red spots on the tongue and in the mouth. These spots develop into sores that break open and spread large amounts of the virus into the mouth and throat. At this time, the person becomes most contagious.

Around the time the sores in the mouth break down, a rash appears on the skin, starting on the face and spreading to the arms and legs and then to the hands and feet. As the rash appears, the fever usually falls and the person may start feeling better.

By the third day of rash, the rash becomes raised bumps.

By the fourth day, the bumps are filled with a thick, opaque fluid and often have a depression in the center that looks like a bellybutton.

Fever often rise again at this time and remains high until scabs form over the bumps.

Pustular Rash

(Duration – about 5 days)

The bumps become pustules which are sharply raised, usually round and firm to the touch as if there's a small round object under the skin. People often say the bumps feel like BB pellets embedded in the skin.

Pustules and Scabs

(Duration – about 5 days)

The pustules begin to form a crust and then scab.

By the end of the second week after the rash appears, most of the sores have scabbed over.

Resolving Scabs

(Duration – about 6 days)

The scabs begin to fall off, leaving marks on the skin that eventually become pitted scars. Most scabs fell off three weeks after the rash appears.

The person is contagious to others until all of the scabs have fallen off.

Scabs resolved

Scabs fell off and the person is no longer contagious.

Homoeopathic Treatment

Some of the medicines with their indications are :

1. **Antimonium tartaricum**
   - Great despondency.

- Thirst for cold water, little and often.
- Desire for apples, fruits and acids.
- Great drowsiness.
- Pustular eruption leaving a bluish-red mark.

2. **Malandrinum**
   - A very effective protection against small pox.
   - Ist effect of vaccinations.
   - Scab on the upper lip, with stinging pain when torn off.

3. **Sarracenia purpurea**
   - Aborts the diseases.
   - Arrests pustulation.
   - Hungry all the time, even after a meal.
   - Sleepy during meals.

4. **Variolinum**
   - A prophylactic of small pox.
   - It aids in the cure of small pox.
   - Morbid fear of small pox.

Other medicines which can be thought of are Ant-c., Apis, Ars., Bell., Bry., Carb-ac., Merc., Nat-m., Puls., Rhus-t., Sulph., Thuj., Zinc.

INFLUENZA (FLU)

Influenza, also known as the flu, is a contagious disease that is caused by the influenza virus. It attacks the respiratory tract in humans. The flu is different from a cold. Influenza usually comes suddenly and may include these symptoms :

- Fever.
- Headache.
- Tiredness.
- Dry cough.
- Sore throat.
- Nasal congestion.
- Body aches.

These symptoms are usually referred to as "flu like symptoms".

Most people who get influenza recover in one to two weeks, but some people will develop life – threatening complications such as pneumonia due to flu. Anyone can get the flu, and serious problems from influenza can happen at any age. People of age 65 years and older, people of any age with chronic medical conditions, and very young children are more likely to get complications from influenza. Pneumonia, bronchitis, and sinus and ear infections are complications of flu. The flu can make chronic health problems worse. e.g., people with asthma may experience asthma attacks while they have the flu, and people with chronic congestive heart failure may have worsening of this condition that is triggered by the flu.

Transmission

The flu is spread, or transmitted, by an infected person through coughing, sneezing, speaking i.e. sending flu virus into the air, where other people inhale the virus. The virus enters the nose, throat or lungs of a person and begins to multiply, causing symptoms of influenza. Influenza may, less often, be spread when a person touches a surface that has flu viruses on it e.g. a door handle and then touches his or her nose or mouth.

Flu is contagious as a person can spread the flu starting one day before he or she feels sick. Adults can continue to pass the flu virus to others for another three to seven days after symptoms start. Children can pass the virus for longer than seven days.

Symptoms start one to four days after the virus enters the body. Some infected persons may have no symptoms. During this time, those persons can still spread the virus to others.

Advice to the Patient
- Rest.
- Drink plenty of liquids.
- Avoid using alcohol and tobacco.
- Take medication to relieve the symptoms of flu.

Influenza is caused by a virus, so antibiotics like penicillin don't cure it. The best way to prevent the flu is to get an influenza vaccine (flu shot) each fall, before flu season.

Aspirin should not be given to a child or teenager who has the flu. It can cause a rare but serious illness called **Reye Syndrome**.

Laboratory Diagnosis

Influenza can include any or all of these symptoms like fever, muscle aches, headache, lack of energy, dry cough, sore throat and possibly running nose. The fever and body aches can last 3-5 days and the cough and lack of energy may last for 2 or more weeks.

Influenza Diagnostic Table

Procedure	Influenza Types Detected	Acceptable Specimens	Time for Results	Point-of-care market
Viral culture	A and B	NP swab, throat swab, nasal wash, bronchial wash, nasal aspirate, sputum	5-10 days[3]	No
Immunofluorescence DFA Antibody staining	A and B	NP swab, nasal wash, bronchial wash, nasal aspirate, sputum	2-4 hours	No
RT-PCR	A and B	NP swab, throat swab, nasal wash, bronchial wash, nasal aspirate, sputum	1-2 days	No
Serology	A and B	paired acute and convalescent serum samples	> 2 weeks	No
Enzyme Linked Immuno Sorbent Assay (ELISA)	A and B	NP swab, throat swab, nasal wash, bronchial wash	2 hours	No

Rapid Diagnostic Tests

Procedure	Influenza Types Detected	Acceptable Specimens	Time for Results	Point-of-care market
Directigen Flu A (Becton-Dickinson)	A	NP swab, throat swab, nasal wash, nasal wash, nasal aspirate	< 30 minutes	Yes
Directigen Flu A+B (Becton-Dickinson)	A and B	NP swab, throat swab, nasal wash, nasal aspirate	< 30 minutes	Yes
FLU OIA (Thermo BioStar)	A and B	NP swab, throat swab, nasal aspirate, sputum	< 30 minutes	Yes
NOW Flu A Test	A	Nasal wash, NP swab[2]	< 30 minutes	Yes
NOW Flu B Test (Binax)	B	Nasal wash, NP swab	< 30 minutes	Yes

Influenza is difficult to diagnose based on clinical symptoms alone because the initial symptoms of influenza can be similar those caused by other infections agents including, but not limited to mycoplasma pneumoniae, adeno virus, respiratory syncytial virus, rhinovirus, parainfluenza viruses and legionella sp.

A number of tests can help in the diagnosis of influenza. But, tests are not required for all patients. For some patients tests are most useful when they are likely to help in the diagnosis and treatment decisions. During a respiratory illness outbreak, however, testing for influenza can be very helpful in determining if influenza is the cause of outbreak. Appropriate samples for influenza testing can include a nasopharyngeal or throat swab, nasal wash or nasal aspirates. Samples should be collected within the first 4 days of illness. Rapid influenza tests provide results within 24 hours and viral culture provides results in 3-10 days. Most of the rapid tests can be done in a physician's office where approximately >70% are sensitive for detecting influenza and approximately >90% are specific. Thus, as many as 30% of samples that would be positive for influenza by viral culture may give a negative rapid test result. And some rapid test results may indicate influenza when a person is not affected with influenza.

Serum samples also can be tested for influenza antibody to diagnose recent infections. Two samples should be collected per person. One sample within the first week of illness and second sample 2-4 weeks later. If antibody levels increase from the first to the second sample, influenza infection has likely occurred. Because of the length of time needed for a diagnosis of influenza by serologic testing, other diagnostic testing should be used if a more rapid diagnosis is needed.

During outbreaks of respiratory illness when influenza is suspected, some samples should be tested by both rapid tests and by viral culture. The collection of some samples for viral culture is essential for determining the influenza subtypes and strains causing illness and for surveillance of new strains that may be included in the next year's influenza vaccine. During outbreaks of influenza – like illness, viral culture also can help to identify other causes of illness in absence influenza.

Influenza Vaccine (Flu shot)

Much of the illness and death caused by the flu can be prevented by a yearly flu shot. People in high risk groups and people who are in close contact with those at high risk should get a flu shot every year.

A flu shot can be given to anyone who wants to avoid the flu. People who provide important community service should consider getting a flu shot so that their services are not disrupted during a flu outbreak.

Pregnant Women

Pregnancy can increase the risk for complications from flu and pregnant women are more likely to be hospitalized from complications of the flu than nonpregnant women of the same age. In previous world wide outbreaks of the flu, deaths among pregnant women were associated with the flu. Pregnancy can change the immune system in the mother, as well as affect her cardio-vascular system. These changes may place pregnant women at an increased risk for complications from the flu.

Because the flu shot is made from inactivated viruses, many experts consider flu shots safe during any stage of pregnancy. However, since miscarriages most often occur in the first trimester of pregnancy, experts traditionally do not give a flu shot during the first trimester to avoid a coincidental association with miscarriage.

Pregnant women of 2nd or 3rd trimester of pregnancy, during the flu season should get a flu shot. Pregnant women who have medical problems that increase their risk for complications from the flu should get a flu shot before flu season, without considering the stage of pregnancy.

Breast Feeding Mothers

It is safe to give a flu shot to mother breast feeding as a flu shot can not cause flu either in mother or her baby.

Healthy Children Aged 6-23 Months

Children aged 6-23 months are substantially at an increased risk for influenza-related hospitalizations. Influenza vaccination of all children in this age group is encouraged when feasible.

Homoeopathic Treatment

Some other medicines like Caust., Influenzinum, Merc., Ph.-ac., Pyrog., etc. can be considered for the treatment of influenza.

Respiratory Infections

Arsenicum album
- Great anguish and restlessness.
- Thin watery excoriating discharge.
- Great thirst but drinks little at a time.
- Craves acids, coffee and milk.
- High temperature.
- Worse after midnight.
- Better from heat.

Baptisia tinctoria
- Mental confusion.
- No appetite
- Constant desire for water.
- Adynamic fever.
- Sore & bruised back & extremities.

Bryonia alba
- Irritable.
- Excessive thirst.
- Bitter taste.
- Stools large, dry hard.
- Stitches and stiffness in the lumbar region.
- Chills with external coldness, dry cough stitches.

Gelsemium sempervirens

Phosphorus

Rhus toxicodendron

MENINGOCOCCAL MENINGITIS

Epidemiology of Disease due to *Neisseria Meningitides*

Agent – *Neisseria meningitides*
- Gram-negative diplococcus.
- Capsular polysaccharide antigens differentiated into serogroups A, B, C, X, Y, Z, 29-E, and W 135.
- Serogroups A, B, and C are associated with epidemics.
- Subtyping identified certain strains (clones) associated with

increased virulence and epidemic potential (e.g. serogroup A, III-1; serogroup B, ET-5).

Reservoir
- Humans.
- Asymptomatic carriage in nasopharynx common.

Mode of Spread
- Person-to-person by direct contact through respiratory droplets of infected people.
- Most cases acquired through exposure to a symptomatic carriers, relatively few through direct contact with patients having meningococcal infection.

Host Factors
- Risk of invasive disease due to *N. Meningitides* higher in children, decreases with age.
- All humans susceptible, but disease risk higher in persons with terminal complement deficiency and splenectomy.

Incubation Period
- 1-10 days, usually < 4 days.

Magnitude of the Problem

Neisseria meningitis was first identified as the causative agent of bacterial meningitis by **Weichselbaum** in 1807. However, clinical meningococcal disease was described by **Vieusseux** in 1805 during an outbreak in the vicinity of Geneva, Switzerland. During the 20th century, major outbreak were noted during world war I and II. In the African continent, epidemic meningitis has been known to occur for a long time. It was reported from the West Coast of Africa by **G. William** in 1909 and has occurred from then onwards. In the Sudan, cerebrospinal meningitis is present from time immemorial. However, the disease probably did not appear in the Northern Savanna of Africa before the 1880s.

Since world war II, epidemic meningitis caused by group A meningococcus has been infrequent in developed countries with a temperate climate, whereas meningococcal disease in its epidemic form continued periodically to devastate sub-Saharan territories of Africa. At least 340,000 cases with 53,000 deaths occurred in the 10 years between 1951-1960 in the countries of this region.

Major epidemics of meningococcal meningitis in 1971-1997

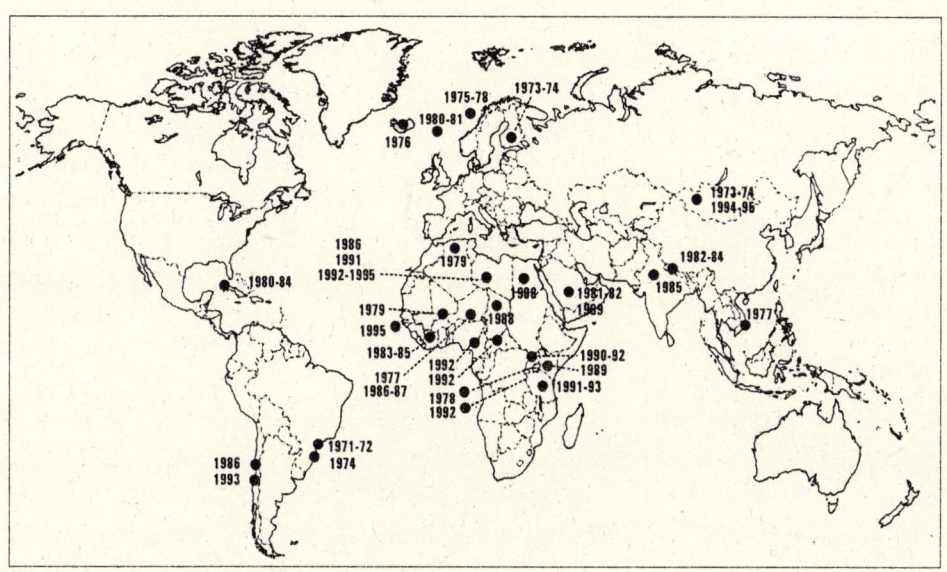

The word "epidemic" used in the context of meningococcal disease, may refer to different events throughout the world. In comparison to explosive epidemics in the African meningitis belt are rather moderate than, European epidemics and recent epidemics in the Americas since their highest incidence is usually lower than the endemic incidence in African countries. Thus, epidemic conditions can be defined, for a given country, as an acceptable incidence rate requiring emergency control measures.

Risk Factors for Epidemics

Risk factors for invasive disease and for outbreaks are not completely understood. A combination of conditions are necessary for epidemic to occur. These include : immunological susceptibility of the population, special climatic conditions, low socioeconomic status and transmission of a virulent strain. Acute respiratory tract infections may also contribute to the development of meningococcal disease epidemics.

Serogroups, Serotypes of the Meningococcus

The risk of epidemic meningococcal disease differs among serogroups Serogroups A, B and C can cause outbreaks. Other serogroups have so far not been associated with outbreaks.

Nasopharyngeal Carriage

Neither the meningococcal carriage rate nor the serogroup specific carriage rate can be used to predict epidemics. Carriage rates, can range between 1% and 50% according to age, socioeconomic status, and predominant strain circulating in the area, but do not seem to vary with season or herd immunity. Although an increasing carrier rate an increase the risk of illness occurring in non immune persons, there is no constant or close relationship between the carrier rate and the incidence of disease. In the course of serogroup A meningococcal epidemics, carriage rates increase. However, surveillance for nasopharyngeal carriage is not recommended as a useful public health tool.

Waning Immunity

Humoral immunity is an essential factor in the prevention of meningococcal disease. Natural infection protects against disease caused by the same serogroup. The risk of acquiring. Meningococcal disease decreases with the age. Waning herd immunity to a particular strain in a population may be necessary for an outbreak to occur and loss of herd immunity against group A meningococci may contribute to the regularity of the epidemic cycles in the sub-Saharan Africa. Development of herd immunity due to widespread carriage should limit meningococcal transmission, and may help to end an epidemic wave.

Environmental Factors

Climate play an important role in the seasonal upsurge of meningococcal disease. In sub-Saharan Africa spread of infection may be enhanced by drought and dust-room. Meningococcal epidemics generally stop with the onset of rains. Low absolute humidity and dust may enhance meningococcal invasion by damaging the mucosal barrier directly or by inhibiting mucosal immunal defences. Unfavorable climate conditions may lead to the crowding of people in poorly ventilated dwellings, where spread of virulent meningococci is optimal.

Demographic Factors

Travel and migration facilitate the circulation of virulent strains inside a country or from one country to another country. The gathering of susceptible people is an important risk factor for outbreaks as exemplified in military communities where many outbreaks have occurred, particularly among new recruits. Large population movements such as pilgrimage, play a major role in the spread of infection and disease. The outbreak which occurred in Mecca in 1987, at the end of the pilgrimage period, caused more cases among pilgrims than among the Saudi population. In many countries, returning pilgrims caused the occurrence of cases of meningococcal meningitis in their immediate communities. Specially by virulent strain of serogroup A meningococcus imported by returning pilgrims. Other large population displacements, e.g. refugees, may pose similar risks.

Socio Economic Factors

As shown in several outbreaks, poor living conditions and over crowded housing are linked with a higher incidence of meningococcal disease.

Concurrent Infections

Upper respiratory tract infections may contribute to some meningococcal outbreaks. Both in temperate and tropical climates. During a group A meningococcal epidemic in Chad in 1988 patients with meningococcal meningitis were about 23 times more likely than matched control patients to have nasopharyngeal shedding of respiratory pathogens, including Mycoplasma hominies, adenoviruses, parainfluenza viruses, rhinoviruses and respiratory syncytial virus.

Viral Meningitis

Viruses are the main causes of acute aseptic meningitis syndrome defined as acute meningitis with CSF lymphocytic pleocytosis for which there is no apparent cause after initial evaluation and routine staining and culture of CSF. The disease is rarely serious and recovery is usually complete. There are no specific treatment or specific control measures.

Viral meningitis occurs worldwide in sporadic and epidemic forms. The incidence during non-epidemic conditions is rarely known. Seasonal variations can be observed and depend on the causative agent. Enteroviruses are the most common cause of epidemics of viral meningitis and they occur generally in late summer or early winter periods, affecting mainly infants and young children. Mumps virus is another important agent of viral meningitis in non-immunized populations. Outbreaks of aseptic meningitis in late winter may be mainly due to mumps. The most affected in these outbreaks are children in the age group 5-9 years.

Arboviral meningitis outbreaks, e.g. – West Nile virus may occur under special favoring conditions such as periods of increased vector activity.

Clinical Features

Symptoms and Signs

Acute meningitis is characterised by a sudden onset of intense headache, fever, nausea, vomiting, photophobia and stiff neck. In addition, neurological signs can be observed, such as lethargy, delirium, coma and/or convulsions. However, infants may have illness without sudden onset and stiff neck.

Meningococcal septicemia is difficult to recognise outside an epidemic : abrupt onset, fever and shock occur. Irregularly petechial rash or purpura may not be obvious initially and meningeal symptoms are usually absent.

Physical Examination

Physical examination should include an examination for :
- Meningeal rigidity : Stiff neck, Kerning's or Brudzinski's signs.
- Neurological signs such as decreased awareness, localizing neurological symptoms are unusual.
- Purpura, sometimes extensive and necrotic, usually localized in the extremities or generalized, cutaneous or mucosal are often associated with meningococcal disease. Purpura is a basic symptoms of meningococcaemia.
- Blood pressure and symptoms of shock. Shock associated with purpura indicates fulminating meningococcaemia, the most severe form of meningococcal disease.
- Focal infections such as arthritis, pleuritis or pneumonia, pericarditis, episcleritis.

Laboratory Investigations

Lumbar Puncture and CSF Examination

Lumbar puncture is necessary to confirm the diagnosis of purulent meningitis and to identify the meningococcus.

Lumbar puncture must be done as soon as meningitis is suspected prior to starting antibacterials. It requires minimal expertise, but careful asepsis is necessary. Fundoscopic examination to rule out papilloedema should be performed when feasible but should not be a prerequisite for lumbar puncture.

Cerebrospinal fluid is usually turbid or purulent (but may occasionally be clear or bloody). Basic routine examination feasible in most laboratories consists of :

(a) Measurement of white blood cell count : white cell count is usually above 1,000 cells/mm^3 (< 3 in normal CSF) with > 60% polymorphonuclears cells;

(b) Measurement of protein level : > 0,80 g/l in normal CSF);

(c) Gram stain, showing Gram-negative diplococci (intra- or extracellular) in 80% of cases not previously treated (Annex 1). If Gram stain is not feasible, it can be replaced by methylene blue stain.

Additional investigations performed on CSF usually include :

- Measurement of glucose concentration (<0.40 g/l).
- Bacterial culture on appropriate media and identification and serogrouping of Neisseria meningitides.
- Rapid antigen detection techniques, to identify directly not only meningococcal infection, but also the causative serogroup. Latex agglutination is the procedure most commonly used. Other techniques are co-agglutination, countercurrent immuno electrophoresis and ELISA.
- Antibiogram testing of sensitivity to antibacterials.

Neisseria meningitides or meningococcus is a Gram-negative diplococcus, non-motile, non-sporulating, usually encapsulated and pilated.

- The meningococcus is a fragile organism, susceptible to cold and drying. It is cultivated on enriched media, such as Mueller-Hinton or chocolate agar.
- Capsular polysaccharide antigens differentiate nine serogroups. Serogrouping is performed either after culture, by agglutination on colonies, or directly on CSF, by latex agglutination.
- Subtyping using new sophisticated procedures is carried out only in some reference laboratories (See Annex 12 for WHO Collaborating Centres).

Other Laboratory Investigations

Blood cell counts may show an increase of polymorphonuclear cells. In severe purpuric cases marked thrombocytopaenia may be observed along with signs of disseminated intravascular coagulopathy.

Blood cultures are often positive. When purpura is present, microscopic direct examination and culture of a specimen of pus or tissue fluid may be useful when haemoculture cannot be performed.

Management

Principles

- Meningococcal disease is potentially fatal and should always be viewed as a medical emergency.
- Admission to a hospital or health care centre is necessary for diagnosis and treatment.
- Antimicrobial therapy is essential and should be combined with supportive treatment.
- As contagiousness of patients is moderate and disappears quickly following antimicrobial treatment, isolation of patient is not necessary.

Antimicrobial Therapy

Timing

Antimicrobial treatment must be instituted as soon as possible. Lumbar puncture should be performed, if possible, prior to the administration of antibiotics, which should be given immediately after the puncture, without waiting for laboratory results. Treatment of a suspected case of meningococcal disease with an antibiotic should not be delayed when lumbar puncture cannot be done on initial presentation. If the lumbar puncture yields blood but the clinical picture suggests meningitis, then antimicrobial treatment should be initiated immediately. This is also the case if the CSF looks clear but the symptoms and signs are suggestive of meningococcal septicemia, initiation of antimicrobial therapy without any delay may be life saving.

Choice of Antimicrobials

Many antimicrobials are active against meningococci in vitro, but only those that penetrate the cerebrospinal space sufficiently should be used. Either parenteral penicillin or ampicillin is the drug of choice. Chloramphenicol is a good and inexpensive alternative. The third generation cephalosporins, ceftrianone and ceftotaxime are excellent alternatives but are considerably more expensive. On the other hand, ceftriaxane can be administered once a day and for a short period as two days. This should be taken into account when comparing the total costs

Respiratory Infections

of treatment with this antibiotic and with a 5 day regimen of ampicillin. Although oral cotrimoxazole is inexpensive and has good CSF penetration. Sulfa resistant strains have become common and sulfa drugs are not recommended unless sulfa sensitivity testing has been done. In unfavorable conditions, the drug of choice is oily chloramphenicol.

Route of Administration

The intravenous route is recommended. However, a series of clinical studies have shown the use of intramuscular chloramphienicol in oil to be as efficacious as intravenous ampicillin for meningococcal disease. Penetration of chloramphenicol into the cerebrospinal space is good even after oral administration. In patients where the intramuscular (1M) or intravenous (IV) route is not possible, oral administration is acceptable. Higher than normal doses are then advisable.

Antimicrobials to treat bacterial meningitis

Agent (generic name)	Route	Dose adults	Dose children	Duration (1) (days)	Cost (2)
Penicillin G	IV	3-4 MU q. 4-6 h	400,000 U/kg	≥ 4	low
Ampicillin or Amoxicillin	IV	2-3 g q. 6 h	250 mg/kg	≥ 4	moderate
Amoxicillin	Oral	2-3 g q. 6 h	250 mg/kg	≥ 4	high
Chloramphenical	IV	1 g q. 8-12 h	100 mg/kg	≥ 4	moderate
Chloramphenical (oily)	IM	3 g single dose	100 mg/kg	1-2	low
Cefotaxime	IV	2 g q. 6 h	250 mg/kg	≥ 4	very high
Ceftriaxone	IV	1-2 g q. 12-24 h	50-80 mg/kg	≥ 4	very high
Ceftriaxone	IM	1-2 g single dose	50-80 mg/kg	1-2	high

Duration of Therapy

A seven day course is still the rule for the treatment of meningococcal disease in most developed countries. However there is good evidence that for meningococcal meningitis a four day course of penicillin G is as effective as longer course of any other antimicrobials. The long acting form of chloramphenicol is also been known to be effective.

Supportive Therapy

Fluid and electrolyte balance should be monitored and fluid replaced accordingly. If the patient is unconscious or vomits, and if an intravenous line cannot be placed, a nasogastric tube should be inserted.

When required, an anticonvulsants, or antiemetics may be administered by an appropriate route.

Increased intracranial pressure probably plays a key role in meningitis mortality. When facilities are available, barbiturate anesthesia with the use of a ventilator seems the best way of decreasing the pressure. Routine use of dexamethasone cannot be recommended for treatment of meningococcal meningitis at this time.

Severe forms of the disease including coma, shock and purpura fulminans should be treated in an intensive care unit or by well-trained physicians. Feeding by the oral or nasogastric route to maintain nutritional status and nursing care, including prevention of bedsores, are important components of supportive care.

Outcome

In meningococcal meningitis the case-fatality rate usually is around 10% among patients who are appropriately treated. In meningococcal septicemia, the case fatality rate may exceed 50%.

Few datas on permanent sequelae of bacterial meningitis are available. In the Gambia, 12% of patients who survived meningococcal meningitis were left with a moderate or severe neurological abnormality. Hearing impairment was the most frequent sequela (6%). Many permanent sequelae remain undetected. It is thus recommended that whenever possible, hearing should be tested one to three months later, or at the earliest age the child is able to cooperate sufficiently. In addition, if possible, a developmental assessment should be performed a year later to decide any subsequent mental handicap condition in the child.

Homoeopathic Treatment

Accoding to A.P. report, *Belladonna, Calcarea carbonica* and *Tuberculinum* proved efficacious in treatment of meningitis.

Some of the homoeopathic medicines with their few indications are:

Apis Mellifica :
- Bores head into pillow, screams out.
- Thirstless.
- Craving for milk.
- Screams and sudden starting during sleep.

Belladonna :
- Boring of head into the pillow, drawn backwards and rolls from side to side.

- Constant moaning.
- Less of consciousness.
- Aversion to meat and milk.
- Great thirst for cold water.
- Starting on closing the eyes or during sleep.

Helleborus niger :
- Complete unconsciousness.
- Involuntary sighing.
- Bores head into the pillow; beats it with hands.
- Screams suddenly in sleep. Cri encephalique.
- Horrible smell from mouth.

Stramonium :
- Devout, earnest, beseeching and ceaseless talking.
- Raises head frequently from the pillow.
- Aversion to water.
- Violent thirst.
- Awakens terrified; screams with fright.

Zincum metallicum :
- Forehead cool; base of brain hot.
- Rolls head from side to side. Bores head into the pillow.
- Ravenous hunger around 11 a.m.
- Screams out loudly at night in sleep without being aware of it.

Others drugs which can be thought of are : *Arn., Cic., Cupr., Phos., Rhus-t.*, etc.

Prevention

Meningococcal disease is potentially preventable through vaccination and/or chemoprophylaxis in special circumstances.

Prevention of Transmission

Transmission of N. meningitides occurs from person to person, usually from a nasopharyngeal carrier rather than from a patient, through contact with respiratory droplets or oral secretions. The prevalence of nasopharyngeal carriage is variable and does not correlate with the risk of an outbreak. Contagiousness rapidly disappears in patients after starting an antibiotic therapy. Since the meningococcus is relatively susceptible to temperature changes and desiccation the organism is not transmitted through shared equipment or material. Thus :

- Neither isolation of the patient nor disinfection of the room, bedding or clothes are necessary.
- Identification of carriers by nasopharyngeal culture is not recommended. Carriage studies are not useful in predicting an outbreak, or in guiding decisions about prophylaxis.

Vaccination

Four specific antigens related to serogroups A, C, Y and W135 are currently available. They are distributed in freeze – dried form, injectable by IM route, either as bivalent AC vaccine, or quadrivalent A, C, Y, W135 vaccine, containing 50 mg. of each antigen.

These polysaccharide vaccines are generally very well tolerated but may induce some mild adverse reactions in 10-20% of recipients, for the 2-3 days following the vaccination.

Chemoprophylaxis

Chemoprophylaxis has been considered for control of meningococcal disease but it has several limitations, and its use should be limited to special circumstances. The aim of chemoprophylaxis is to prevent secondary cases by eliminating nasopharyngeal carriage. To be effective in preventing secondary cases, chemoprophylaxis must be initiated as soon as possible.

Chemoprophylaxis is only effective in eradicating nasopharyngeal carriage when systemic antibiotics are used. Topical chemoprophylaxis and topical disinfection are of no value. Among potentially useful agents, the antibiotic most often recommended is rifampicin, administered in a two day course. Ciprofloxacin and ceftriaxone are very efficient but expensive. Alternatives are a five day course of spiramycin or minocycline. Penicillins and chloramphenicol are not recommended since they are ineffective.

Antimicrobials for chemoprophylaxis of meningococcal disease

Generic name	Dose adults	Dose children	Route	Duration	Cost
Rifampicin	600 mg/12h.	10 mg/kg/12h.	oral	2 days	moderate
Spiramycin	1 mg/12h.	25 mg/kg/12h.	oral	5 days	moderate
Ciprofloxacin	500 mg	–	oral	Single dose	high
Ceftriaxone	250 mg	–	IM	Single dose	high

Special Circumstances

Special circumstances erist for which chemoprophylaxis is appropriate.

In non-epidemic settings, chemoprophylaxis should be restricted to close, contacts of a case, such as :
- Household members.
- Institutional contacts who shared sleeping quarters, boarding – school pupils, room mates, etc.
- Nursery school or child care centre contacts.
- Others who have had contact with the patient's oral secretions through kissing or sharing food and beverages.

In addition, in areas where household contacts routinely receive prophylaxis, chemoprophylaxis should also be given to the patients with meningococcal disease on being discharged from the hospital provided the patient's illness was treated with an agent which does not eliminate the organism from the nasopharynx.

Mass chemoprophylaxis to prevent/control epidemics is not recommended.

Acute Respiratory Infections (ARI)

Most children have about 46 acute infections each year. Children with respiratory infections account for a large proportion of patients seen by health workers in health centres. These infections tend to be even move frequent in urban communities than in rural areas.

Respiratory infections are the infections in any area of the respiratory tract, including the nose, middle ear, throat (pharynx) windpipe (trachea), air passages (bronchi or bronchioles) and lungs.

Many areas of the respiratory tract can be involved, and there can be a wide variety of signs and symptoms of infection. These include : cough, difficult breathing; sore throat; running nose; ear problems.

Fever is also common in acute respiratory infections. Fortunately, most children with these respiratory symptoms have only a mild infection such as cold or bronchitis. They may cough because nasal discharge form a cold drip down to the back of the throat or because of a viral infection of the bronchi (bronchitis). They are not seriously ill and can be treated at home by their families without antibiotics.

However a few children have an acute infection of lungs (pneumonia). If they are not treated with antibiotics, these children may die, either from a lack of oxygen or from a bacterial infection of the blood stream called as septicaemia. About one quarter of all children less than 5 years of age who die in developing countries do so because of pneumonia. Pneumonia and diarrhoea are the two most common causes of death in children. Many of deaths from pneumonia occur in young infants of less than 2 months of age.

Therefore, treatment can greatly reduce deaths in children suffering from pneumonia. In order to treat these children, the health worker must be able to carry out the difficult task of identifying the few, very sick children among the children who are not having serious respiratory infections.

Asking the Mother

Ask the mother the following questions :
- How old is the child?
- Is the child coughing? For how long?
- Age between 2 months to 5 years, is the child able to drink?
  The child should only be regarded as "not able to drink" if he or she is not able to drink at all. This includes the child who is too weak to drink when offered fluids is notable to suck or swallow or who repeatedly vomits and keeps nothing.
  Children who are breast fed may have difficulty sucking when their noses are blocked. However, if they are not severely ill, they can still breast-feed if their noses are blocked.
- Age less than 2 months, has the young infant stopped feeding well?
  This question is similar to the one listed above. The difference between the two question, however, is that the sign in the older child is not able to drink at all. In the young infant, the sign is taking less than half of the usual amount of breast milk or formula. Mothers can estimate changes in the amount of milk taken from the length of time the child sucks.
- Has the child had fever? For how long?
- Has the child had convulsions?
  Ask the mother if the child has had convulsions during the current illness.

What to Look and Listen for?

This section describes how to look at and listen to a child to find out whether the child has signs of difficult breathing such as chest indrawing, fast breathing, stridor or wheeze.

Respiratory Infections

It is especially important to look at and listen to the child's breathing only when the child is quiet and calm. It is not possible to count the breathing rate accurately or assess other signs of difficult breathing in a child who is frightened, crying or angry. To calm the child, give him something to play with, ask the mother to breast feed the child, or suggest they wait in another room until the child's calms down.

Breathing Rate

Look for breathing movement anywhere on the child's chest or abdomen. If you are not able to see this movement easily, ask the mother to lift the shirt and then count.

As children get older, their breathing rate slows down. Therefore, the cutoff you will use to determine if a child has fast breathing will depend on the age of the child.

If the child age is :	Then he/she has fast breathing if the count is :
• Less than 2 months	60 breaths per minute or more.
• Between 2 months upto 12 months	50 breaths per minute or more.
• Between 12 months upto 5 years	40 breaths per minute or more.

Chest Indrawing

The child has chest indrawing if the lower chest wall goes in when the child breathes in. Chest indrawing occurs when the effort required to breathe in is much greater than normal.

Stridor

Look to see when the child is breathing in. A child with stridor makes a harsh noise when he breaths in. Stridor occurs when there is a narrowing of the larynx, trachea or epiglottis which interferes with the air entering the lungs.

Wheeze

A child with wheezing makes a soft whistling noise or shows signs that breathing out is difficult. Wheezing is caused by a narrowing of the air passages in the lungs. The breathing out phase takes longer than normal and requires effort.

Abnormally Sleepy or Difficult to Wake

An abnormally sleepy child is drowsy most of the time when he or she should be awake and alert.

Body Temperature

A temperature of 38° C or above is regarded as fever. Below 35.5° C is an abnormally low body temperature called as hypothermia.

Severe Malnutrition

Look for :
- Severe marasmus, which is characterised by severe muscle wasting and a lack of subcutaneous fat, so that the child looks like skin and bones.
- Kwashiorkor, which is characterised by a generalized swelling of the body (oedema), dry flatting skin and weak, thin hair.

Classifying the Illness of the Child aged between 2 Months upto 5 Years

It means making decisions about the type and severity of disease. This is done by answering questions about the signs during the assessment. Each child should be put into one of the four categories :
- Very serious disease.
- Severe pneumonia.
- Pneumonia (not severe)
- No pneumonia : cough or cold.

Each disease classification has a corresponding treatment plan which should be followed after the child's illness has been classified. There are three general plans of treatment, although there will be minor variations depending on the child's age, whether the child has fever or is wheezing and whether referrals are feasible.

Severe Disease

- Does the child has danger signs? A child who has any danger sign is classified as having very severe disease.

Danger signs for the child aged 2 months upto 5 years of age are :
- Unable to drink.
- Convulsions.
- Abnormally sleepy or difficult to wake.
- Stridor when calm.
- Severe malnutrition.

Respiratory Infections

Unable to Drink

A child who is not able to drink could have severe pneumonia, bronchiolitis, sepsis, an infection of brain, a throat abscess, or other problems. Oxygen, antibiotics and other medicines are life saving for some of these children.

Convulsions, Abnormally Sleepy or Difficult to Wake

A child with these signs may have severe pneumonia resulting in too little oxygen being taken in, sepsis, cerebral malaria or meningitis. Meningitis can develop as a complication of pneumonia or it can occur on its own.

Stridor in Calm Child

If a child has stridor when calm, the child may be in danger of a life-threatening obstruction of the airway from swelling of the larynx, trachea or epiglottis.

Severe Malnutrition

A severely malnourished child is at a high risk of developing and dying from pneumonia. In addition, the child may not show typical signs of illness.

Treatment

A child who is classified as having very severe disease is very ill, and should be referred urgently to a hospital.

- Give the first dose of antibiotic before the child leaves the health center. Treat fever and wheezing if present.
- If there is falciparum malaria in the area and the child has any fever or a history of fever with convulsions, is abnormally sleepy or difficult to wake, or is not able to drink, then these signs indicate that the child may have cerebral malaria, which can be fatal if it is not treated quickly. Follow the guidelines of the national malaria programme for treatment of this condition.

Deciding Factors for Pneumonia

The child without danger signs is classified as having either **severe pneumonia, pneumonia**, or **no pneumonia** : cough or cold.

The most important signs to consider when deciding if the child has pneumonia are :

- The child's breathing rate.
- Whether or not there is chest indrawing.

Severe Pneumonia

A child with chest indrawing usually has severe pneumonia. Chest indrawing occurs when the lungs become stiff and the effort required to breathe in is much greater than normal.

A child with chest indrawing may not have fast breathing. If the child becomes tired, and if the effort needed to expand the lungs is too great, then the breathing slows down. Therefore, chest indrawing may be the only sign that the child has severe pneumonia. In such a case the child is at higher risk of death from pneumonia than the child with the fast breathing without chest indrawing.

A child classified as having severe pneumonia might have other signs like :
- Nasal flaring, when the nose widens as the child breathes in.
- Grunting, the short sounds made with the voice when the child has difficulty in breathing.
- Cyanosis, a dark bluish or purplish colouration of skin, caused by hypoxia. If the tongue is cynosed, the child should be given oxygen.

Treatment

A child who is classified as having severe pneumonia should be referred urgently to a hospital.
- The child should receive the first dose of antibiotic.
- Fever and wheezing, if present should be treated.

Pneumonia (not severe)

A child who has no chest indrawing and fast breathing is classified as having pneumonia (not severe).

Treatment

In developing countries, pneumonia is often caused by bacteria. The child classified as having pneumonia should be treated at home with an antibiotic.
- Infections of the respiratory tract may be caused by bacteria or viruses.
- Bacteria are killed by antibiotics.

Antibiotic treatment can thus prevent many deaths from pneumonia if given early enough in an infection.

Antibiotics do not kill bacteria. Although pneumonia can be caused by virus, there is no reliable way to distinguish viral from bacterial pneumonia. For this reason, children should be given an antibiotic whenever they have signs of pneumonia.

- The mother should be given instructions on home care including when to return if child is getting worse and how to give the antibiotic.
- Mother should also be advised to return with the child in 2 days for reassessment, or earlier if any of the signs occur like :
  ⇨ breathing becomes difficult or fast.
  ⇨ child is not able to drink.
  ⇨ child becomes more sick.

Homoeopathic Efficacy

Some of the homoeopathic medicines with their few indications are :

Antimonium Tartaricum
- Great rattling of mucus, but very little is expectorated.
- Tongue coated, pasty, thick white, with red edges.
- Desire for apples, fruits & acids generally.
- Great drowsiness.
- Worse in evening; from lying down at night.
- Better from sitting erect.

Bryonia alba
- Frequent desire to take a long breath; difficult quick respiration; worse every movement.
- Thirst for a large drought.
- Abnormal hunger, loss of taste.
- Drowsy; starting when falling asleep.
- Cannot sit up; gets faint & sick.
- Better rest, pressure etc.

Ipecacuanha
- Dyspnoea; constant constriction in the chest.
- Tongue usually clean.
- Constant nausea and vomiting.
- Irritable.
- Worse lying down.

Phosphorus
- Tightness across chest; great weight on chest.
- Worse lying on the left side.
- Fan-like motion of nostrils.
- Thirst for very cold water.
- Hungry soon after eating.

Senega
- Rattling in chest.
- Worsing walking in open air, during rest.
- Better bending head backwards.
- Inclined to quarrel.

Some of the other homoeopathic medicines which can be considered are Ant-t., *Ars., Ars-i., Bryonia alba, Carb-v., Chel., Ferr-p., Hep., Ip., Lob., Lyc., Merc., Phosphorus, Seneg., Sep., Sulph., Verat-v.*, etc.

No Pneumonia : Cold or Cough

A child who has no chest indrawing and no fast breathing is classified as having no pneumonia; cold or cough.

Most of the children with a cough or difficult breathing do not have any danger signs or signs of pneumonia. These children have simple cough or cold.

Homoeopathic Efficacy

Some of the homoeopathic medicines which can be thought of are *Acon., Bry., Hyos., Spong., Hep., Dros., Rumx., Ambra grisea, Corallium rubrum*, etc.

Classifying the illness of the young infant (age less than 2 months)

This part describes the procedure to classify illness of the young infant with cough or difficult breathing and identify the appropriate treatment plan. The process is similar to the one described for the child aged 2 months upto 5 years.

Young infants have special characteristics that must be considered when their illness is classified. They can become sick and die very quickly from serious bacterial infections are much less likely to cough with pneumonia, and frequently the only non-specific signs such as poor

Respiratory Infections

feeding, fever or low body temperature. Further, mild chest indrawing is normal in young infants because their chest wall bones are soft.

The presence of these characteristics means that the health worker will assess, classify and treat young infants differently from the older children. The differences between the two age groups are presented in detail. Briefly the most important differences are :

- Some of the dangerous signs are different. In a young infant a danger sign include "stopped feeding well, fever or low body temperature" and wheezing. The sign of severe malnutrition is not a danger sign in young infants, although it is so in older children.
- A young infant must have severe chest indrawing to be classified as having severe pneumonia. A child aged 2 months up to 5 years is classified as having severe pneumonia if there is any chest indrawing that is clearly visible.
- The cut off for fast breathing is quiet different. A young infant has fast breathing when he or she is breathing 60 times per minute or more than 60. The cut offs for fast breathing in children aged 2 months up to 5 years are 50 times per minute or more if the children are aged 2 months up to 12 months or 40 times per minute or more if they are aged 12 months upto 5 years.
- Any pneumonia in young infants is considered to be severe. Young infants with pneumonia should be referred immediately to a hospital. Older children can be classified as having "pneumonia" or "severe pneumonia" in which they should be referred urgently to a hospital.

Essential Skills and Knowledge

By the end of this chapter, one should be able to :
- Classify the illness of a young infant with cough or difficult breathing based on signs found during the assessment.

Classification	Corresponding signs
Very severe disease	Stopped feeding well, convulsions, abnormally sleepy or difficult to wake, stridor when calm, wheezing, fever or low body temperature.

Severe pneumonia	Fast breathing or severe chest indrawing.
No pneumonia : Cold or Cough	No fast breathing and no severe chest indrawing or danger signs.

- Select appropriate treatment for the young infants based on the above classification & refer or advise the mother to give him/her home care.

The treatment include :
- Give an antibiotic.
- Advise the mother to give home care.
- Treat wheezing.
- Treat fever.

An Antibiotic

WHO recommends treating pneumonia by giving one of the following antibiotics for 5 days :

- Co-trimoxazole.
- Amoxycillin.
- Ampicillin.
- Procaine penicillin.

If the child cannot take an oral antibiotic, give a parenteral antibiotic such as procaine penicillin and refer the child as quickly as possible.

First Dose of an Antibiotics

The child needs to receive the first dose of an antibiotic in the health centre before being referred to a hospital or sent home to continue treatment. (If the referral time is less than an hour, such as in an urban area, it may not be necessary to give first dose at the health centre). If the child is to be treated at home by the mother, you should use this opportunity to show her how to give the antibiotic.

Instructions to the Mother

1. Explain carefully to the mother that how much of the antibiotic to be given, how often to give and when to give it. Write this information down for her, If she cannot read, draw a simple and understandable picture.

Respiratory Infections

2. Give the mother enough antibiotics for 5 days. Explain to her that she must give the antibiotics for 5 days. Finish the 5 days treatment even if the child seems better.
3. Make sure that the mother understands all the instructions and are easy to carry out. There are several ways to do this. Ask the mother to repeat the instructions. Then listen to her and correct the mistakes she makes.
4. Advise the mother how to give the home care.
5. Ask her to bring the child back to be reassessed in 2 days, or sooner if condition of the child worsens. It is required to reassess the child to see whether the child is improving with the antibiotic.

Reassessment after 2 days

The mother of any child receiving an antibiotic for pneumonia should bring the child back in 2 days, or sooner if the child worsens. During reassessment, one should follow the same procedures as for assessing a child with cough or difficult breathing for the first time.

Use the information about the child's signs to decide whether the child is :

- worse
- same or
- improving.

The child has **worsened** if he or she has more difficulty in breathing, is not able to drink, has chest indrawing, or has other danger signs. Refer the child urgently to a hospital.

The child has **improved** if he or she is breathing more slowly, has less fever or is eating better. The cough may still be present. Tell the mother to finish the 5 days treatment.

If the child,s condition is **same** as at the last assessment, ask the mother whether the child has been given the antibiotic as told to her. That the child may not have receive any of the antibiotic, or received too low or too infrequent a dose. If so, then he can be given antibiotics again.

If the child received antibiotic change to another antibiotic (if you have another appropriate alternative available for childhood pneumonia) for another 5 days.

- If the child was taking co-trioxazole switch on to ampicillin, amoxycillin or procaine penicillin.

- If the child was taking ampicillin, amoxycillin or procaine penicillin, switch to co-trioxazole.
- If you do not have another appropriate antibiotic available refer the child to the hospital.

Home Care

Home care is very important for a child with an acute respiratory infection due to its beneficial effects. Good home care means that the mother will :
- Feed the child to prevent weight loss as it can lead to malnutrition.
- Increase the amount of fluids in the child's diet to prevent dehydration. It can weaken the child to make the child even more sick.
- Soothe the child's sore throat and relieve the cough with a safe remedy.
- Most importantly watch for the signs that the child is getting worsened; return quickly to the health centre if they occur.

Teach the mother how to provide home care, and to ensure that she understands why it is important. If this child has a simple cough or cold; explain why the child will not get an antibiotics.

Feed the child
- Feed the child during illness. Children older than 4-6 months of age shoud be given foods rich in nutrients and energy. Depending on the age of the child these should be mixtures of the cereals, vegetables or pulses or mixtures of cereals and meat or fish. Increase the energy content of the food by adding vegetable oil. Encourage the child to eat as much as he or she wants. If the child is less than 4-6 months old or has not started taking soft foods, encourage the mother to breast feed frequently.

Increase fluids
- Offer the child extra to drink. Children with respiratory infection can lose more fluids than usual, especially when they have a fever. Tell the mother to give the child more fluids than usual. Examples of suitable fluids are : breast milk, water, formula or cow's milk, rice water or water in which other cereals have been cooked, home made soups, fresh fruit juices and yoghurt based drinks.

Respiratory Infections

Increase breast feeding
- If the child is exclusively breast-fed advise the mother to breast feed more frequently than usual.

Bad Throat and Cough
The mother can soothe the child's throat and relieve the cough by giving tea sweetened with sugar or honey, as a safe home made cough syrup or soothing remedy. However commercial medicines are often expensive and usually no more effective than home remedies.

Wheezing
Treat wheezing by using bronchodilater.

Fever
Fever is common in acute respiratory infections. The method of treating fever in a child aged 2 months upto 5 years will depend on whether the fever is high or low.

Fever High
- The child will feel better and eat better if the fever is lowered with paracetamol. It is harder for a child with pneumonia to breathe when he or she has a high fever.
- Tell the mother to give paracetamol every 6 hours in appropriate dosage until the child's temperature drops below 39° C. Give the mother enough paracetamol for 2 days.

Fever Low
- Advise the mother to give the child more fluids than usual. Paracetamol is not needed.

TUBERCULOSIS
TB is one of the most important killer of the present world. It has a very high prevalence.

Epidemiology

Agent
Myco-bacterium tuberculosis.

Source of Infection
The reservoir is almost always a case of pulmonary tuberculosis with sputum positivity.

Mode of Transmission
(i) Inhalation of droplets nuclei.
(ii) Ingestion.
(iii) Surface implantation.

Incubation Period
4 to 12 weeks usually.

Diagnosis

Tuberculin Test
This is a test for delayed hypersensitivity of tissue in response to tubercular proteins :

(A) Principles

Tuberculin is a extract from tubercle bacilli, having tubercular protein and other constituent. When this tuberculin is injected in small amounts —

(i) In a normal healthy animal then it results in a negligible inflammatory response.

(ii) In an animal who already has a previous tubercular infection 4-6 weeks earlier; leads to induration, oedema, erythema and pseudopodia formation at the site of injection with 48-72 hours. This is positive tuberculin reaction indicating existence of hypersensitivity to tuberculo-protein.

(B) Material

(i) Old Tuberculin (O.T.) — Used by Koch. A concentrated filtrate of tuberculous broth culture 6 weeks old on synthetic media.

(ii) Purified Protein Derivative (P.P.D) — Obtained by precipitation of proteins from O.T by trichloroacetic acid or half saturated solution of $(NH_4)_2 SO_4$.

Strength of Tuberculin
(i) Old tuberculin :

0.1 ml of 1 in 10,000 dilution = 1 T.U. (Tuberculin Unit)

0.1 ml of 1 in 1000 dilution = 10 T.U.

0.1 ml of 1 in 100 dilution = 100 T.U.

(ii) P.P.D = 0.0001 ml = 5 T.U

Respiratory Infections

Types of Tuberculin Test

(i) Intradermal method (Mantoux test) – Most commonly used, most accurate and reliable.

(ii) Multiple puncture – A layer of concentrated P.P.D (100,000 T.U/ml) is applied to skin and six intra dermal picks are made by a "Heaf gun". It is more rapid test, but not so easily standardised as Mantoux test.

(iii) Tine test – A test disc containing P.P.D is pressed on the forearm and a positive result is indicated by papules with induration of 2 mm or more.

(iv) Others — Subcutaneous (Koch).
  — Cutaneous scarification (Von-Pirquet).
  — Patch or jelly method (Volmer).
  — Optithalmic (calmetle).

Mantoux Test

(a) 0.1 ml of 1 in 10,000 dilution of O.T in normal saline is injected intradermally on flexor surface of one forearm. A similar dilution of normal saline is injected into the other arm as control.

(b) The results are read after 48-72 hours.

(c) The negative test is indicated by no change or negligible inflammatory change at the site of inoculation.

(d) A positive test is indicated by an induration (not less than 10 mm in diameter) with or without erythema, oedema and pseudopodia formation.

These local reactions may be accompanied by focal reactions (flaring up of already present tuberculous lesions) or general reactions – fever, malaise, prostration, etc.

Reading

Longitudinal diameter or induration :
- Less than 10 mm – Test is negative
- 10 mm or more – Test positive
- More than 15 mm – Strongly positive.

An immediate reaction which passes off within 48 hours is considered negative.

(e) If the test is negative after 48-72 hours, the test is repeated using 1 in 1000 dilution (10 T.U) and if this is negative, a further test with 1 in 100 dilution (100 T.U) is attempted. If this too, gives a negative result the patient is considered to be mantoux negative. A repeatedly negative result for a period of 6 weeks even on using gradually higher concentration of tuberculin, usually rules out the diagnosis of tuberculosis.

Interpretation of Tuberculin Test

(a) Tuberculin positive :
1. It indicates presence of tuberculous infection in the body, either past infection at least 4-6 weeks old or active disease.
2. In a child below three years age indicates active tuberculosis.
3. In a serial study, if there is a conversion from tuberculin negative to positive, it indicates active tuberculosis.
4. It indicates a potential state in the host, in which active disease can be caused without further exposure.
5. It indicates delayed hypersensitivity to tubercle bacilli.
6. False positive test :
   - Transient positive reactions, which disappear within 48 hours.
   - In warm climates, shows the presence of other mycobacteria.

(b) Tuberculin negative :
1. It means that the individual has never had any contact with tubercle bacilli, past or present.
2. Individual has got no immunity to tuberculosis, so that there is more susceptibility to infection.
3. The test may be considered negative, if results are repeatedly negative for a period of 6 weeks even on using higher concentration of tuberculin.
4. False negative reactions :
   - Due to loss of ability to express cell mediated immunity e.g. acute miliary tuberculosis or over-whelming tuberculosis, sarcoidosis, hodgkins disease, lepromatous leprosy. Immunosuppressive drugs like corticosteroids and cytotoxic agents, old age, gross malnutrition, intercurrent infection like measles, whooping cough and rheumatoid disease.
   - Last trimester of pregnancy – due to interaction of placental hormones.
   - If the test is done too early (before 4 weeks of infection).

5. Significance of Tuberculin test :
   - Early diagnosis particularly in children.
   - Mass surveillance.
   - Before giving B.C.G (Screening Test).
   - After giving B.C.G (To test efficacy of B.C.G.).
   - Defferential tuberculin test with antigens from the other mycobacteria helps in distinguishing tubercle bacilli from a typical mycobacteria.

Revised National TB Control Programme
Objectives
(a) **Overall**
   i) To reduce mortality and morbidity from tuberculosis.
   ii) To interrupt the chain of transmission of infection.

(b) **Operational**
   i) To cure at least 85% of all newly detected cases of pulmonary tuberculosis with supervised short course chemotherapy.
   ii) To detect at least 70% of the estimated incidence of smear positive pulmonary tuberculosis cases.

However, effort at increasing case detection would be made only after achieving 85% cure rate in the already detected cases.

Strategy
To achieve the above objectives of the revised NTP, the following strategy is being developed :
1. To change the current practice of radiological diagnosis to diagnosis by sputum microscopy.
2. To treat all smear positive cases and seriously ill sputum negative cases with *short course chemotherapy* directly supervised in the intensive phase and appropriately supervised in the continuation phase, through involvement of peripheral health functionaries.
3. To make available the required antitubercular drugs in appropriate blister combipacks, uninterruptedly to all peripheral areas.
4. To strenghten the capability of district tuberculosis centre and state TB demonstration and training centres for effective implementation, monitoring and evaluation of the programme including cohort analysis of patients under treatment.

5. Strenghtening supervision beyond district level.
6. Augmenting training capabilities both at national and state levels.
7. Introducing a professionally managed Information, Education & Communication (IEC) campaign.
8. To involve NGOs and private medical practitioners.
9. Operational research.

The revised strategy is in line with the recommendations made by WHO. Khatri (Ind J. Tub 1999, 46, 157) reviewed the results of treatment of first 100,000 patients put on treatment from October 1993 to March 1999. The quality of diagnosis was stated to be good, and treatment success was achieved in :

- 79% of both new smear positive and smear negative cases.
- 88% of patients with extra pulmonary tuberculosis.
- 67% of retreatment of smear positive patients.

Case finding methods under RNTCP

1. Sputum smear examination for AFB : 3 sputum specimens are examined – 1 spot, 2nd early morning, 3rd also spot sample when the patient brings 2nd sample. These are preferably collected within 2 days. Staining by **Z-N technique is done**.
2. X-Ray chest : This is unreliable, but is useful in sputum –ve cases or when only 1 sputum sample out of 3 is positive in chest symptomatics of miliary or extra pulmonary TB with history of contacts with infectious cases.
3. Culture : Useful to confirm the diagnosis in smear negative but X-ray positive symptomatics. Valuable for epidemiological surveillance and treatment planning for resistant/failure cases.
4. Tuberculin test : Important only in young children where a positive test (10 min. or more reaction) indicates likelihood of a recent infection.
5. Defaulter : A patient who interrupted treatment for 2 months or more after receiving ATT for 1 month or more.
6. Cured : A smear positive patient who has completed treatment and had negative sputum smears on at least 2 occasions, one of which was at completion of treatment.
7. Treatment completed : Sputum smear +ve case who has completed treatment with –ve smear at the end of initial phase but none at the end of treatment.

8. Chronic case : A patient who remains smear +ve after completing a retreatment regimen.

Case Definitions

Smear-positive Pulmonary Tuberculosis

TB in a patient with at least 2 initial sputum smear examinations positive for AFB or TB in a patient with one sputum positive and X-ray consistent with TB, or TB in a patient with one sputum positive and culture positive for *M.tuberculosis.*

Smear-negative Pulmonary Tuberculosis

TB in a patient with symptoms suggestive of TB with at least 3 sputum examinations negative for AFB, and X-ray consistent with active tuberculosis or diagnosis based on positive culture but negative AFB sputum examinations.

Extra-pulmonary Tuberculosis

TB of organs other than the lungs, such as the pleura, lymphnodes, abdomen, genitourinary tract, skin, joints and bones, tubercular meningitis, etc. Diagnosis should be based on one culture-positive specimen from the extra-pulmonary site, or histological evidence, or strong clinical evidence consistent with active extra-pulmonary TB.

Note : *Pleurisy is classified as extra-pulmonary TB.*

A patient with both pulmonary and extra-pulmonary TB should be classified as pulmonary TB.

Types of Cases

New : A patient who has never had treatment for tuberculosis or has taken anti-TB drugs for less than one month.

Relapse : A patient declared cured of TB by a physician, but who reports back and is found to be sputum positive.

Treatment after default : A patient who received ATT for one month or more from any source and who returns to treatment after having defaulted i.e., not taken drugs consecutively for two months or more.

Failure : A smear-positive patient who remains smear positive at 5 months or more after starting treatment. It also includes a patient who was initially smear-negative but who becomes smear-positive during treatment.

Determine the category of treatment based on the following table :

Category of Treatment	Type of Patient	Regimen*
Category I	New sputum smear positive PT Seriously ill smear-negative PT Seriously ill extra-pulmonary	2(HRZE)^3 4(HR)^3
Category II	Smear positive Relapse Smear positive Failure Smear positive Treatment after	2(HRZES)^3 1(HRZE)^3 5(HRE)^3
Category III	Smear negative, not seriously ill Extra pulmonary not seriously ill	2(HRZ)^3 4(HR)^3

Homoeopathic efficacy

Some of the medicines which can be thought of are :

Agar., Ars-i., Calc., Calc-p., Hep., Iod., Kali-c., Kali-s., Lyc., Psor., Puls., Senec., Sil., Spong., Stann., Sulph., Ther., Tub., Zinc.

Few Homoeopathic medicines with their indications are :

1. **Arsenicum iodatum :**
   - Hoarse racking cough.
   - Profuse purulent expectoration.
   - Intense thirst; water is immediately ejected.
   - Emaciation with good appetite.

2. **Calcarea carbonica :**
   - Bloody expectoration with a sour sensation in the chest.
   - Suffocating spells.
   - Aversion to meat, boiled things.
   - Desires indigestible things – chalk, coal, pencils, egg, salt and sweet.
   - Thirst for cold drinks.

3. **Phellandrium aquaticum :**
   - Offensive expectoration.
   - Everything tastes sweet.
   - Generally middle lobes affected.
   - Cough compels him to sit up.

Respiratory Infections

4. Tuberculinum
- Very susceptible to changes in weather.
- Hard, hacking cough.
- Averse to meat.
- Desire for cold milk.
- Poor sleep.

Sputum Collection and Examination

Three sputum samples are collected from all the patients presenting the symptoms of tuberculosis. The three samples are collected over two days – spot on the first day, and one early morning and one spot on the second day. This is equally sensitive as the collection of early morning specimens on three days. Sputum examination is of central importance in the RNTCP, and thus ensuring proper collection, transportation and examination of sputum is of critical value in the success of the programme. Microscopy is more objective and reliable than X-Ray. Inter-observer variation is much less with microscopy than with X-Ray. AFB microscopy also provides information on infectiousness of the patient and allows prioritization of cases. It is fair to say that sputum smear AFB positivity provides "good" evidence of tuberculosis while X-Ray does not. A systematic evaluation by National TB Institute, Bangalore, of well functioning district TB centres found that nearly 70% of the cases diagnosed and put on treatment on the basis of X-Ray, did not have tuberculosis at all.

If the slide has	Results	Positive(grading)	No. of fields to be examined
More than 10AFB/Field	Positive	3+	20
1-10AFB/Field	Positive	2+	50
10-99AFB/100 Fields	Positve	1+	100
1-9AFB/100 Fields	Scanty	Record exact no.	200
NoAFB in 100 Fields	Negative	–	100

Diagnosis of Tuberculosis : A Simple Flowchart

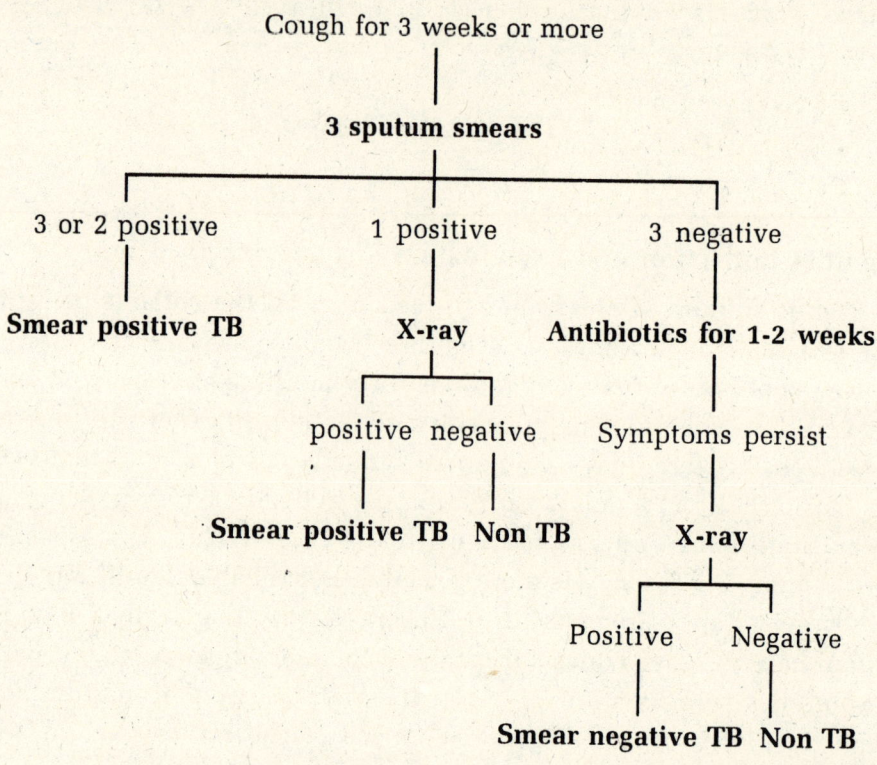

CHAPTER-5

INTESTINAL INFECTIONS

TYPHOID FEVER

Epidemiology

Agent : Salmonella typhi. It is a gram –ve bacillus.

Reservoir : Man is the natural reservoir either as case or carrier.

Cases are infectious as long as bacilli appear in stools or urine.

Carriers can be temporary or chronic. In most chronic carrier the bacilli persists in gall bladder and biliary tract.

Incubation Period : 10-14 days usually, but it is variable.

Transmission

Salmonella typhi lives only in humans. Persons with typhoid fever carry the bacteria in their blood stream and intestinal tract. In addition, a small number of persons, called carriers, recover from typhoid fever but continue to carry the bacteria, but ill persons and carriers shed S. typhi in their faeces (stool).

A person can have typhoid fever if he eats food or drinks beverages that have been handled by a person who is shedding S. typhi or if sewage contaminated with the bacterium gets into the water used for drinking or washing food. Therefore, typhoid fever is more common in areas where hand washing is less frequent and water is likely to be contaminated with sewage. Once S. typhi bacteria are eaten or drunk, they multiply and spread into the blood stream. The body reacts with fever and give forth signs and symptoms.

Prevention

Two basic actions for protection from typhoid fever :
1. Avoid risky food and drinks.

2. Get vaccinated against typhoid fever.
   - Mineral water should be used. Otherwise water should be boiled.
   - Ice used in the drinks should be made from bottled or boiled water.
   - Avoid raw vegetables and fruits that cannot be peeled.
   - Vaccination is the best method be get protected from typhoid, but typhoid vaccines lose effectiveness after several years.
   - Taking antibiotics will not prevent typhoid but they will only treat it.

Clinical Features
Signs and Symptoms
Persons with typhoid fever usually have a sustained fever as high as 103° to 104°F [39° to 40°C]. They may also feel weak or have stomach pains, headache.

Lab. Diagnosis
It is done either by culture or serological tests. Culture can be done from blood, faeces or urine. Serological test include widal test.

Widal Reaction
This test is based on the presence of antibodies against the H and O antigen in high numbers. Two types of tubes are used, **Dreyer's** agglutination tube for the H agglutination. Felix tube for the O agglutination. Equal volumes of diluted serum and H and O antigens are mixed in Dreyer's agglutination & **Felix** tube respectively and incubated in water bath at 37° C for 12 hours. To check the agglutination, control tubes having antigen and normal saliva are used. H agglutination leads to the formation of loose, cottony dumps whereas O agglutination forms discoid arrangement.

The test is useful only after 1 week because agglutinin starts appearing in the blood only after 1 week. After 4th week the titres, starts decreasing. A titre of 1/100 or more for O agglutinins and 1/200 for H agglutinins is concidered significant. Other tests are hemagglutination, ELISA, etc.

FIRST WEEK
1. Leucocyte count shows lymphopenia.
2. Blood culture is positive +++.

Intestinal Infections

3. Agglutination ± (widal test).
4. Stool culture ±.
5. Urine culture ±.

2nd WEEK

1. Agglutination +++ (widal test).
2. Stool culture ±.
3. Blood culture ±.
4. Urine culture ±.

3rd–4th WEEK

1. Agglutination ++.
2. Stool culture +.
3. Urine culture +.
4. Blood culture –.

In some cases, patients have a rash of flat, rose coloured spots. The only way to know for sure if an illness is typhoid fever is to have samples of stool or blood tested for the presence of Salmonella typhi.

Treatment

For the treatment of typhoid, antibiotics are prescribed. Three most commonly prescribed antibiotics are ampicillin, trimethoprim – sulfamethoxazole and cipro-floxacin. Persons given antibiotics usually begin to feel better within 2 to 3 days and death occurs rarely.

However, persons who do not get treatment may continue to have fever for weeks or months, and as many as 20% may die from complications of the infection.

Even if symptoms seem to be away, the person may still be carrying S. typhi bacteria and the illness could return or it can pass to other persons also.

If a person has been treated for typhoid fever, it is important to take care of some of the steps :

- Keep taking the prescribed antibiotics for as long as the doctor has asked to take them.
- Wash hands carefully with an antibiotic soap and water after using the bathroom, and do not prepare or serve food for the other people.

Homoeopathic Efficacy

Some of the homoeopaths have highly recommended Baptisia tinctoria, Typhoidinum, Bryonia alba and Hhyoscyamus niger for treatment of typhoid.

Other drugs which can be considered are Ars., Gelsemium sempervirens, Acidum muriaticum, Absinthium, etc.

POLIOMYELITIS

Poliomyelitis is caused by an RNA virus called polio virus. There are 3 serotypes 1, 2 and 3.

Man is the only known reservoir of infection.

Host Factors

The most vulnerable age is between 6 month – 3 years.

Mode of Transmission

Faecal-oral route is the main route of transmission but infection can occur via droplets.

Incubation period

7 to 14 days.

Clinical Spectrum

Four types :
(1) Inapparent illness.
(2) Minor illness.
(3) Non paralytic polio.
(4) Paralytic polio.

POLIO ERADICATION

Polio eradication

It is the interruption of transmission of indigenous wild polio virus and not solely the eradication of paralytic poliomyelitis.

Criteria for Eradication

(1) No case of Poliomyelitis caused by wild polio virus for 3 consecutive years.
(2) No wild polio virus identified world wide through sampling of communities & environment.

Intestinal Infections

Strategies of Polio Eradication
(1) High coverage & routine immunization if (100) % children new borns (2).
(2) Conducting IPPI rounds.
(3) Acute Flaccid Paralysis (AFP) surveillance actions.
(4) Conducting 'mopping up' immune when polio is reduced to focal transmission.
  4 States → 1 State → 1 District → 1 Tehsil.

Some Drawbacks of Routine Immunization Programme
- In Delhi – Coverage 70-80%.
- Wide variation between different areas in JJ cluster, unauthorised and resettlement colonies having poor coverage.
- Many missed opportunities for immunization children attending OPDs/Hospitals/Health Centres for minor ailment.
- 'O' dose often not given to new borns.

Supplementary Immunization Activities
- NIDs → Covers entire country especially in Bimarro states.
- Sub National Immunization days (SNID's).
- Mopping up Immunization → Focal transmitted area.

NID/SNID
Simultaneous administration of OPV to all children :
- 0-59 months of age.
- Over a short period of time.
- In a large geographical area, regardless of previous immunization status.

Usually 2 rounds separated by 4 to 6 weeks. Popularly known as PPI in India.

4 Rounds	Sept. – last week.
2 NID	Nov.
2 SNIDs	Feb.

Limitation of PPIs
1. Coverage not uniform.
2. Overall coverage figures mask pocket of poor package.

3. Nearly 10% children left out may be more in some area.
4. Large susceptible pool left out especially in high risk areas.

Reason for Non-immunization during PPI
1. Child out of home (accompanying working parents).
2. No one available in household to take child to PPI post.
3. Lack of interest on motivation to take child to PPI post.
4. Fear/Mistrust of vaccination.
5. Child too small/sick.

Intensification

Quantitative	Qualitative
1. Adding more rounds.	1. House-to-house search for the missed and vaccinating.
2. Adding more days in each round to ensure completeness of the activity.	2. Intensive planning.
	3. Intensive supervision & monitoring.

IPPI Benefits
- Overcome the shortcoming of PPI.
- Directs the resources to the area which need most.

Schedule of IPPI
Day 1 – Vaccination post based.
Day 2 – House-to-House vaccination.
Day 3 – House-to-House continues till no child is left unvaccinated.

1 Worker = 500 Houses × 5 days.
[last day of month is convenient < 7'O' clock] or after noon time.

Surveillance for Global Polio Eradication
- T/–ve of wild virus.
- Identify area of transmission.
- Direct immunisation activities.
- AFP surveillance in < 15 years.
- Sudden onset of flaccid paralysis.

Intestinal Infections

- No or obvious cause for flaccid paralysis is found or paralytic illness at any age of life.

AFP → PM
→ GBS
→ Transverse myelitis.
→ Traumatic Neuritis.

Non AFP → Hypokalemen   – Om
→ Trauma   – Vascular lesions.
→ Securing.
→ Acute Rheumatic fever.
→ Synovitis.

AFP Surveillance

For a each AFP case :
- 2 stool sample, collected at least 24 hours.
- Apart & in 14 days of onset of AFP. (after 14 days → virus may not be the in stool)
- Outbreak responding Immunization (Active case search).
- As easily as possible after case pacific ideally & in 12 hours.
  1 Round in be 17 to 19.
  Cover all under 5 children.
  At least 500 children.
  Collect 2 stool sample.

Mopping up Immunization

One of is strategies of Polio eradication focal area transmission.
- Target area remaining & evidence of wild virus.
- Massive, active, House-to-House immunization of high quality.
- Meticulous is planning.
- 4-6 weeks interval.
- 0-59 month.

1998	1999	2000	2001
1934 case	1126 case	265 case	81 case

Uttar Pradesh → 67
Bihar → 11

FOOD POISONING

Botulism

Botulism is a rare but serious paralytic illness caused by a nerve toxin that is produced by the bacterium *Clostridium botulinum*. There are three main kinds of botulism :

1. **Food borne botulism** is caused by eating foods that contain the preformed botulism toxin.
2. **Wound botulism** caused by toxin produced from a wound infected with Clostridium botulinum.
3. **Infant botulism** is caused by consuming the spores of the botulinum bacteria, which then grow in the intestines and release toxin.

All forms of botulism can be fatal and are considered medical emergencies. Food borne botulism can be especially dangerous because many people can be poisoned by eating the contaminated food.

Agent

Clostridium botulinum is the name of a bacteria commonly found in soil. These rod-shaped organisms grow best in low oxygen conditions. They produces spores which allow them to survive in a dormant state until exposed to conditions that can support their growth. There are seven types of botulism toxin designated by the letters A to G; only types A, B, E and F cause illness in humans.

Clinical Picture

The classical symptoms of botulism include double vision, blurred vision, drooping eyelids, slurred speech, difficulty in swallowing, dry mouth and muscle weakness. Infants with botulism appear lethargic, feed poorly, are constipated, and have a weak cry and poor muscle tone. These all are symptoms of the muscle paralysis caused by bacterial toxin. If untreated, these symptoms may progress to cause paralysis of the arms, legs, trunk and respiratory muscles. In food borne botulism, symptoms generally begin 18 to 36 hours after eating a contaminated food, but they can occur as early as 6 hours and as late as 10 days.

Diagnosis

Physicians may consider the diagnosis if the patients history and physical examination suggest botulism. However these clues are usually not enough to allow a diagnosis of botulism. Other diseases such as Guillian – Barre syndrome, stroke and myasthenia gravis can appear similar to botulism and special tests may be needed to exclude these other conditions. These tests may include a brain scan, spinal fluid examination, nerve conduction test (electromyography or EMG), and a Tensilon test for myasthenia gravis. The most direct way to confirm the diagnosis is to demonstrate the botulinum toxin in the patient's serum or stool by injecting serum or stool into mice and look for signs of botulism. The bacteria can also be isolated from the stool of persons with food borne and infant botulism. These tests can be performed at some state health department laboratories and at CDC.

Treatment

The respiratory failure and paralysis that occur with severe botulism may require a patient to be on a breathing machine for weeks, plus intensive medical and nursing care. After several weeks, the paralysis slowly improves. If diagnosed early, food borne and wound botulism can be treated with an antitoxin circulating in the blood. This can prevent patients from worsening, but recovery still takes many weeks. Physicians may try to remove contaminated food present in the gut by inducing vomiting or by using enemas. Wounds should be treated, usually surgically, to remove the source of the toxin – producing bacteria. Good supportive care in a hospital is the main stay of therapy for all forms of botulism. Currently, antitoxin is not routinely given for treatment of infant botulism.

Homoeopathic Treatment

Some of the recommended medicines are *Ars., Carb-v., Nux-v., Puls.,* etc.

Complications

Botulism can result is death due to respiratory failure. However, in the past 50 years the proportion of patients with botulism who die has fallen from about 80% to 50%. A patient with severe botulism may require a breathing machine as well as intensive medical and nursing care for several months. Patients who survive an episode of botulism poisoning may have fatigue and shortness of breath for years and long term therapy may be needed to aid recovery.

Prevention

Botulism can be prevented. Food-borne botulism has often been due to home – canned foods with no acid content, However, outbreaks of botulism from more unusual sources such as chopped garlic in oil, chile peppers, tomatoes, improperly handled baked potatoes wrapped in aluminium foil and home – canned or fermented fish. People who do home canning should follow strict hygienic procedures to reduce contamination of foods. Oils infused with garlic or herbs should be refrigerated. Because the botulism toxin is destroyed by high temperatures, persons who eat home – canned food should consider boiling the food for 10 minutes before eating to ensure safety. Instructions on safe home canning can be obtained from county extension services or from the Department of Agriculture. Honey can contain spores of Clostridium botulism and this has been a source of infection for infants less than 12 months old & they should not be fed honey. Honey is safe for children of 1 year of age and older. Wound botulism can be prevented by promptly seeking medical care for infected wounds and by not using injectable street drugs.

Public education about botulism prevention is an ongoing activity. Information about safe canning is widely available for consumers. If antitoxin is needed to treat a patient, it can be quickly delivered to a physician anywhere in the country. Suspected outbreaks of botulism are quickly investigated, and if they involve a commercial product, the appropriate control measures are coordinated among public health and regulatory agencies. Physicians should promptly report suspected cases of botulism.

CHAPTER-6

ARTHROPOD BORNE DISEASES

MALARIA
Members of the genus Plasmodium are collectively known as malarial parasites because they cause a febrile disease called malaria.

In man i.e. the intermediate host, they invade the reticuloendothelial system and in female Anopheles mosquito, i.e. definitive host, they reside in the salivary glands.

Species
- Plasmodium vivax.
- P. Malariae.
- P. falciparum.
- P. ovale.

Life Cycle of Plasmodium
It completes its life cycle in two phases :
(1) A-sexual or Endogenous phase in human.
(2) Sexual or Exogenous phase in mosquito.

A sexual phase takes place in man. It is divided in three phases :
(a) Pre-erythrocytic phase.
(b) Exo-erythrocytic phase.
(c) Erythrocytic phase.

LIFE CYCLE OF PLASMODIUM IN HUMAN
Pre-erythrocytic Phase
When an Anopheles mosquito, in which malaria parasites are present, bites a healthy man, it leaves some sporozoites in the blood of man with the saliva of mosquito. Each sporozoite is sickle-shaped and about 14 μ long. These sporozoites come into the blood stream of man. After about half an hour they leave the circulatory system and reach parenchymatous cells of the liver.

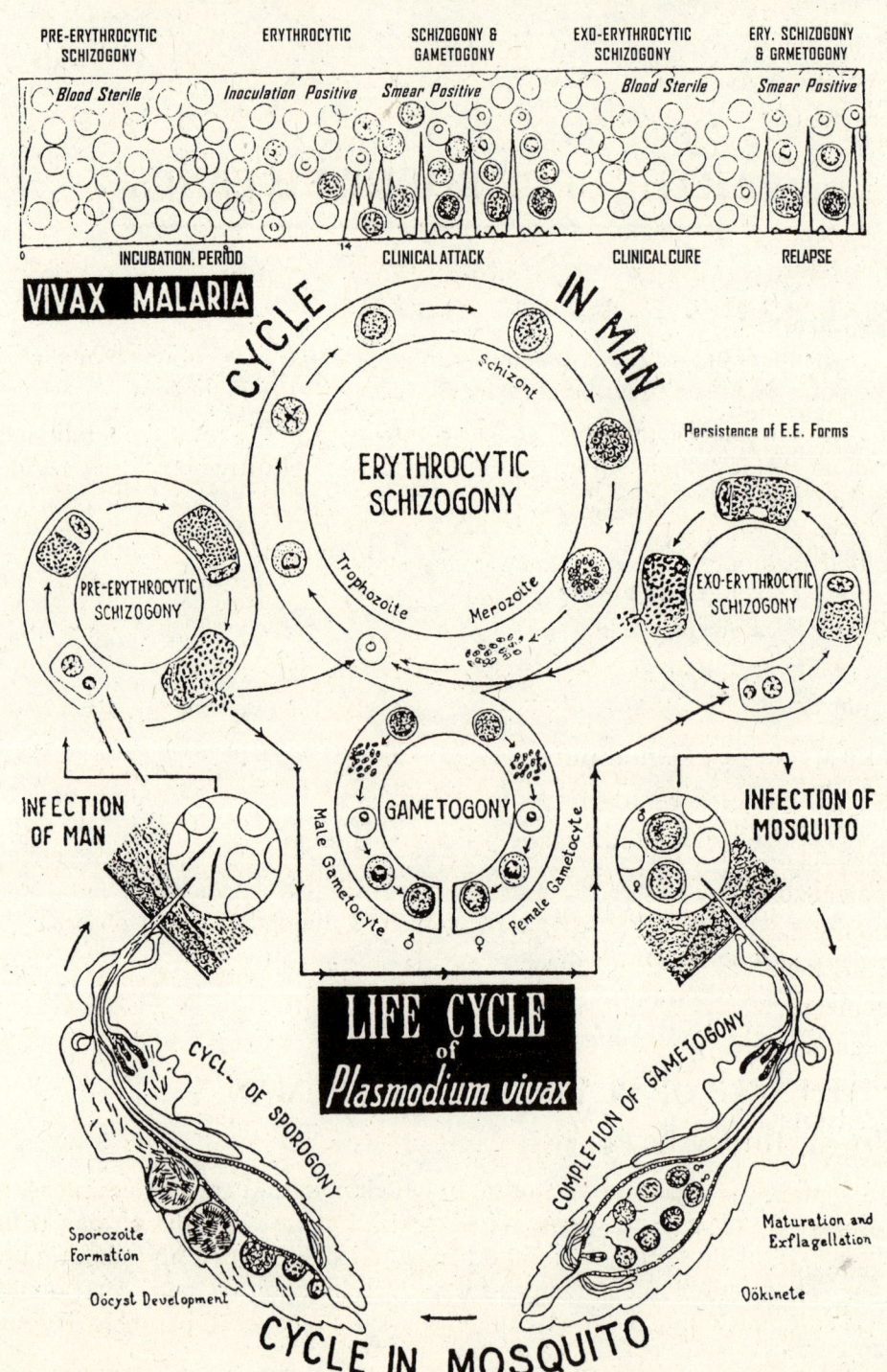

Liver Schizogony

In the parenchymatous cells of liver they grow and form **schizonts**. After sometime the nucleus of schizont divides into about 1,000 small nuclei. A little cytoplasm around each nuclei and thus 1,000 mcrozoites are formed which are also called **cryptozoites**. The nucleus of schizont divides by multiple fission. This division is called liver schizogony. The wall of schizont and liver cell bursts due to great numbers of the cryptozoites in them and all the cyptozoites go into the sinusoides of the liver.

Exo-erythrocytic Phase

The cyptozoites of the pre-erythrocytic phase which are released in the liver sinusoides attack new liver cells and they again form schizonts. These again under go multiple fission and form many **cryptozoites** which are called **metacryptozoites**. This phase is known as exoerythrocytic phase. After two or more such phases some metacryptozoites come into blood circulation and attack the red blood corpuscles.

Erythrocytic Cycle

Meta-eryptomerozoites start growing in the RBCs obtaining their food from them. They are round in shape and soon a non-contractile vacuole is formed. This stage is called signet-ring stage. With further growth the vacuole disappears and it assumes amoeba like form. It starts feeding on haemoglobin and grows rapidly. This is known as trophozoite stage. After feeding on haemoglobin they form a yellowish brown substance called **haemozoin**. As the trophozoite increase in size, it becomes round and completely fills red blood corpuscles. This is known as **schizont**. The RBC becomes weak and loses its normal shape due to growth of the schizont within it. It swells in size and becomes light in colour with its regular shape. In its remaining cytoplasm several small, orange or yellow coloured granules are formed which are known as **Schuffner's dots**. Multiple fission takes place in schizont and its nucleus divides into many small nuclei around each of which a little cytoplasm gathers. In this manners 6 to 36 merozoites are formed in each schizont. After sometime schizont bursts liberating the merozoites in the blood. These merozoites attack fresh red blood corpuscles. This process is repeated many times and innumerable RBCs destroyed.

LIFE CYCLE OF PLASMODIUM IN MOSQUITO

The sexual or exogenous phase takes place in female Anopheles. It is divided into two stages.
- Gametogamy.
- Sporogamy.

Gametogamy

After many sexual cycle some merozoites increases in size within the RBC and form gametocytes. Some of these are small and are known as **microgametocyte**, while others are large and are called as **macrogametocytes**. Have a clear cytoplasm with a central nucleus.

Females or macrogametocytes are round and their cytoplasm is laden with food. The nucleus is ecentric, placed on one side. Male or microgametocytes have clear cytoplasm with central nucleus.

If the female anopheles mosquito bites a man having this stage of plasmodium, then along with merozoites some gametocytes are also sucked up with blood and reach the stomach of mosquito where their development takes place. The nucleus of microgametocytes divides into 6 to 8 small nuclei around each of which a little cytoplasm collects forming long flagellated structure known as microgametes. This process is called exflagellation Macrogametocyte undergoes little changes. It increases in size and its nucleus divided into two. One of the nuclei moves out along with some cytoplasm and form the polar body. In the remaining larger part, a small conical structure is formed which is known as reception zone. Thus a macrogamete is formed from one macrogametocyte only.

Fertilization

Microgamete is attracted towards the macrogametes and enters the latter in its reception zone. This nucleus and cytoplasm of both the gametes fuse and forms a zygote. This process is called as fertilization.

The zygote remains inactive for sometime after which it lengthens and becomes motile like worm. This motile zygote is known as **ookinete** or vermicule. The ookinete after passing through stomach muscles settles in the outermost layer where it forms a protective covering or cyst around itself. Such structures are called **oocysts** and this process is known as **oocystation**. Fifty to five hundred oocysts are found in the stomach of a female mosquito.

Sporogony

The oocyst now increase about five times in its size and its nucleus divides into many small nuclei. Simultaneously by several vacuoles are formed in the cytoplasm and the nuclei gather around them. A little cytoplasm collects around each nuclei forming elongated structures called sporozoite. A single oocyst may contain about 1,000 sporozoites. This process of formation of sporozoites in the wall of the stomach is known as sporogony. After sometime the wall of the oocyst brusts due to much pressure and the sporozoites are set free in the body cavity of the mosquito. Soon after this, sporozoites enter the salivary glands of the mosquito which becomes infective. When this mosquito bites a healthy man the sporozoites enter his blood along with the saliva. Thus the life history of malarial parasite is completed.

Pathogenicity

It causes malaria characterised by febrile paroxysms, anaemia and splenomegaly.

Types of Fever

The febrile paroxysm synchronises with the erythrocytic schizogony of the malarial parasite.
  (a) With in a 48 hour cycle the fever recurs every third day (tertian fever).
  (b) With a 72 hour cycle the fever recurs every fourth day, (quartan fever).

Lab Diagnosis of Malaria

Main diagnostic examination is microscopical examination of a blood film. This show the plasmodium unless an anti-malarial drug has been administered prior.

In a well stained film, if parasites are numerous, the species can be easily identified but the possibility of mixed infection should always be remembered.

Other methods of diagnosis :
  1. Blood Count – The significant change in chronic malaria is moderate leucopenia with monocytosis.
  2. Cultural examinations.
  3. Serological Tests – Complement fixation test, Immuno- fluorence, etc.

Measurements of Malaria

Classical — Spleen rate.
Average enlarged spleen.
Parasite rate.
Parasite density index.
Infant parasite index.
Proportional case rate.

Currently used indices — Annual parasite incidence.
Annual blood examination rate.
Annual falciparum incidence.
Slide positivity rate.
Slide falciparum rate.

Vector indices — Human blood index.
Sporozoite rate.
Mosquito density.
Man-biting rate.
Inoculation rate.

$$\text{Annual Blood Examination Rate, (ABER)} = \frac{\text{No. of slides examined}}{\text{Total population}} \times 100 \text{ (for July)}$$

$$\text{Annual Parasite Incidence, (API)} = \frac{\text{Continued cases during 1 year}}{\text{Population under surveillance}} \times 100$$

$$\text{Total parasite infestation rate} = \frac{\text{No. of +ve persons}}{\text{Population}} \times 100$$

$$\text{Specific parasite rate} = \frac{\text{No. of parasites detected}}{\text{Total no. of +ve persons}} \times 100$$

TREATMENT OF MALARIA (AS PER NAMP)
*Uncomplicated Malaria
Presumptive Treatment (PT)

Chloroquine   sulphadoxine = 25mg 1kg.
                     primaquine = 0.75mg 1kg.

Low Risk Area

It comprises of a single dose of Chloroquine phosphate 10mg/kg. body weight to all suspected malaria cases.

	Chloroquine Phosphate	
Age in Years	Mg. base	No. of Tablets (150 mg)
< 1	75	½
1-4	150	1
5-8	300	2
9-14	450	3
15 & above	600	4

High Risk Area

As per revised drug policy of NAMP, presumptive treatment of all suspected malaria cases, at *Sub-centre level* and above, in "high risk areas" is as follows :

Adults :

Day 1 — Chloroquine base 600 mg + Primaquine 45 mg
Day 2 — Chloroquine base 600 mg
Day 3 — Chloroquine base 300 mg

Children :

Day 1 — Chloroquine base 10 mg + Primaquine 0.75 mg/kg
Day 2 — Chloroquine base 10 mg/kg
Day 3 — Chloroquine base 5 mg/kg

Note : Presumptive treatment at Fever Treatment Depots or Drug Distribution Centres, i.e. below the level of sub-centre consists of single dose of chloroquine (10 mg/kg) only and no primaquine is given.

Radical Treatment

Low Risk Area

Plasmodim vivax

Adults :

First day : Chloroquine base 600 mg base + Primaquine 15 mg
2nd-5th day : Primaquine 15 mg daily

Children :

First day : Chloroquine 10 mg/kg body weight + Primaquine 0.25 mg/kg body weight
2nd-5th day : Primaquine 0.25 mg/kg body weight

Plasmodim falciparum

In "Low Risk Areas" where presumptive treatment with 600 mg chloroquine alone (adult dose) has been given and later found positive for P. Falciparum, they should be given complete radical treatment with a single dose of chloroquine 600 mg base alongwith 45 mg of primaquine.

High Risk Area

Plasmodium vivax

In high risk areas where presumptive treatment with 1500 mg Chloroquine base and 45 mg Primaquine (Adult dose) has been given, Chloroquine need not be administered again, but Primaquine 0.25 mg/kg body weight (15 mg daily for adults) must be given for 5 days.

Plasmodium Falciparum

In "High Risk Areas", fever cases are given presumptive treatment with 1500 mg. Chloroquine (over 3 days) and 45 mg Primaquine (adult single dose). Therefore, further radical treatment with primaquine is not required if they are found positive for P. Falciparum microscopically, as the same has already been administered.

Note : Infants and Pregnant women are not to be given Primaquine.

Chloroquine Resistant P. Falciparum Cases

The radical treatment of P. Falciparum cases in chloroquine resistant areas which are under alternate drug schedule, and in specific cases not responding to chloroquine, second line of treatment must be given in a single dose of Sulphalene/Sulphadoxine (1500 mg) + Pyrimethamine (75 mg) (3 tablets in adults) followed by Primaquine (45 mg).

Children are given Sulfalene/Sulfadoxine 25 mg/kg + Pyrimethamine 1.25 mg/kg + Primaquine 0.75 mg/kg body weight as single dose.

Note : Sulfadoxine/Sulfalene and Pyrimethamine combination is ineffective against P. vivax.

Homoeopathic Approach and Treatment

Hahnemann has clearly stated intermittent fever to which are apparently non-febrile, typical, periodically recurring morbid states, observed in individual cases, always belong to chronic diseases, mostly psoric and very occasionally complicated with syphilis (§ 234).

Some of the drugs with reliable indications are :

1. **Natrium muriaticum**
   - Fever, paroxysmal < 11 a.m.
   - Fever with dry tongue with thirst.
   - Constipation.
   - Anaemia.
   - Hot patient.
   - Desire salt, bitter.

2. **Arsenicum album**
   - Fever < mid day/mid night.
   - Restlessness.
   - Chilly.
   - Thirst for small quantity of water at short interval.
   - Desire warm drinks.
   - Aversion to sweet.

3. **Cinchona officinalis**
   - Paroxysmal fever
   - Anticipatory chill
   - Chilly patient
   - Anaemia
   - Desire sour food
   - Irritable
   - Spleen enlarged

4. **Chininum sulphuricum**
   - Fever < afternoon 3-5 p.m.
   - chilliness
   - Anaemia
   - Severe frontal headache

5. **Arsenicum sulphuratum rubrum**
   - Fever < mid day/mid night
   - Hot patient
   - Aversion to sweet
   - Thirst for small quantity of water of small interval.

6. **Eupatorium perfoliatum**
   - Fever < morning hours
   - Chilliness preceded by thirst

- Aching bones & soreness of body
- Headache not relieved after fever
- Bitter taste in mouth with thirst.

Some of the mother tinctures with their indications are :

1. **Azadirachta indica**
   - Afternoon fever
   - Sweat an upper part of body
   - Fever with aching pain.

2. **Alstonia scholaris**
   - Malarial fever with diarrhoea/dysentry/indigestion.
   - Anaemia
   - Diarrhoea < after eating.

3. **Nyctanthes arbortristis**
   - Fever with thirst before andy during chill and heat stage.
   - Sweat stage most marked.
   - Constipatioin.

4. **Gentiana chiarata**
   - Chill with nausea and bitter vomitting.
   - Desire for hot drinks in heat stage.

WHAT IS ROLL BACK MALARIA?

ROLL BACK MALARIA (RBM) is a global partnership founded in 1998 by the World Health Organization (WHO), the United Nations Development Programme (UNDP), the United Nations Children's Fund (UNICEF) and the World Bank with the goal of halving the world's malaria burden by 2010 – estimated to be greater than 300 million acute illnesses and 1 million deaths per year. The RBM partnership includes national governments, civil society and non-governmental organizations, research institutions, professional associations, UN and development agencies, development banks, the private sector and the media. The strength of RBM is the diverse strengths and expertise of its many partners.

RBM was founded in response to a growing concern by governments, particularly in Africa, about the continuing and increasing burden of disease and death due to malaria. RBM is being built on the shoulders of recent successful efforts in malaria-affected countries and regions to improve and support capacity to scale up action against malaria.

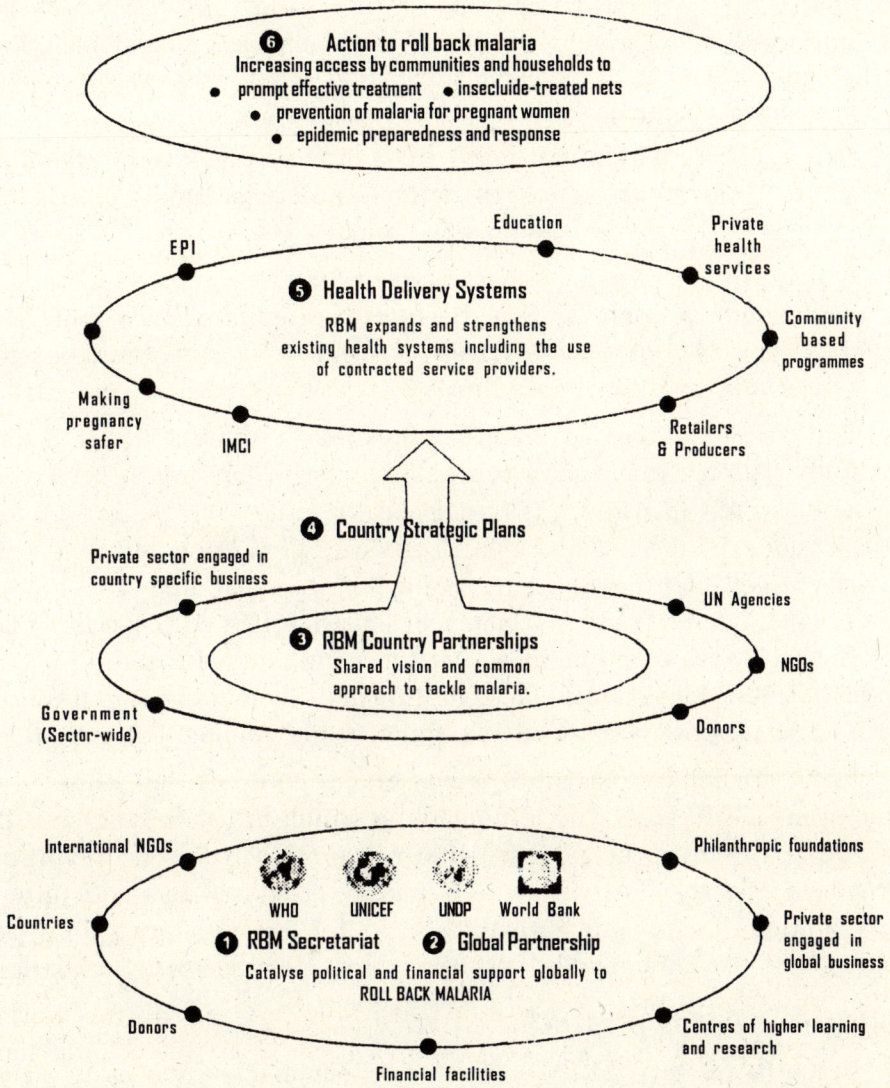

The RBM partnership supports efforts to tackle malaria wherever it occurs. However 90% of the malaria burden is in Africa, south of the Sahara. In addition, almost everywhere that malaria occurs, but particularly in Africa, the burden of disease and death falls mainly on two vulnerable groups : young children and pregnant women. As a result, the focus of RBM and its greatest challenges are in reducing the burden of malaria in these two vulnerable groups in the African region.

RBM is seeking to :

- Expand the use of interventions which are already known to be effective in tackling malaria. This includes prompt access to effective treatment, promotion of insecticide-treated mosquito nets and improved vector control, prevention and management of malaria in pregnancy and improving the prevention of and response to malaria epidemics and malaria in complex emergencies;

- Support work which will result in even more effective interventions in the near future, such as better medicines and longer-lasting insecticide-treated mosquito nets; and
- Encourage the research necessary for even better interventions to be developed and deployed in the future – including new and better drugs and insecticides, as well as malaria vaccines and possibly genetically modified mosquitoes that will not transmit malaria.

Political commitment is essential for RBM. In Abuja, Nigeria, in April 2000 delegations from 44 African nations met in the largest ever Head-of-State summit focussed on a single health issue. The African leaders, who endorsed RBM's goal for 2010 in the Abuja Declaration, also set interim targets and drew up a plan of action for expanding access to and use of effective interventions. One year later, the first Africa Malaria Day re-affirmed that commitment across the continent with public events, education campaigns and a demonstration of the commitment of resources and action against malaria in the spirit of the **Abuja Declaration**.

RBM corporate partners have also demonstrated their own commitment and generated a momentum which brings more companies into the partnership every year. RBM corporate partners are helping to expand access to effective interventions by providing services, through contributions to research directly and indirectly, and through support to RBM's efforts to reduce the cost of established and newer interventions.

RBM's four Pillars of Action

ROLL BACK MALARIA is promoting four main strategies to pursue its goal of halving the world's burden of malaria by 2010. The strategies are evidence-based (shown to be effective), outcome-focussed and cost-effective.

- **Prompt access to treatment** : All people, especially young children, must receive prompt treatment with effective drugs. RBM is working to ensure that people seek treatment promptly when they or their children have malaria symptoms and to educate health workers and shopkeepers (who sell anti-malarial drugs) to recognize and correctly treat malaria. Mapping drug resistance, encouraging and supporting countries to change their treatment policies when necessary and promoting the development and use of new drugs, particularly combination drugs which slow the development of resistance, are essential to the success of this strategy.

- **Insecticide-treated mosquito nets (ITNs)** : A substantial body of evidence shows that in malarious areas, ITNs reduce deaths in young children by about 20% and that for every 1,000 children under five protected by ITNs about six lives are saved each year. Sleeping under an ITN is the most effective method for individuals and families to avoid malaria. Social marketing programmes, encouraging local mosquito net industries and persuading governments to abolish taxes and tariffs on ITNs, are helping bring down the cost of an ITN while the recent development of long-lasting insecticide-treated nets may eliminate the need for regular re-treatment.

- **Prevention and control of malaria in pregnant women** : Pregnant women and their unborn children are particularly vulnerable to malaria, which is a major cause of perinatal mortality, low birth weight and maternal anaemia. As well as sleeping under ITNs, intermittent treatment doses of effective anti-malarial drugs, given to all pregnant women at risk of malaria, is highly effective in reducing the consequences of malaria during pregnancy.

- **Malaria epidemic and emergency response** : Epidemics can occur when malaria attacks vulnerable populations with little or no immunity. In such situations, people of all age groups are at risk of death or severe disease. Factors which may precipitate a malaria epidemic fall into two categories : natural (climatic variations, natural disasters), and man-made (conflict and war, agricultural projects, dams, mining, logging). The RBM partnership is working to improve the prediction, detection of and response to epidemics as well as developing tools and strategies to prevent or limit the impact of malaria in complex emergencies.

NATIONAL MALARIA ERADICATION PROGRAMME

National Malaria control programme (NMCP) was launched in India in April 1953. It was based on indoor residual spraying with DDT (1 g per sq. metre of surface area) twice a year in endemic areas where spleen rates were over 10%. The NMCP was in operation for 5 years (1953-58). The result of the programme were highly successful in that the incidence of malaria had declined sharply from 75 million cases in 1953 to 2 million cases in 1958, an estimated 80% reduction of the malaria problem, it also paid rich dividends to the country in different fields like agriculture, land projects and industry. Encouraged by these spectacular results government of India in the ministry of health changed the strategy from malaria control to eradication, and launched the more ambitious National Malaria Eradication Programme (NMEP) in 1958. According to international standards, the programme was divided in to preparatory, attack, consolidation and maintenance phases.

In the beginning, malaria eradication programme was highly successful. But very soon setbacks appeared in the form of focal outbreaks. The resurgence had grown to epidemic proportions. The annual incidence of malaria cases in India escalated from 50,000 in 1961 to a peak of 6.4 million cases in 1976.

Revised Strategy

Considering the resurgence of malaria as well as the situation in the neighboring countries, the government of India in the ministry of health appointed several task forces and expert committees on malaria to review the situation. Based on their recommendations, a modified Plan of Operation (MPO) to control malaria was evolved, and put into operation from April 1977.

Modified Plan of Operation

1. Objectives

The Modified Plan of Operation under the NMEP came into force from 1st April 1977 with the following objectives :

- to prevent deaths due to malaria.
- to reduce malaria morbidity.
- to maintain agricultural and industrial production by undertaking intensives anti-malarial measures in such areas.
- to consolidate the gains so far achieved.

Flexibility in the policies according to the epidemiological situation and local conditions is an essential feature in this programme.

2. Reclassification of Endemic Areas

The report of the consultative committee of experts indicated that in order to stabilize the malaria situation in the country, areas with Annual Parasites Incidence 2 and above should be taken up for spray operations. This led to the abolition of the earlier phasing of the anti-malaria units as attack, consolidation and maintenance phase areas, and reclassification of areas according to Annual Parasites Incidence.

3. Areas with API more than 2

(a) **Spraying** : All areas with API2 and above are brought under regular insecticidal spray with 2 rounds of DDT, unless the vector is refractory. Where the vector is refractory to DDT, 3 rounds of malathion are recommended. Areas refractory both to DDT and malathion are to be treated with 2 rounds of synthetic pyrethroids dosage applied are 1.0, 2.0 and 0.25g per sq. meter surface respectively. BHC has been discontinued since 1.4.1997 in view of its adverse environmental effects. Whenever an honest effort has been made to spray insecticides systematically, malaria has either been brought down, or at least kept at low levels.

(b) **Entomological Assessment** : This is done by entomological teams. They carry out susceptibility tests and suggest appropriate insecticide to be used in particular areas.

(c) **Surveillance** : The collection and examination of blood smears is a key element of the Modified Plan of Operation. Active and passive surveillance activities are carried out fortnightly in all areas with API2 and above.

(d) **Treatment of Cases** : Great emphasis is laid on the presumptive and radical treatment of cases.

4. Areas with API less than 2

(a) **Spraying** : These areas will not be under regular insecticidal spraying. However, "focal spraying" is to be undertaken only around P. falciparum cases detected during surveillance.

(b) **Surveillance** : As these areas will not be under regular spraying, active and passive surveillance operations will have to be carried out vigorously every fortnight.

(c) **Treatment** : All detected cases should receive radical treatment as prescribed.

(d) **Follow-up** : Follow-up blood smears are to be collected from all positive cases on completion of the radical treatment and thereafter at monthly intervals for 12 months.

(e) **Epidemiological Investigation** : All malaria positive cases are to be investigated. This may include mass surveys.

5. Drug Distribution Centres and Fever Treatment Depots

With the increasing number of malaria cases, the demand for antimalarial drugs has increased tremendously. It became cleat that drug supply only through surveillance workers and medical institutions was not enough. This led to the establishment of a wide network of Drug Distribution Centres and Fever Treatment Depots. Drug distribution centres are only to dispense the anti-malarial tablets as per NMEP schedules. Fever treatment deposits collect the blood slides in addition to the distribution of anti-malarial tablets. About 3.57 lakhs of such centres are functioning all over the country in rural areas. These centres are manned by voluntary workers from the community.

6. Urban Malaria Scheme

As the cities grow, urban malaria poses an increasing problem. In New Delhi, water storage tanks on roof tops which were poorly maintained, were found to be breeding places for *Anopheles stephensi* which is a major vector for malaria. The urban malaria scheme was launched in 1971 to reduce or interrupt malaria transmission in towns and cities. The methodology comprises vector control by intensive antilarval measures and drug treatment. The urban component of NMEP covers 181 cities and towns including New Delhi, Mumbai, Calcutta and Chennai. So far it has been implemented in 131 towns.

7. P. falciparum Containment

Within the Modified Plan of Operation, an additional component known as "P. falciparum containment programme" has been introduced from October 1977, through the assistance of Swedish International Development Agency (SIDA). The specific purpose of this component is to prevent or contain or control the spread of falciparum malaria.

Currently the programme is operating in North East India, and some areas in the States of Orissa, Bihar, West Bengal, Andhra Pradesh, Madhya Pradesh, Gujarat, Maharashtra and Rajasthan. Four zones have been established to tackle the problem in these districts. Under this programme, special inputs have been provided to strengthen the supervision of field operations.

8. Research

Six monitoring teams are now working in different parts of the country to identify P. falciparum sensitivity to chloroquine. One team is working on testing alternative drugs wherever chloroquine-resistance has been detected. Studies by Indian council of medical research have revealed chloroquine-resistant foci in several States – Orissa, Assam, Bihar, Maharashtra, North Eastern States, UP, Andhra Pradesh, Delhi, Madhya Pradesh, Andaman and Nicobar Islands.

9. Health Education

In the modified plan of operation, due emphasis has been given to the health education of the public to enlist their cooperation in malaria control activities.

10. Reorganization

Before the implementation of the modified plan of operation, the NMEP unit was on population basis, which in many places did not conform to the administrative boundaries. This has now been remedied and anti-malaria units have been reorganised in conformity with the geographic boundaries of the district making the District Health Officer (DHO) responsible for the implementation of the programme. The existing unit officers have been designated as District Malaria Officers (DMOs) and are posted at the district headquarters. They have been entrusted with the operational and evaluation aspects of the programme. The DMO is usually assisted by Asst. Malaria Officers. In the modified plan of operation, laboratory services are decentralised to minimise the time lag between collection of blood smears and their examination. Laboratory technicians have been posted at each primary health centre. Entomological teams have been attached to all the 72 zones in the country. The chief medical officers, and the medical officers of primary health centres have to play a key role in the execution of the programme. The programme which was vertical before is now horizontal and integrated with the general health services from the district level to the periphery and gradually surveillance workers are being replaced by multi-purpose workers.

Surveillance

Surveillance in malaria is aimed at case detection through laboratory services, and providing facilities for proper treatment. The timely collection and examination of blood smears is a key element in the modified plan of operation. If all the detected cases are given radical treatment, it will certainly lead to a depletion of the human reservoir. Surveillance in malaria is of 2 types – active and passive.

Active Surveillance

This is carried out by paid workers known as "surveillance workers" who are now being replaced by the multipurpose workers (MPWs). Each surveillance worker (or MPW) is allotted a population of 10,000 or approximately 2,000 houses and for every 4 surveillance workers, there is a surveillance inspector (health assistant). For difficult terrain areas, there is one surveillance worker for a population of 8,000 and one surveillance inspector for 32,000 population (5).

The surveillance worker will visit each house in his area once a fortnight and enquire; (a) whether there is a fever case in the house, including guests or visitors in the house, and (b) whether there was a fever case in the house between his previous visit and the present visit. If the answer to either of these two questions is "yes", the surveillance worker/MPW collects a blood film (thick and thin on the same slide) and administers a single dose (600 mg for an adult and proportionate doses for others) of chloroquine according to the prescribed NMEP schedule. This is known as "presumptive treatment". The surveillance worker/MPW makes necessary entries in the stencil or house card about his visit and dispatches stides (primary health centre) for microscopic examination. He is required to collect the blood slides from the sub-centres and fever treatment depots and send these to the laboratory. If the blood film is reported positive for malaria parasite, the surveillance worker/MPW returns to the patient and administers a course of radical treatment for malaria, as prescribed.

Passive Surveillance

The search for malaria cases by the local health agencies such as the primary health centres, sub-centres, hospitals, dispensaries and local medical practitioners is known as "passive surveillance". Their contribution to case detection is by no means small, because cases of fever which escape the net of active surveillance workers are screened by the passive surveillance agencies. The passive agencies collect blood smears from all fever cases and also from those with history of smears from all fever cases and also from those with history of recent fever. After the collection of blood smear, a single dose treatment for malaria is administrated as is done under the active surveillance programme. The blood smear, a single dose treatment for malaria is administered as is done under the active surveillance programme. The blood slides are collected by the local surveillance worker/MPW and sent to the unit examination are communicated to the local surveillance worker/MPW for institution of radical treatment.

Parameter of Malaria Surveillance

By definition surveillance also implies the continuing scrutiny of occurrence and spread of a disease, that are pertinent to effective control, included in these are the systemic collection and evaluation of field investigation, etc. The following parameters are widely used in the epidemiological surveillance of malaria :

(a) Annual parasite incidence (API);
(b) Annual blood examination rate (ABER);
(c) Annual falciparum incidence (AFI);
(d) Slide positively rate (SPR);
(e) Slide falciparum rate (SER).

Malaria Control through Primary Health Care

A new approach to malaria control was approved by WHO in 1978, i.e. implementation of malaria control in the context of the primary health care strategy. This is because several anti-malarial activities, including drug distribution, can be carried by of the most peripheral level of primary health care system with community participation, where such system has been developed. Malaria control within the framework of PHC demands national commitment, community participation and intersectoral cooperation. Strategies and approaches are being adjusted to control malaria through primary health care.

The 1994 resurgence of malaria compelled the government of India to appoint an expert committee on malaria to identify the problem areas and to suggest specific measures against the different paradigms of malaria. Thus Malaria Action Programme (MAP) was evolved and guidelines were distributed to all the states for prediction, early detection and effective response to malaria outbreaks at district level. It necessitated the need to strengthen the health promotion malaria component of the programme by observing "Anti-Malaria Month" before the onset of monsoon i.e. during the month of June to create awareness in the community regarding malaria and its prevention (7).

The anti-malaria activities have been intensified with additional inputs in 100 selected districts of the states of Andhra Pradesh, Bihar, Gujarat, Maharashtra, Madhya Pradesh, Rajasthan and Orissa. In 19 cities/towns in these states and in the states of Karnataka, Tamil Nadu and West Bengal, an enhanced malaria control project with world Bank support has been launched on 30th September 1997. The total cost of the project is about Rs. 891 crore spread over a period of 5 years.

The expert committee on malaria has recommended the inclusion of all urban areas with more than 50,000 population and reporting slide positively rate of 5 per cent and above under urban malaria Scheme and introduction of active surveillance under this scheme.

LYMPHATIC FILARIASIS

It involves infection with nematodes of 3 species W. bancrofti, B. timori, B. malayi.

The pathology associated with lymphatic filariasis results from a complex interplay of the pathogenic potential of the parasite, the immune response of the host and external bacterial and fungal infections.

While genital damage and lymphoedema/elephantiasis are the most recognizable clinical entities associated with lymphatic filarial infections, there are much earlier stages of lymphatic pathology and dysfunction whose recognition has only recently been made possible through ultrasonographic and lympho scintigraphic techniques. e.g. ultrasonography has identified massive lymphatic dilatation around and for several beyond the adult filarial worms which though are in continuous vigorous motion, remain 'fixed' at characteristic sites within lymphatic vessels.

Vectors

Culex, Anopheles and Aedes serve as the vectors for the W. bancrofti which causes lymphatic filariasis.

Mansonia, Coquilletlida and Anopheles mosquitoes serve as the vectors of the Brugia malaya and B. timori.

Incubation Period

It is the interval from invasion of larvae to the clinical manifestations development. It is commonly 8 to 16 months or longer.

Clinical Features

There are chronic, acute and 'asymptomatic' presentations of lymphatic filarial disease as well as a number of syndromes associated with these infections that may or may not be caused by the parasites.

Chronic Manifestations

Hydrocoele, even though found only with W. bancrofti infections is the most common clinical manifestation of lymphatic filariasis. It is uncommon in childhood but is seen more frequently post-puberty and with a progressive increase in prevalence with age. In many endemic communities, 40-60% of all adult males have hydrocoele. It is often seen that micro-filariae circulats in the blood. Though the mechanism of the fluid accumulation in the tunica vaginalis is still unknown, direct ultrasonographic evidence indicates that in bancroftian filariasis, the scrotal lyphatics are the preferred site for localization of the adult worms and their presence may stimulate not only the proliferation of lymphatic endothelium but also a transudation of 'hydrocoele fluid' whose chemical constituents are similar to those of serum. The localization of adult worms in the lymphatics of the spermatic cord leads to a thickening of the cord that is palpable on physical examination of most patients. The hydrocoeles can become massive but still occur without lymphoedema or elephantiasis developing in the penis and scrotum, since the lymphatic drainage of these tissues is separate and more superficial.

Life Cycle of W. bancrofti

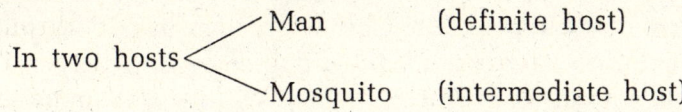

In two hosts
- Man (definite host)
- Mosquito (intermediate host)

Development of Microfilariae Mosquito

When female **culex pipines fatigans** takes a blood meal from a human carrier containing microfilariae, the further developmental changes of the microfilariae take place in the gut of the mosquito in the following ways :

(i) Sheathed microfilariae ingested by the mosquito during its blood meal collect round the anterior end of the stomach. They cast off their sheath quickly, penetrate the gut wall within an hour or two and then it goes to the thoracic muscles and there it starts growing.

(ii) In the next 2 days, the organism changes to thick short, sausage shaped form with a short spiky tail measuring about 124-250 μm in length and 10-17 μm in breadth.

(iii) In 3 to 7 days time the larva grows rapidly, moulds once or twice and its length at the end of this stage is about 225-355 μm in length by 15-30 μm in breadth (second stage larva).

(iv) On the 10th-11th day the metamorphosis is complete.

There is atrophy of tail and digestive system, genital organs and body cavity are fully developed. This is *third stage larva*, size 1500-2000 μm × 18-23 μm. It is injective to man and enters the proboscis sheath of mosquito on 14th day.

Entrance into Man and Development into the Adult Worm

When the infected mosquito bites a human being, the third stage larvae are not directly infected into the blood stream like malarial parasites but are deposited on skin near the site of puncture. The third stage larvae reaches the lymphatic channels, settles down and begin to grow in adult form. In a period of about 5 to 18 months they become sexually mature. The males fertilise the females and gravid females give rise to larvae. New generation of microfilaria is produced which passes either through the thoracic duct or the right lymphatic duct to the venous system and pulmonary capillaries and then to peripheral. Thus, it completes its life cycle.

Pathogenicity

There is irregular fever, enlargement of lymphatic glands, lymphangitis, hydrocele, elephantiasis of legs, scrotum and vulva and rarely arms and breast. If the pre-erotic glands are blocked the condition of true chyluria may arise i.e. urine having chyle. Frequently, when the lymphatics of kidneys ureter or bladders are blocked, it leads to cellular degeneration of the walls of lymphatics.

Elephantiasis

The affected skin becomes markedly thickened due to a process of hyperplasia and hypertrophy which is caused by an irritant action of high protein content of the tissue fluid. Due to the inflammatory process, the tissue fluid cannot drain out due to lymphatic obstruction and the condition is known as elephantiasis.

Lab. Diagnosis

It includes the examination of blood for the detection of microfilariae. Due to nocturnal periodicity of micro-filariae, the blood from the patient should be taken during night between 10.00 p.m. to 2.00 a.m.

The blood should be examined in a following ways :

(1) **Examination of fresh blood** : It can be done by putting fresh drop of blood from the patient, on a clean slide with cover slip and examine under the microscope.

(2) **Thick smear** : It may be made from the blood collected from a suspected case on a clean slide and can be examined under microscope after staining it with leishman's stain.

(3) **Concentration Method** : In this method 5 ml of blood is collected from the vein of the patient in 10 ml of citrated saline. Next morning the blood is dehaemoglobinised by adding 1% saponin solution in the normal saline drop by drop till the haemolysis is complete. Then a drop of heparin is added and the sediment of the blood is examined under the microscope after contrifuging it at 2000 revolution per minute for 2-5 minutes.

Arthropod Borne Diseases

Direct finding of micro filariae
(i) In the peripheral blood.
(ii) In the chylous urine.
(iii) In the exudate of lymph varix.
(iv) In the hydrocele fluid.

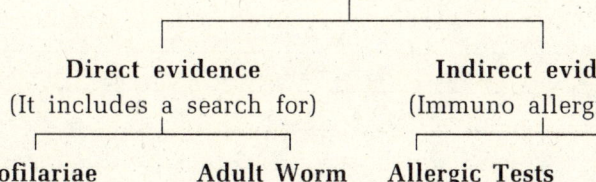

Key to Diagnosis of Filariasis

Direct evidence (It includes a search for)

Indirect evidence (Immuno allergic test)

Microfilariae
(A sheathed microfilaria having tail tip free from nuclei) there presence can be found out by the following methods.

Adult Worm
(i) In the biopsied lymph node
(ii) Calcified worm by X-ray.

Allergic Tests
(i) Blood examination
(ii) Intradermal Test – an immediate hypersensitivity reaction.

Immunological tests and complement fixation tests.

D/d for various micro filariae
Tail nuclei not up to end : W. bancrofti
Tail nuclei up to end : Loa loa.
Terminal nuclei : W. malai

Until recently, diagnosis of filariae infection depended on the direct demonstration of the parasite in blood or skin specimens using relatively cumbersome techniques and having to take into account the periodicity of microfilariae in the blood. Alternative methods based on detection of Anti-bodies by immuno-diagnostic tests did not prove satisfactory since they both failed to distinguish between active and past infections and had problems with specificity owing to their cross reactivity with common gastrointestinal parasites and other organisms.

Antigen Detection

Circulating filariae antigen (CFA) detection should now be regarded as the gold standard for diagnosing Wuchereria bancrofti infections. The specificity of these assays is near complete and the sensitivity is greater than that achievable by the earlier parasite detection assays. Essentially all individuals with microfilariaemia also have detectable circulating antigen, as well as do a proportion of those amicrofilariaemic individuals with clinical manifestations of filariasis but no circulating microfilariae. In addition, some individuals who appear normal also have detectable circulating antigen that disappears after effective treatment with DEC for these cryptic infections. Two commercial configurations of this assay are available, one based on ELISA methodology that yields semi-quantitative results and the other based on a simple card test, yielding only qualitative answers. Thus, this new diagnostic approach is equally applicable to clinical or field evaluation of bancroftian filariasis infections. Unfortunately, no such test is currently available for brugian filariasis.

Control Measures

(a) Chemotherapy (b) Mosquito control

(a) Chemotherapy : DEC is the drug of choice. It is given as 6 mg/kg body weight per day for 6 days in a week orally and the duration of therapy is 2 weeks i.e. total dose of 72 mg of DEC/kg body weight.

(b) Mosquito Control :

(i) Anti-larval measures : Larvicidal oil, larvicides, deweeding of pistia ploughing.

(ii) Anti adult measures : Chemical control pyre thrown spraying.

(iii) Personal protection : Using mosquito nets, repellants, etc.

Homoeopathic Therapeutics

Some of the medicines with their indications are :

1. **Hydrocotyle**
   - Skin turns like elephant hide.
2. **Apis mellifica**
   - Skin red, hot, shining with oedema.
   - No thirst.
   - Heat aggravates.
3. **Natrium muriaticum**
   - Oedema
   - Desire salt, bitter.
   - Aversion hot drinks.
   - Dislike sympathy.

Other medicines which can be considered are :

Calcarea fluorica, Silicea, Thuja occidentalis, Natrium sulph, Medorrhinum, etc.

Prevention

Filarial infection can be acquired only from vector borne infective larvae. Therefore, prevention of infection can be achieved either by decreasing contact between humans and vectors or by decreasing the amount of infection the vector can acquire by treating the human host.

Population

Efforts at filariasis control in populations through reducing the numbers of mosquito vectors have proven largely ineffective. Even when good mosquito control can be put into place, the long life span of parasite (4-8 years) means that the infection remains in the community for a long period of time, generally longer than intensive vector control efforts can be sustained. More recently, with the advent of extremely effective single-dose, once yearly, 2 drug treatment regimens an alternative approach has been taken in an initiative being launched through the World Health Organisation to utilize a strategy of yearly mass treatment of all "at risk" population to eliminate lymphatic filariasis as a public health problem by decreasing microfilariae in the population, there by interrupting transmission and preventing infection.

Individuals

Contact with infected mosquitoes can be decreased through the use of personal repellents, bed nets or insecticide impregnated materials. Alternatively, suggestive evidence from animal models and some limited experience in human populations indicates that a prophylactic regimen of DEC could be effective in preventing the acquisition of infection.

Vector Control

1. Anti-larvae system
   (i) Chemical
      Larvicidal oil, pyrosene oil, organophosphorus larvicides e.g. temephos, fenthion, weekly application.
   (ii) Control of breeding of mansonia.
      Mechenical removal.
      Use of herbicides.
      Environmental management as control breading.
2. Antiadult measures.
3. Personal prophylaxis
      Nets
      Screening of house.
      Repellants.

Integrated Vector Control

Health Care

NFC Programm, 1955

1. **Objectives**
   (i) To carry out survey to find.
   - Prevalance.
   - Types of infection.
   - Their vectors.

   (ii) Training of staff.

   Set-up for NFCP.

   (i) Regional filaria Training & Research Centres.
   Calcutta.
   Rajasthan.
   Varanasi.

   (ii) State Headquarter Bureau.

   (iii) Filaria Control Units. 206 FLU to evaluate different control methods. One FCU attached to 3 lakh population. So far 47 million covered with protection (nearly 15% population).

   (iv) Antilarvae operation.

   Monitoring the breeding places for larve/inf.

2. **Filaria Survey Unit (FSU)**
   Sample survey in an area endemic for filaria.
   Filaria Clinic : Detection of carrier & cases attach to medical collage.
   No. of distt. in endemic area = 300.
   15-20 lakh population of 1 Distt.
   (594) 600 Distt. in India. So ½ of India is endemic.
   No. of Distt. served – 238
   No. of found endemic – 175.

3. **Activities of NFCP**
   - Problem delimitation in unserveyed area.
   - Control in urban areas thorough anti larval and anti parasitic.
   - In rural areas detection & treatment of infectious cases & filaria cases.

CHAPTER-7

CONTACT INFECTIONS

LEPROSY

Leprosy is a chronic infectious disease caused by Mycobacterium leprae, an acid fast rod shaped bacillus. The disease mainly affects the skin, the peripheral nerves, mucosa of the upper respiratory tract and also the eyes, apart from some other structures. Leprosy has afflicted humanity since time immemorial. It once affected every continent and left behind a terrifying image in history and human memory of mutilation, rejection and exclusion from society.

Leprosy struck fear into human beings for thousands of years. It was well recognized in the oldest civilizations of China, Egypt and India. A cumulative total of number of individuals who over the millennia have suffered its chronic course of incurable disfigurement and physical disabilities can never be calculated.

Since ancient times, leprosy has been regarded by the community as a contagious, mutilating and incurable disease. There are many countries in Asia, Africa and Latin America with a significant number of leprosy cases.

It is estimated that there are between one and two million people visibly and irreversibly disabled due to past and present leprosy who require to be cared for by the community in which they live. When M. leprae was discovered by G.A Hansen in 1873, it was the first bacterium to be identified as causing disease in man. However, treatment for leprosy only appeared in the late 1940s with the introduction of dapsone and its derivatives, leprosy bacilli resistant to dapsone gradually appeared and became widespread.

In 1997, there were an estimated 1.2 million cases in the world, most of them concentrated in South-East Asia, Africa and the Americas. The number of new cases detected world wide each year is about half a million.

Microbiology of Mycobacterium Leprae

The aetiological agent of leprosy is Mycobacterium leprae. It is a strongly acid fast rod shaped organism with parallel sides and rounded ends. In size and shape it closely resembles the tubercle bacillus. It occurs in large numbers in the lesions of lepromateus leprosy, chiefly in masses within the lepra cells, often grouped together like bundles of cigar or arranged in a palisade. Chains are never seen. Most striking are the intracellular and extracellular masses, known as globi, which consist of dumps of bacilli in capsular material. Under the electron microscope, the bacillus appears to have a great variety of forms. The commonest is a slightly curved filament 3-10 m in length containing irregular arrangements of dense material sometimes in the shape of rods. Short rod-shaped structures can also seen and also dense spherical forms. Some of the groups of bacilli can be seen to have a limitating membrane.

It is believed that only leprosy bacilli which stain with carbot fuchsin as solid acid-fast rods are viable and that bacilli which stain irregularly are probably dead and degenerating. The differences are valuable pointers in biopsy. In patients receiving standard multi drug therapy (MDT), a very high proportion of bacilli are killed within days, which suggests that many of the manifestations of leprosy, including reactions of the erythema nodosum type, which follow initial treatment, must be due in part to antigens from dead organisms rather than living bacilli. We therefore, need drugs which will help the body to dispose off dead but still intact leprosy bacilli. Two indices which depend on observation of M. leprae in smears from skin or nasal smears are useful in assessing the amount of infection, and the viability of organisms and also the progress of the patient under treatment. They are the morphological index and the bacteriological index.

The Bacteriological Index (BI)

This is an expression of the extent of bacterial loads. It is calculated by counting six to eight stained smears under the 100 X oil immersion lens, in a smear made by picking the skin with a sharp scalpels and scraping it; the fluid and the tissue obtained are spread fairly thickly on a slide and stained by the Ziehl-Neelsen method and decolorized (but not completely) with 1% acid alcohol. The results are expressed on a logarithms scale.

1+ At least 1 bacillus in every 100 fields.
2+ At least 1 bacillus in every 10 fields.

3+ At least 1 bacillus in every fields.
4+ At least 10 bacilli in every fields.
5+ At least 100 bacilli in every fields.
6+ At least 1000 bacilli in every fields.

The bacteriological index is valuable because it is simple and is representative of many lesions but is affected by the depth of the skin lesions, the thoroughness of the scrape and the thickness of the film.

A more accurate and reliable index of the bacillary content of a lesion is given by the logarithmic index of biopsies (LIB). These indices help to assess the state of patients at the beginning of treatment and to assess progress.

The Morphological Index (MI)

This is calculated by counting the number of solid staining acid-fast rods. Only the solid staining bacilli are viable. It is not unusual for solid staining M. leprae to reappear for short periods in patients being successfully treated with drugs. It is important to recognize that measurement of MI is liable for observer variations and therefore not always reliable.

Diagnosis of leprosy

It is most commonly based on the clinical signs and symptoms. These are easy to observe and elicit by any health worker after a short period of training. In practice, most often persons with such complaints report on their own to the health care centre. Only in rare instances there is a need to use laboratory and other investigations to confirm a diagnosis of leprosy.

In an endemic country or area, an individual should be regarded as having leprosy if she or he shows one of the following cardinal signs :

1. Skin lesion consistent with leprosy and with definite sensory loss, with or without thickened nerves.
2. Positive skin smears.

The skin lesion can be single or multiple, usually less pigmented than the surrounding normal skin. Sometimes the lesion is reddish or copper-coloured. A variety of skin lesions may be seen but macules (flat), papules (raised), or nodules are common. Sensory loss is a typical feature of leprosy. The skin lesion may show loss of sensation to pin prck and/ or light touch. Thickened nerves, mainly peripheral nerve trunks constitute another feature of leprosy. A thickened nerve is often accompanied by other signs as a result of damage to the nerve. There may be loss of sensation in the skin and weakness of muscles supplied by the affected nerve. In the absence of these signs, nerve thickening by itself, without sensory loss and/or muscle weakness is often not a reliable sign of leprosy.

Positive Skin Smears

In a small proportion of cases, rod-shaped, red-stained leprosy bacilli, which are diagnostic of the disease, may be seen in the smears taken from the affected skin when examined under a microscope after appropriate staining.

A person presenting with skin lesions or with symptoms suggestive of nerve damage, in whom the cardinal signs are absent or doubtful should be called a 'suspect case' in the absence of any immediately obvious alternate diagnosis. Such individuals should be told the basic facts of leprosy and advised to return to the centre if signs persist for more than 6 months or if at any time worsening is noticed. Suspect cases may be also sent to referral clinics with more facilities for diagnosis.

Classification of Leprosy

Leprosy can be classified on the basis of clinical manifestations and skin smear results. In the classification based on skin smears, patients showing negative smears at all sites are grouped as Pauci bacillary leprosy (PB) while those showing positive smears at any site are grouped as having Multi bacillary leprosy (MB). However, in practice, most programmes use clinical criteria for classifying and deciding the appropriate treatment regimen for individual patients, particularly in view of the non-availability or non-dependability of the skin smear services. The clinical system of classification for the purpose of treatment includes the use of number of skin lesions and nerves involved as the basis for grouping leprosy patients into multi bacillary (MB) and pauci bacillary (PB) leprosy.

While classifying leprosy, it is particularly important to ensure that patients with multi bacillary disease are not treated with the regimen for the pauci bacillary form of the disease.

(MDT) Multi Drug Therapy

The drugs used in WHO-MDT are a combination of rifampicin, clofazimine and dapsone for MB leprosy patients and rifampicin and dapsone for PB leprosy patients. Among these rifampicin is the most important anti leprosy drug and therefore is included in the treatment of both types of leprosy.

Treatment of leprosy with only one anti-leprosy drug result in development of drug resistance to that drug. Treatment with dapsone or any other anti-leprosy drug used as mono-therapy should be considered as unethical practice.

Rifampicin : The drug is given once a month. No toxic effects have been reported in the case of monthly administration. The urine may be coloured slightly reddish for a few hours after its intake, this should be explained to the patient while starting MDT.

Clofazimine : It is the most active when administered daily. The drug is well tolerated and virtually non-toxic in the dosage used for MDT. The drug causes brownish-black discolouration and dryness of skin. However, this disappears within few months after stopping treatment. This should be explained to patients starting MDT regimen for MB leprosy.

Dapsone : The drug is very safe in the dosage used is MDT and side effects are rare. The main side effect is allergic reaction, causing itchy skin rashes and exfoliative dermatitis. Patients known to be allergic to any of the sulpha drugs should not be given dapsone.

Homoeopathic efficacy

Some of the homoeopathic medicines which are efficacious in leprosy are – Ars., Bad., Carb-an., Elae., Crot-h., Hydrc., Nat-c., Nuph., Sec., Sulph., etc.

Multi Bacillary Leprosy

For adults the standard regimens is :
Rifampicin   : 600 mg. once a month.
Dapsone   : 100 mg. daily.
Clofazimine : 300 mg. once a month and 50 mg daily.
Duration   : 12 months.

Pauci Bacillary Leprosy

For adults the standard regimens is :
Rifampicin : 600 mg. once a month.
Dapsone   : 100 mg. daily.
Duration   : 6 months.
Single skin lesion Paucibacillery leprosy.

Single Skin Lesion Pauci Bacillary Leprosy

For adults the standard regimens is a single dose of :

Rifampicin : 600 mg.
Ofloxacin   : 400 mg.
Minocycline : 100 mg.

Lepromin Test

In this test intradermal reaction to lepra bacilli antigen (LEPROMIN) is observed. Lepromin is prepared by boiling and emulsifying lepromatous tissue rich in lepra bacilli.

Procedure

0.1 cc lepromin is injected intradermally. In a positive reaction an erythema and induration develops in 24-48 hrs. It is called early reaction of Fernandez. It is followed by late reaction of Mitsuda, starts within 1-2 weeks and is characterized by an indurated skin nodule, which increases and shows ulceration. It is a measure of cell mediated Immunity induced by injected lepromin.

Uses

(i) To classify the leprosy.

(ii) To assess the prognosis and effectiveness of treatment.

(iii) It gives the measure of immunity of a person against lepra bacilli.

(iv) To identification of lepra bacilli.

CHAPTER-8

EPIDEMIOLOGY OF NON-COMMUNICABLE DISEASES

ACCIDENTS
Events without a cause, random events, etc.
Accidents evokes a feeling of chance, misfortune & helplessness.

Injury
Bodily lesion at organic level resulting from accidental exposure to energy (mechanical, thermal, electrical, chemical or radiant) interacting with the body in amount or rates that exceeds the threshold of Physiological tolerance.

It could be from an insufficiency of vital element (drowning, strangulation, freezing, etc.).

- Acute or chronic.
- Intentional & unintentional.

Result
- Pain, mental stress, depression.
- Disabilities.
- Disruption of family & social structure.
- Financial loss : Physical, medical cost, rehabilitative expenses, production loss, etc.

Injury = Preventable.

International Classification of Injuries

A. *Unintentional*
- RTA (Road Traffic Accidents).
- Poisoning.
- Falls, fires.
- Drowning, Firearms.

B. Intentional
- Self inflicted.
- Homicide.
- War.

Magnitude of Problem

World – 10,000 people die from injuries. It is estimated that 5-8 m worldwide died from injuries in 1998. Corresponding to every person that dies several thousands more injured with permanent sequalae.

Injuries rank 10th leading cause of death.
  5-14 years it is 3rd.
  15-44 years – 2nd.

India – Every 2nd min. – injury
  9 min. – death due to injury.

- Seventh leading cause.
- In age group of 5-44 years, it is 3rd leading cause.
- RTA most common.
- Drowning & self inflicted are the next common causes.

Causation of Injury

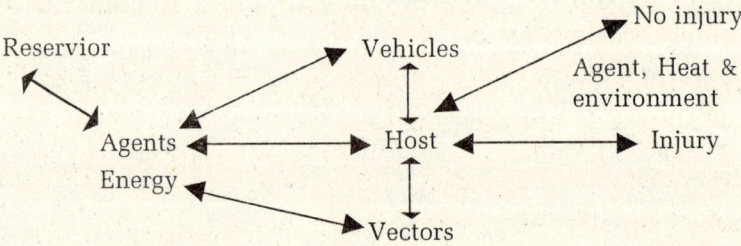

Injury – Damage to the host, ranging from blunt trauma in tissues & organs due to penetrating wounds.

Reservoir – Place in environment where agent is usually found.

Agent – Energy which causes injury to the host & energy source is reservoir.

Host Response

Haddon Matrix 1963 – According to it injuries are divided as per time factor :

A. **Pre-event** : Period before the event occur & including all factor that influence the potential exposure e.g. use of alcohol, before driving a motor cycle.

B. **Event** : Injury phase workers phase that effect energy transmission during the event, such as presence of energy absorbing material.
C. **Post event** : Response to event.

According to national crime rate bureau, traffic causes more death and death due to fall are very few.

Road Traffic Injuries (RTI)
- Bicycle related crush & pedestrian injuries are most common followed by scooter injuries.
- Young age group is mostly affected.
- Use of helmet reduces head injuries by 75%-85%.
- Inspite of this we rarely see bicyclist wearing helmet.
- Helmet or bicycle helmet legislation is a must.
  * Compulsory for all age particularly very young & old.
  * Standard helmet must be used.
  * Location where riders must wear helmet.
  * Enforcement of law.
  * Community programme for promotion of helmet.
  * School based programme.
  * Easy provision of providing timely medical help to victim.

Teenage driving behaviour (Ref. Higson 1993) :
  * Excessive speed.
  * Running red lights.
  * Making illegal turns.
  * Not wearing safety belts.
  * Riding with an intoxicated driver.
  * Driving after drug or alcohol.

Other Factors
- Traffic flow & speed limit. Chances of accident.
- Designs of the motors as per the safety to the pedestrian, bicycle peddlers & also drivers – construction, smoothness, crossing light, etc.
- Emergency system – Centralized accident & trauma services (CATs), Ist aid, linkage & hospitals.
- Public awareness, media involvement, phone : 1099, 102.
- Insurance

Injuries in Hospital Staff
- Needle & sharp instrument injuries.
- Slips & falls
- Electrical.
- Collapse of building, etc.
- Leakage of anaesthetic gas.
- Inter personal violence between relatives of patient & doctors or other staff.
- Others.

Needle prick injuries in surgical, orthopedic, gynaecological, etc. are maximum

Skip & fall injuries are maximum emergency cases.

Prevention of occupational injuries
- Barriers (e.g. fences).
- Avoiding children labour (legally or otherwise).
- Wearing protective equipments & safe clothing.
- Workers, education and training.
- Labeling & clearly indicating the danger signs at appropriate places.
- Limited working hours.
- Safety measures enforcement through various legislation.
- Ergonomics.
- Research in better designs.

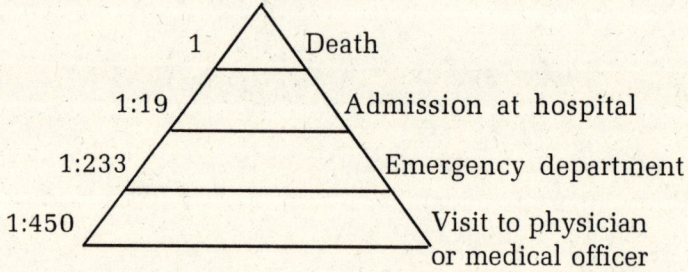

Violence
Swift & intense force; act of commission cashing injury (in physical, dental & social)

Cause
- Social discontentment, disharmony.
- Rivalries & conflict (political, religion & ethnic.).
- Illiteracy.
- Injustice & exploitation.

Preventive measures through
- Political commitment.
- Religious tolerance.
- Ethnic understanding.
- Government – law enforcement & Policies.
- Non-Government organisation & voluntary groups.
- Mass media.
- School.
- Film industries.
- Health sector – Principal of triage.

Suicide
Self-inflicted injuries are most common & one of the most fatal.

Pychological
- Overwhelming effects of rage & guilt.
- Other psychiatric causes.
- Alcohol.

Biological

Prevention
- Community participation.
- An agency must be identified to coordinate with various concerned agencies.
- Relevant community resources should be identified.

Other Steps
- Identify the factors that increase the risk.
- Determine the factors which are modifiable e.g. earthquakes.

BLINDNESS
Factors for increased rate of blindness :
1. Increasing population.
2. Poor access to health care.
3. Under utilizations of sources.
4. Malnutrition especially in younger patients.
5. Occupation.
6. Lack of awareness.
7. Environment.
8. Poor hygiene.
   66.7% of blindness is preventable/avoidable.

Cataract
- 1.2 – 1.5 million people are affected in a year.
- Age : > 60 years (developed) > 40 years (developing).
- Sex : More in females.
- Socioeconomic status – low.
- Exposure to UV rays, etc. are risk factors.

Nutritional Blindness
- 0.4% in Asia.
- Poor awareness.
- Diet-malnutrition.
- Measles.
- Worms.
- Drought, early withdrawal of breast milk.

Glaucoma
- Age more than 40 years.
- Increased intra ocular tension, loss of visual fluid. OAG = CAG.

Trachoma
- 400-600 million people are affected worldwide.
- 2 million turn blind due to trachoma.
- Age less than two years.
- Females more than males are affected.
- (Low)   (High)
  Jammu & Kashmir   Rajasthan
  Maharashtra   Punjab
  Tamil Nadu
  Kerala
  West Bengal.

Factors
- Poor housing
- Overcrowding.
- Inadequate water supply.

Age related macular degeneration
- Age more than 50 years
- Females more than males are affected.
- 1 million people are affected.
- More in smokers.

Onchocesciasis – uncommon in India, Africa.
Ocular – Corneal opacity.
   5.25% – patients varies according to regions.
Measles – 75% blind in Africa.
  - Does not directly causes blindness.
  - Lack of vitamin A deficiency.

Blindness Control
Primary prevention :
1. Eye health promotion & specific protection.
   - Education about hygiene.
   - Proper nutrition.
   - Injury avoidance.
2. Essential dry provision – Vit. A solution, drugs.
3. Specific protection – Vit. A
   Measles vaccine.
   Safe water supply.
   Sanitation improvement.

Secondary prevention :
1. Early diagnosis & treatment.
2. History of diminution of vision, headache, halo around light, discharge, Bitots spots, leprosy.

Tertiary prevention :
1. Decrease the disability limitation → less.
2. Vocational, physical rehabilitation.
3. NIVH (National Institute for Visually Handicap), Dehradun → Training blind. Sikandrabad.

National Programme for Control of Cataract
General Objects :
1. Improve quality of cataract surgery.
2. Strengthen capacity for high quality and low cost eye care of involving skilled persons NGO's, public sector collaboration, etc.
3. Increase the coverage of eye care delivery in under privileged population as in rural & private areas.

Specific Objects :
1. Achieve 11.03 million cataract operation (94-2001) in 2 states.
2. Upgrade ophthalmic department in 7 states medical college.
3. Upgrade district hospitals (IOL implantation, ECCE facility).

4. Establish at least one district mobile unit.
5. Set up District Blindness Control Society in each district.
6. Upgrade subdivisional/CHC hospitals.
7. Upgrade PHC block.
8. Appointment of registered ophthalmic surgeons (700 operation/year/s).
9. Appointment of registered allied manpower.
10. Trained ophthalmic manpower in approved centre.
11. Improved IEC.
12. Quality assurance – Grievance Committee.
13. Seek cooperation – private/voluntary sectors.

Strategies :
1. Provide high skill of care.
2. Incorporate technological advancement for skill upgradation.
3. Develop for collaboration with NGO, public sector, etc.
4. General demand by IEC.
5. Function as team – one surgeon and 2 nurses in 1 O.T. In one district hospital – 2 OA/Surgeon. In CHC, PHC – 1 O.A/mobile unit. Develop technical standards.
6. Diagnostic survey.
   – Surgical standards.
   – Treatment of unilateral cases, ECCE/IOL.
7. Maintain visual quality outcome by :
   – Assessing no. of surgeries (50 surgery/camp.).
   – Payments to NGOs, based on records.
   – Monitor patients satisfaction.
8. Establish grievance committee – C/o by patients for treatment & assistance.

Organization :

Primary care
MO, OA.
Health assistant under health worker supervision
Primary health worker
(2yrs.-5yrs. work in community sub centre, community.

Secondary care
District hospitals.
Sub district hospitals.
CHC.

Tertiary Care :
RIO (Regional Institutes of ophthalmology).
Medical colleges.

CHAPTER-9

DEMOGRAPHY & FAMILY PLANNING

DEMOGRAPHY

Definition

It is the scientific study of human population. It is mainly concerned with changes in size of population, composition and distribution of population.

The demographic processes which modify the above three phenomenon associated with population are – (1) Births (2) Deaths (3) Marriages (4) Migration (5) Social factors.

The various sources of demographic statistics are census, vital event registration, national sample surveys, etc.

Demographic Cycle

Population varies in size over the period of time. It passes through a number of distinct stages, with each stage showing variation in size of population. These stages constitute what is known as demographic cycle. It has 5 stages :

(i) **High stationary** : This stage is characterised by a high birth rate and a high death rate. They both nullify each other's effect, as a result of which the population size remains stationary e.g. in India before 1920 there was lack of health care facilities, poor standard of living.

(ii) **Early expanding stage** : It is marked by high fertility pattern but the death rate tends to decline. It is indicative of improved health care services. The population size starts building up. It is a common feature of developing countries.

(iii) **Late expanding stage** : The improvements in public health system continues as a results of which death rate declines further and birth rate shows downward trend. Net result is increasing population size.

RELATION BETWEEN GROWTH RATE AND POPULATION

Rating	Annual rate of growth%	Number of years required for the population to double in size
Stationary population	No growth	
Slow growth	Less than 0.5	More than 139
Moderate growth	0.5 to 1.0	139-70
Rapid growth	1.0 to 1.5	70-47
Very rapid growth	1.5 to 2.0	47-35
"Explosive" growth	2.0 to 2.5	35-28
-------"-------	2.5 to 3.0	28-23
-------"-------	3.0 to 3.5	23-20
-------"-------	3.5 to 4.0	20-18

India at present is in this stage. The Crude Birth Rate is 26.4 and Crude Death Rate is 9 in India. This stage is an indicative of improved family planning services to curb on the high fertility.

(iv) **Low stationary stage** : Here, there is substantial decline in both birth and death rate, as a result of which the population size becomes stationary and growth rate appears close to zero. It is a feature of developed countries.

(v) **Declining stage** : The death rate becomes more in comparison to birth rate as a result population size decreases e.g. Hungary, Germany, etc.

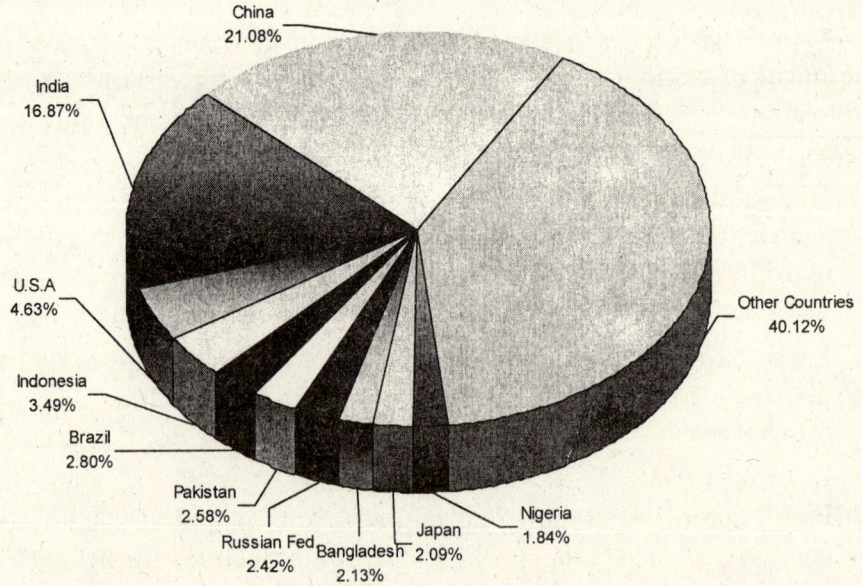

CRUDE BIRTH AND DEATH RATES IN SELECTED DEVELOPED AND DEVELOPING COUNTRIES IN 1999

	Crude birth rate	Crude death rate
India	25	9
Bangladesh	28	9
Pakistan	35	7
Sri Lanka	18	6
Thailand	16	7
Myanmar	21	9
Nepal	34	10
China	16	7
Japan	10	8
Singapore	14	5
UK	12	11
USA	14	8

TRENDS IN INCREASE OF POPULATION OF SEAR COUNTRIES (IN THOUSANDS)

Country	1985	2000	2005 (Projected)
India	767940	1008937	1082184
Bangladesh	99310	137439	139911
Bhutan	1451	2085	2313
DPR Korea	18942	22268	25416
Indonesia	167332	212092	226938
Maldives	184	291	355
Myanmar	37544	47749	53479
Nepal	16503	23043	27439
Sri Lanka	16060	18924	19858
Thailand	51128	62806	52612
Total	**1176394**	**1535634**	**1640505**

CENSUS INDIA – UPDATE

Sl. No.		1991	2001
1.	Total Population	846 million	1027 million
2.	Decadal Growth rate	23.8 %	21.34 %
3.	Sex-ratio	927	933
	Highest : Kerala	1040	1058
	Lowest : Haryana	874	861
4.	Population Density	273	324
5.	Literacy rate (%)	52.2	65.4
	Male	64.1	75.8
	Female	39.1	54.2
	Highest : Kerala	90.5	90.9
	Lowest : Bihar	38.5	47.5
6.	Population (0-6 years)		157.86 million
	Sex-ratio (0-6 years)		927
	Lowest : Punjab		793

RURAL HEALTH INFRASTRUCTURE

No. of Districts : 593
No. of Blocks : 5428
No. of Villages : 5,87226 PHC – 21854 (1996). Sub centre – 132730.

	National Norms		Achievements (30.6.99)	
	General	Hilly/Tribal	1/Population	Total number
Sub Centre	5,000	3,000	4,579	1,37,271
PHC	30,000	20,000	27,364	22,975
CHC	1,20,000	80,000	2.14 Lakh	2,935

GOALS FOR HEALTH FOR ALL BY 2000 A.D

S. No.	Indicator	Current Level		Goals - 2000
1.	Infant mortality rate	70	(1999)	Below 60
	Perinatal mortality rate	42.5	(1994)	< 35
2.	Crude Death Rate	8.7	(1999)	9.0
3.	Pre School child (1-5 years) Mortality rate	23.7	(1994)	10.0
4.	Maternal Mortality Rate	4.08	(1997)	Below 2
5.	Life expectancy at birth (estimated in years) Male	62.4	(1996-2001)	64
	Female	63.4	(1996-2001)	64
6.	Babies with birth weight below 2500 gms (%)	30.0	(1997)	10
7.	Crude birth rate	26.1	(1999)	21.0
8.	Effective Couple Protection (percentage	48.0	(1999)	60.0
9.	Net reproduction rate (NRR)	1.48	(1981)	1.0
10.	Growth Rate (annual)	1.74%	(1999)	1.20
11.	Family Size	2.9	(1999)	2.3
12.	Percentage mothers receiving antenatal care	65.0	(1999)	100.0
13.	Deliveries by trained attendants	42.0	(1999)	100.0
14.	Immunization status (% coverage)	Current Level		Goals for 2000 AD
	TT (Preg. Women)	67	(1999)	100.0

	Infants:			
	BCG	67.5	(1999)	100.0
	DPT 3	46.4	(1999)	100.0
	OPV 3	58.8	(1999)	100.0
	Measles	50.2	(1999)	100.0
	Fully Immunized	42.0	(1999)	
15.	Leprosy – percentage of disease arrested cases out of those detected	109.6%*	(2000)	80.0
16.	TB – percentage of disease arrested cases out of those detected	84.0	(2000)	90.0
17.	Blindness due to Vit. A Deficiency	1.4	(1991)	0.3

* During 1999-2000 number of discharged cases was 5.7 lakh against new case detection of 5.2 lakh cases.

Demographic Trends in India

From the first census (1871), the population of India has risen from 203 million to 685 million in 1981, 845 million in 1991 and 1027 million in 2001. India is thus the most heavily populated country after China. 16% of the world population is living which occupies only 2.4% of the earth surface. India's relative population increases since 1871 which may be split into phases. In first phase, which is characterized by the British imperial health service shows a strongly fluctuating course, indicating an altogether medium-sized population increases only. The level of birth rates and death rates is decisive for this, the balance of which determine the population development. The high values of both of these demographic indicators are perfectly in line with those of the third world especially in the case of the death rate. The reasons of high death rates are famines, diseases and epidemics with heavy tool of lines. The two census period 1891/1901 and 1911/1921 even had the effect of bringing about a population decrease amounting to no less than 41 million i.e. 14.5% in the first case. The devastating influenza epidemic of 1918 cost 18.5 million lives.

The British imperial government brought improvement in health services in India through medicine, hygiene, nutrition and education. The government improved the public health services, controlled infectious tropical diseases and provided better access to medicine and medical care.

POPULATION OF INDIA, 1901-2001

Year	Total population (in million)	Average annual exponential growth rate (%)
1901	238.4	
1911	252.1	0.56
1921	251.3	(-)0.03
1931	279.0	1.04
1941	318.7	1.33
1951	361.1	1.25
1961	439.2	1.96
1971	548.2	2.20
1981	683.3	2.22
1991	843.9	2.14
2001	1027.0	1.93

BIRTH AND DEATH RATES IN INDIA

Year	Birth rate	Death rate
1941-1950	39.9	27.4
1951-1960	41.7	22.8
1961-1970	41.2	19.0
1971-1980	37.2	14.8
1981	33.9	12.5
1991	29.5	9.8
1995	28.3	9.0
1996	27.5	9.0
1997	27.2	8.9
1998	26.4	9.0
1999	26.1	8.7

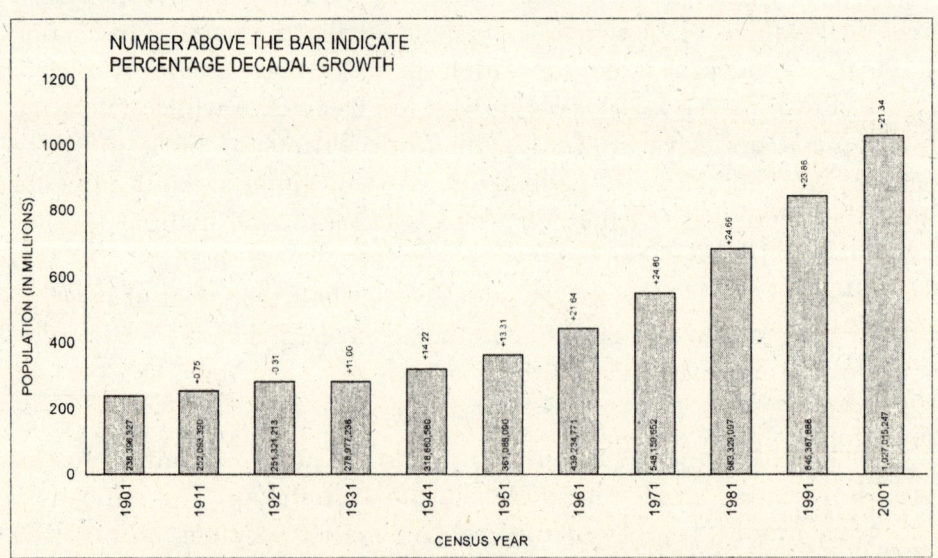

Decadal growth of population in India 1901-2001

Demography and Family Planning

During the second phase i.e. after independence (1947) the rapid population growth led to a sudden increase in the population which became known as the **"population explosion"** on account of its very magnitude. This is expressed in the doubling of the population from 361 to 1027 million between 1951 to 2001. India's relatively rapid population growth is thus identical to that of most developing countries.

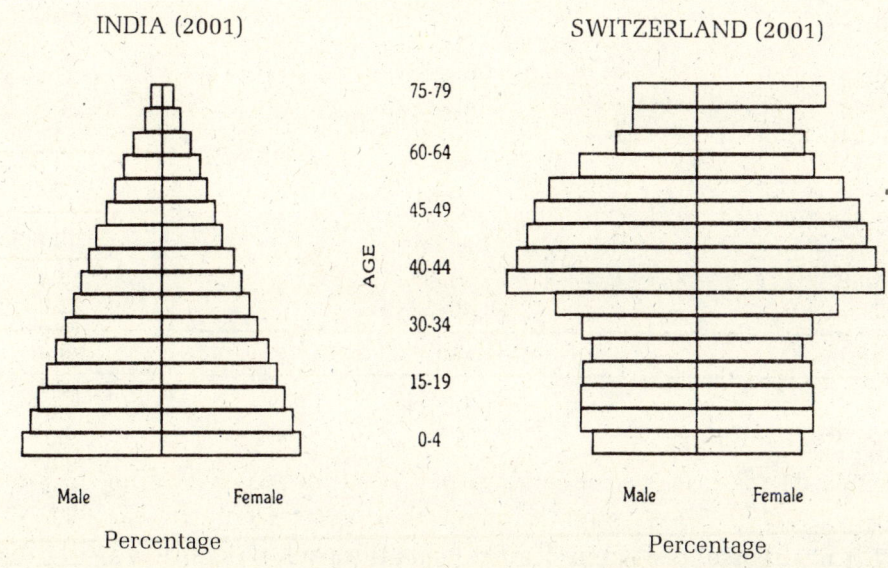

Percentage distribution by age of the population of India and of the population of Switzerland

Age and Sex Composition

In graphic representation, the age structure of the Indian population shows the typical form of developing countries. A pyramid indicative of a particularly greatly dynamic population. Indian population is increasing at the rate of 2.1%. The broad base, on the other hand, demonstrates a large proportion of children and young adults (42.1% below 15 years); the tapering apex shows the small proportion of old people (only 4.7% over 60 years of age). How young the Indian population really is, shown by the fact that every second Indian is under 18 years old. As a consequence of the large families, the proportion of the population capable of employment (15-59 years) is only 53.2%, and hence comparatively low. Thus, the production potential dependent upon labour is more likely to be limited than indicated by the labour market.

F-12A

PERCENT DISTRIBUTION OF POPULATION BY AGE AND SEX FROM THE NFHS-2, INDIA, 1998-99

Age	Male	Female
0-4	11.2	11.1
5-9	12.8	12.4
10-14	12.1	11.8
15-19	10.4	10.3
20-24	8.5	9.3
25-29	7.8	8.7
30-34	6.7	7.1
35-39	6.6	6.4
40-44	5.1	4.7
45-49	4.5	4.2
50-54	3.4	3.1
55-59	2.6	3.3
60-64	2.9	3.0
65-69	2.0	2.0
70+	3.3	2.8
Total	100.0	100.0

Sex-ratio

It is defined as 'no. of females per 1000 males'. According to latest census 2001 it is 933 slightly better then 1991 where it was 927. But still it is adverse to women. Kerala leads the pack with sex-ratio of 1058.

Literacy

India still has an alarmingly high proportion of illiterate people and a comparatively small number of literate ones. Although the 43.7 million illiterate persons include 60 million children below the school age, subtracting them from the total, still leaves every second Indian of school age, an illiterate.

In 1991, there was a spatial amplitude in the literacy rate which varied between 69% (Kerala) and a depressing 20% (Arunachal Pradesh). The grounds for this rate are to be found in the regionally varying number and upkeep of the educational institutions.

The striking gradient also exists between urban and rural areas, with the large number and better development of schools in town resulting in a higher literacy rate (59.7% in 1971) than in the villages (only 27.4%). A comparison of the two sexes reveals a particularity low literacy rate among women. In 1981 the percentage of literate women was only 25% while in case of men it was 47%.

Population Density

'Number of persons living per square km.'. The population growth in India led as well to a rapid increase in the average density of population (1951 : 117 inhabitants/km², 1981 : 221 inhabitants/km²). The population density provides a graphic expression of the regionally very natural endowments as well as of the unequal agricultural potential of the Indian sub-continent.

Urbanization

The twin processes of urbanization and rural exodus are responsible for the rural-urban population development. The two phenomena are examined here on a quantitative basis. In India, towns are classified into six classes on the basis of population number :

Number of inhabitants		Class
100,000 and more	–	I
50,000 – 100,000	–	II
20,000 – 50,000	–	III
10,000 – 20,000	–	IV
5,000 – 10,000	–	V
5,000 and above	–	VI

The urban population development in India, already indicated by the large increase in the total number of towns from 1834 in 1901 to 3245 in 1991, receives emphatic documentation through the increase of urban population from 26 to 150 million (i.e. by 500%). The greater part of the urban population now lives in large cities. Between 1901 and 1981, their number grew from 24 to 216, the number of their inhabitants jumped from 7 to 94 million.

A significant role in the rapid urban population development in India has been played by the 'metropolitan areas'. Their number has risen to 12 with a total of 42 million inhabitants, accounting for 27% of urban population. The growth rate of metro cities is altogether the highest in India. Every metro city, with the exception of Kolkata, exceeds the growth rate of the urban population as a whole and is higher than the all-India growth rate (71%). Their rapid population increase is, therefore, only partly due to the surplus of births, partly due to the gains through migration. In the period 1971-81, million cities of India showed a population growth from 29.597 to 42.160 million inhabitants accounting for a rise of 12.563 million (42.4%), exactly twice as much as natural growth rate (21.2%) of India.

RANKING OF MOST POPULOUS STATES BY POPULATION SIZE 2001

Rank	State	Population 1.3.2001 (million)	Per cent to total population of India 1.3.2001
1.	Uttar Pradesh	166.05	16.17
2.	Maharashtra	96.75	9.42
3.	Bihar	82.87	8.07
4.	West Bengal	80.22	7.81
5.	Andhra Pradesh	75.72	7.37
6.	Tamil Nadu	62.11	6.05
7.	Madhya Pradesh	60.38	5.88
8.	Rajasthan	56.47	5.50
9.	Karnataka	52.73	5.14
10.	Gujarat	50.59	4.93

Fertility

Fertility is a term most often used by demographers to describe the reproductive capacity of the women. Actually fertility or natality means 'bearing of children'. It measures total number of children a women has during her reproductive period (15 to 45 years), e.g. a total fertility rate of 4 signifies that on average a woman would gives birth to 4 children.

Various factors affecting fertility are :

1. Education.
2. Socio-economic conditions.
3. Religion.
4. Caste
5. Age at marriage.
6. Family planning.
7. Duration of married life.
8. Birth spacing.
9. Nutritional status.
10. Customs and beliefs.
11. Industrialization.

Demography and Family Planning

FERTILITY INDICATORS 1994 – ALL INDIA

Indicator	Rural	Urban	Combined
General Fertility Rate (GFR)	128.6	89.7	118.2
General Marital Fertility Rate (GMFR)	162.5	195.2	153.3
Total Fertility Rate (TFR)	3.8	2.7	3.5
Total Marital Fertility Rate (TMFR)	5.1	4.3	4.9
Gross Reproduction Rate (GRR)	1.8	1.2	1.7

Various fertility related statistics are given below :

1. **General Fertility Rate (GFR)**

    The number of live births per 1000 women in the reproductive age group (15-44 or 49 years) in a given year.

    $$GFR = \frac{\text{Number of live births in an area during the year}}{\text{Mid - year female population are (15 - 44 or 49 years) in the same area in the same year}} \times 1000$$

2. **General Marital Fertility Rate**

    The number of live births per 1000 married women in the reproductive age-group (15-44 or 49 years) in a given year.

3. **Age Specific Fertility Rate**

    The number of live births in a year to 1000 women in any specified age-group.

    $$ASFR = \frac{\text{Number of live births to mothers of a specified age group}}{\text{Mid - year female population of the same age - group}} \times 1000$$

AGE-SPECIFIC FERTILITY RATES – ALL INDIA (1997)

Age group	Urban	Rural	Total
15-19	0.032	0.061	0.054
20-24	0.178	0.242	0.226
25-29	0.152	0.200	0.188
30-34	0.071	0.122	0.109
35-39	0.029	0.063	0.055
40-44	0.012	0.030	0.026
45-49	0.003	0.009	0.008
TFR 15-44	2.36	3.59	3.29
TFR 15-49	2.38	3.63	3.32

4. Age Specific Marital Rate

The number of live births in a year to 1000 married women in any specified age-group.

5. Total Fertility Rate

The average number of children a woman would born if she were to pass through her reproductive years bearing children at the same rates as the women now in each age-group.

TFR = Sum of ASFRs

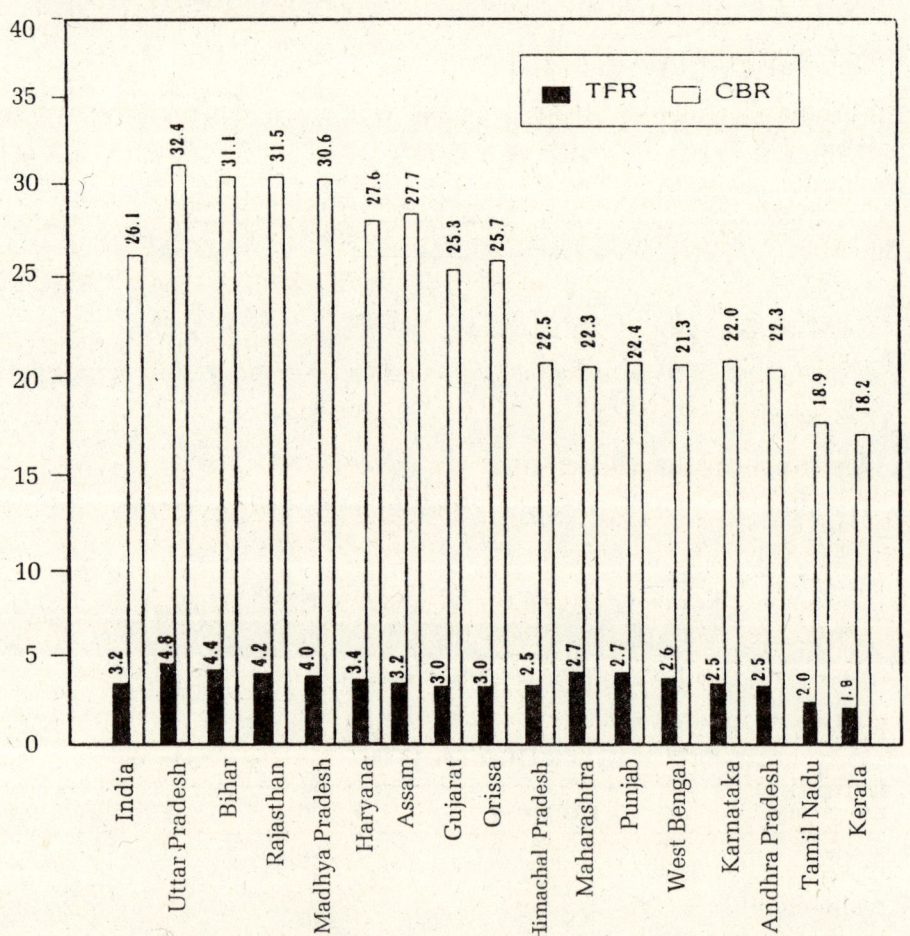

Crude birth rate (1999) and Total fertility rate (1998) for major states

6. Total Marital Fertility Rate

Average number of children that would be born to a married women if she experiences the current fertility pattern throughout her reproductive span.

Demography and Family Planning

7. **Gross Reproduction Rate (GRR)**
   Average number of girls that would be born to a woman if she experiences the current fertility pattern throughout her reproductive span (15-44 or 49 years) assuming no mortality.

8. **Net Reproduction Rate**
   The number of daughters a newborn girl will bear during her lifetime assuming fixed age-specific fertility and mortality rates.

9. **Pregnancy Rate**
   It is the ratio of number of pregnancies in a year to married women in ages (15-44 or 49 years).

10. **Abortion Rate**
    The number of all types of abortion usually per 1000 women of child bearing age (26).

11. **Abortion Ratio**
    This is estimated by dividing the number of abortions performed during a particular time period by the number of live births over the same period.

12. **Marriage Rate**
    The number of marriages in the year per 1000 population :

    (i) Crude marriage rate = $\dfrac{\text{Number of marriages in a year}}{\text{Mid-year population}} \times 1000$

    (ii) General marriage rate = $\dfrac{\text{No. of marriages within one year}}{\text{No. of unmarried persons age 15-49 years}} \times 1000$

FAMILY PLANNING

Definition
WHO defined family planning as a way of thinking and living that is adopted voluntarily, upon the basis of knowledge, attitudes and responsible decisions by individuals and couples, in order to promote the health and welfare of the family group and thus contribute effectively to the social development of a country.

Objectives
- To avoid unwanted births.
- To bring about wanted births.

- To regulate the intervals between pregnancies.
- To determine the number of children in the family.
- To control the time at which births occur in relation to the ages of the parent.

Family Planning Services Provides
- The proper spacing and limitations of births.
- Advice on sterility.
- Screening for pathological conditions related to the reproductive system.
- Genetic counselling.
- Sex education.
- Education for parenthood.
- Premarital consultation and examination.
- Carrying out pregnancy tests.
- The preparation of couples for the arrival of the first child.
- Providing services for unmarried (mothers) women.
- Teaching home economics and nutrition.
- Providing adopted services.
- Marriage counselling.

Family planning was the motto of the national population policy in independent India since the introduction of the first five year plan (1951-56). Family planning programme is perhaps the most effective policy intervention to control fertility and stabilise population size. Since the effect of the programme varies from state to state, the fertility impact also varies from state to state. Contraception is the need of the day to counteract the explosive increase in population.

After independence, family planning was stepped up. The sole aim was the lowering of the birth rate. There was no significant economic or social measure to accompany it.

Religion plays a vital and important role in the life of the people of India. Muslims by-and-large do not adopt the family planning programme. Other factors responsible for the failure of family planning is illiteracy, poverty, etc. Islam like other religions believes that children are the gift of god and advise a proper care to feed, love and educate them.

The family planning methods provided by the programmes are : vasectomy, tubectomy, the IUCD, conventional contraceptives (i.e. condoms, diaphragms, jelly/cream tubes, foam tables and oral pills. In addition, induced abortion is available free of charge, in institutions recognised by the Govt. for this purpose.

Sterilisation is the main method for the family planning programme in India. The number of annual acceptors of this method is far larger than the IUD. The number of conventional contraceptive users relates to the prevalence of such use, rather than to number of new acceptors (statistics on sterilizations and other contraceptive methods. In 1972-73 over three million sterilizations were performed, two thirds of them in camps. During the emergency period (1975-77), almost 11 million sterilizations were performed but later on this programme witnessed virtual collapse.

Methods of Family Planning
- Cafeteria approach – user may make his/her own choice according to individual requirement and preferences.
- Number of children.
- Risks of method.
- Require motivation.
- Privacy to use.

Methods of Family Planning
1. **Terminal method**
   (a) Vasectomy.
   (b) Tubectomy.
2. **Spacing or Nonterminal methods**
   (a) Periodic abstinence.
   (b) Barrier methods like.
      I. Physical :
        (i) Condom.
        (ii) Diaphragm.
      II. Chemical :
        Foam tablet, jellies, creams, suppositories.
      III. Combined :
        Vaginal sponge – not right for fertility age-group.
   (c) Intrauterine devices (IUD) – Most commonly used in females.
   (d) Hormonal methods :
      1. Oral pills.
      2. Depot formulation.

(e) Post conceptional method.
      i. Menstrual induction.
      ii. Manual regulation.
      iii. Abortion.
   (f) Miscellaneous
      i. Male contraception.
      ii. Anti fertility vaccine.
      iii. Natural family planning method.

Qualities of a Good Contraceptive

1. Reliability – 100%.
2. Safety.
3. Reversibility.
4. Low cost.
5. Convenience.
6. Consumer control : Generally meant for use by women. Male contraception device is only condom.
7. Cultural acceptability method – Requiring contact with genital area or producing menstrual irregularities may not be acceptable in certain cultures.

Condom

A condom is a sheath or covering made to fit over man's erect penis also called rubbers, sheaths, skins and prophylactics and known by many different brand names. Most common condoms are made of thin latex rubber. Some condoms are coated with a dry lubricant or with spermicide. Different sizes, shapes and colours may be available.

Condoms help to prevent both pregnancy and sexually transmitted diseases (STDs). Their correct use keep the sperms and any disease organisms in the semen out of contact of the vagina. Condoms also stop any disease causing organisms from entering the penis.

To be highly effective, it must be used correctly every time. Many men do not use condoms correctly or do not use them every time they have sex. Thus, they may risk causing pregnancy, getting STDs or giving STDs to their partners.

It is somewhat effective for preventing pregnancy as the rate of preganancies is 14 per 100 women in the first year of use. However, when correctly used 3 pregnancies per 100 women have been recorded.

Advantages
- It prevents STDs, HIV/AIDs as well as pregnancy, when used correctly, with every act of sexual intercourse.
- It helps protect against conditions caused by STDs – pelvic inflammatory disease, chronic pain and possibly cervical cancer in women, infertility in both men and women.
- Can be used to prevent STD infection during pregnancy.
- Can be used immediately after childbirths and it has no effect on the breast milk unlike the combined oral contraceptives. It also protect against infection in the uterus at a time when such infection occurs easily.
- It is safe and has no hormonal side effects.
- It can be used by the men of all ages.

Disadvantages
- Latex condoms may cause itching in people who are allergic to latex. In addition, some people may be allergic to the lubricants on some brands of condoms.
- May decrease the sensations, making sex less enjoyable for either partners.
- Couple must take time to put the condom on the erect penis before sex.
- It may be embarrassing for some people to purchase, ask a partner to use, put on, take off or throw away condoms.

Vaginal Methods

Vaginal methods are contraceptives that a woman places in her vagina shortly before sex. There are several vaginal methods :

1. Spermicides, including foaming tablets or suppositories, melting suppositories foam, melting film, jelly and cream.
2. Diaphragm, a soft rubber cup that covers the cervix. It should be used with a spermicidal jelly or cream.
3. Cervical cap is like the diaphragm but is smaller. It is not widely available outside North America, Europe, Australia and New Zealand.

Spermicides work by killing sperm or making sperm unmovable towards the egg. Diaphragms block the sperm from entering the uterus and tubes, when sperm could meet an egg.

Advantages

1. Safe and woman controlled methods that almost every woman can use.
2. Help prevent some STDs and conditions caused by STDs – pelvic inflammatory disease (PID), infertility, ectopic pregnancy and possibly cervical cancer. May offer some protection against HIV/AIDs, but this has not been demonstrated yet.
3. It offers contraception when needed. No daily action needed.
4. No side effects from hormones.
5. No effect on breast milk.

Disadvantages

1. Side effects :
   - Spermicide may cause irritation to woman on her partner, especially if used several times a day.
   - Spermicide may cause local allergic reaction in the woman or her partner.
   - Can make urinary tract infections more common.
2. Effectiveness requires availability of the method at hand and taking correct action before act of sexual intercourse.

A woman can begin using a vaginal method any time during her monthly cycle and soon after childbirth, abortion or miscarriage.

The diaphragm and cervical cap generally should not be fitted, however, in the first 6 to 12 weeks after full-term delivery or second trimester, spontaneous or induced abortion, depending on when the uterus and cervix return to their normal sizes. If needed, a woman can use the spermicidal alone or with condoms until then.

Intra Uterine Device (IUD)

An intrauterine device (IUD) usually is a small, flexible plastic frame. It often has copper wire or copper sleeves on it. It is inserted into a woman's uterus through her vagina. Almost all brands of IUDs have two strings or threads, tied to them. The strings hang through the opening of the cervix into the vagina. A provider can remove the IUD by pulling gently on the strings with the forceps.

IUDs work chiefly by preventing sperm and egg from meeting. Perhaps the IUD makes it hard for sperm to move through the woman's reproductive tract, and it reduces the ability of sperm to fertilize the egg.

It can also prevent the egg from implanting itself in the wall of the uterus.

It is very effective as commonly used. And shows a pregnancy rate of only 3 per 100 women.

Commonly used IUDs are :

Copper bearing IUDs (made of plastic wit copper sleeves an/or copper wire on the plastic) e.g. Tch-380A and MLCn-375.

Hormone releasing IUDs, made up of plastic, steadily release small amounts of hormone progresterone or another progestin such as (levonorgestrel) e.g. LNG-20 and progestasert.

Advantages
1. A single decision can lead to effective long-term prevention of pregnancy.
2. Long lasting e.g. the most widely used IUD (outside China), the TCU-380A lasts at least 10 years. Inert IUDs never need to be replaced.
3. They are very effective and require little rememberance.
4. No interference with sex.
5. Increased sexual enjoyment because there is no worry about pregnancy.
6. It can be inserted immediately after childbirth except the hormone releasing IUDs or after induced abortion if there is no evidence of infection.

Disadvantages
1. Common side effects : Menstrual changes
   - Longer and heavier menstrual periods.
   - Bleeding or spotting between periods.
   - More cramps or pain during periods.
2. Other uncommon side effects and complications :
   - Severe cramps and pains beyond the first 3 to 5 years after insertion.
   - Heaving menstrual bleeding or bleeding between periods, possibly contributing to anemia. More likely with the inert IUDs than with copper or hormone releasing IUDs.
   - Perforation or piercing of the wall of the uterus if the IUD is not properly inserted.

3. Does not protect against sexually transmitted diseases (STDs) including HIV/AIDs. Not a good method for women with recent STDs or with multiple sex partners or partner with multiple sex partners.
4. Pelvic inflammatory disease (PID) is more likely to follow STD infection if a woman uses an IUD. PID can lead to infertility.

DMPA

Women receive Depot - medroxyprogesterone acetate injections to prevent pregnancy. It is seen to be very effective. A rate as low as 0.3 per 100 women in the first year of use have been recorded when injections are regularly spaced 3 months apart.

1. It stops ovulation (release of eggs from ovaries).
2. It thickens the cervical mucus, making it difficult for sperm to pass through.
3. It does not disrupt existing pregnancy.

Advantages

1. It is very effective, and results in long term pregnancy prevention, which is reversible. One injection can prevent pregnancy for 3 months.
2. It does not interfere with sex and can be used at any stage.
3. Breast – feeding mothers can feel safe as it does not harm the quantity and quality of breast milk. It can be used by nursing mothers as soon as six weeks after childbirth.
4. It has no estrogenic side effects. It does not increase the risk of estrogen related complications such as heart attack.
5. It helps to prevent endometrial cancer and uterine fibroids. It may also help to prevent ovarian cancer.

Disadvantages

1. Common side of effects like changes in menstrual bleeding in the beginning. Amenorrhoea is a normal effect especially after the first year of use.
2. These injections can cause weight gain; change in diet can prevent weight gain.
3. Headaches, breast tenderness, moodiness, nausea, hair loss, less sex drive and/or acne in some women.
4. Does not protect against sexually transmitted diseases including the HIV/AIDs.

During Menstruation

A woman can start anytime she is reasonable certain that she is not pregnant. If started during the first seven days after the menstrual bleeding starts, and if she is still bleeding, no back up method is needed for extra protection.

Breast Feeding

It can be taken as early as six weeks after childbirth. If women is not breast-feeding after childbirth, it can be taken immediately or in the first six weeks after childbirth. She need not wait for her menstrual period to return. If not reasonably certain about pregnancy, then it is advisable to avoid sex, or use of spermicide until her first periods begin and then start DMPA.

After Miscarriage or Abortion

It can be started immediately or in the first 7 days after either first or second trimester miscarriage or abortion, or later when reasonably certain that she is not pregnant.

Use of DMPA Injectables

1. They are very effective and safe.
2. Change in vaginal bleeding are very normal. It is not harmful and not a sign of danger.

Female Sterilization

Female sterilization provides permanent contraception for women who do not want more children. It is a safe and simple surgical procedure and can usually be done with local anesthesia and light sedation.

A small incision is made by the doctor in the woman's abdomen and the two fallopian tubes are blocked off and cut. These tubes carry eggs from the ovaries to the uterus. With the tubes blocked the woman's egg can't meet the man's sperm. Two procedures are most commonly in use :

(A) Lapraroscopy (B) Mini laparotomy.

The effectiveness of this method depends partially on how the tubes are blocked, but all pregnancy rates are low. Only 0.5 pregnancies per 100 women (1 in 200) have been recorded in the first year after the procedure. Within 10 years, this figure increases to 1.8 pregnancies per 100 women (1 in 55).

Advantages

- Very effective.
- It is permanent. A single procedure leads to lifelong, safe and very effective family planning.
- Nothing to remember, no extra supplies needed and no repeated clinic visits required.
- No interference with sex. Don't affect a woman's ability to have sex.
- No known long-term side effects or health risks.

Disadvantages

It is usually painful for several days after the operation. Certain uncommon complications of the surgery can occur :

- Infection or bleeding at the incision.
- Internal infection or bleeding.
- Injury to internal organs.
- Anaesthetic risk : With local anesthesia alone or with sedation, rare risks of allergic reaction or overdose. With general anesthesia, occasional delayed recovery and side effects. Complications are more severe than with local anesthesia. There is also a risk of overdose.
- Reversal surgery is difficult, expensive and not available in most areas. Successful reversal too is not guaranteed. Woman who may want to become pregnant in the future should choose a different method.

The right time to go female sterilization. A woman can have female sterilization procedure at anytime when :

- She decides that she will never want to be pregnant in future.
- It is reasonably certain that she is not pregnant. These times can include :

    (1) Immediately after childbirth or within 7 days, if she has made a voluntary informed choice in advance.

    (2) Six weeks or more after childbirths.

    (3) Immediately after abortion (within 48 hours) if she has not decided voluntarily in advance.

    (4) Any other, but not between 7 days and 6 weeks post partum.

FAMILY WELFARE PROGRAMME IN INDIA

Introduction

India launched the National Family Welfare Programme in 1951 with the objective of "reducing the birth rate to the extent necessary to stabilise the population at a level consistent with the requirement of the National economy".

The family welfare programme in India is recognised as a priority area, and is being implemented as a 100% centrally sponsored programme. As per constitution of India, family planning is in the concurrent list. The approach under the programme during the first and second five year plans was mainly "Clinical" under which facilities for provision of services were created. However, on the basis of data brought out by the 1961 census, clinical approach adopted in the first two plans was replaced by "Extension and Education Approach" which envisaged expansion of services facilities along with spread of message of small family norm.

IV Five Year Plan

Evolution of FW Programme

In the IV Plan (1969-74), high priority was accorded to the programme and it was proposed to reduce birth rate from 35 per thousand to 32 per thousand by the end of plan. 16.5 million couples, constituting about 16.5% of the couples in the reproductive age group, were protected against conception by the end of IVth Plan.

V Five Year Plan

The objective of the V plan (1974-79) was to bring down the birth rate to 30 per thousand by the end of 1978-79. The programme was included as a priority sector programme during the V Plan with increasing integration of family planning services with those of health, *Maternal and Child Health (MCH)* and nutrition, so that the programme became more readily acceptable. The years 1975-76 and 1976-77 recorded a phenomenal increase in performance of sterilisation. However, in view of rigidity in enforcement of targets by field functionaries and an element of coercion in the implementation of the programme in 1976-77 in some areas, the programme received a set-back during 1977-78. As a result, the government made it clear that there was no place for force or coercion or compulsion or for pressure of any sort under the programme and the programme had to be implemented as an integral part of "Family Welfare" relying solely on mass education and motivation. The name of the programme also was changed to Family Welfare from Family Planning. The change was not merely in nomenclature but essentially in the content of its objectives.

VI Five Year Plan

In the VI Plan (1980-85), certain long-term *demographic goals* of reaching net reproduction rate of unity were envisaged. The implications of this were to achieve the following by the year 2000 A.D.

- Reduction of average size of family from 4.4 children in 1975 to 2.3 children.
- Reduction of birth rate to 21 from the level of 33 in 1978 and death rate from 14 to 9 and infant mortality rate from 127 to below 60.
- Increasing the couple protection level from 22% to 60%.

Year-wise acheivement during the VI Plan period of the four Family Planning Methods was as below :

(figures in 1000)

Year	Sterilisations	IUD Insertions	C.C	Oral Pills
1980-81	2053	628	3718	91
1981-82	2792	751	4439	120
1982-83	3983	1097	5765	183
1983-84	4532	2134	7661	729
1984-85	4085	2562	8505	1290

VII Five Year Plan

The Family Welfare Programme during VII five year plan (1985-90) was continued on a purely voluntary basis with emphasis on promoting spacing methods, securing maximum community participation and promoting maternal and child health care. In order to provide facilities/services nearer to the door steps of population, the following steps/initiatives were taken during the VII Plan period.

- It was envisaged to have one sub-centre for every 5000 population in plain areas and for 3000 population in hilly and tribal areas. At the end of VII plan i.e. 31.3.1990, 1.30 lakhs sub-centres were established in the country.

F - 13B

- The *Post Partum* programme was progressively extended to sub-district level hospitals. At the end of VII plan, 1012 sub-district level hospitals and 870 Health Posts were established in the country.
- The *Universal Immunization Programme* started in 30 Districts in 1985-86 was extended to cover all the districts in the country by the end of the VII plan.
- A project for improving Primary Health Care in urban slums in the cities of Bombay and Madras was taken up with assistance from World Bank.
- *Area Development Projects* were implemented in selected districts of 15 major States with assistance from various donor Agencies.

The achievements of the Family Welfare Programme at the end of the VII plan were :

- Reduction in crude birth rate from 41.7 (1951-61) to 30.2 (SRS : 1990).
- Reduction in total fertility rate from 5.97 (1950-55) to 3.8 (SRS : 1990).
- Reduction in infant mortality rate from 146 (1970-71) to 80 (SRS : 1990).
- Increase in Couple Protection Rate from 10.4% (1970-71) to 43.3% (31.3.1990).
- Setting up of a large network of service delivery infrastructure, which was virtually non-existent at the inception of the programme.
- Over 118 million births were averted by the end of March, 1990.

The approach adopted during the Seventh Five Year Plan was continued during 1990-92. For effective community participation, Mahila Swasthya Sangh at village level was constituted in 1990-91, MSS consists of 15 persons, 10 representing the varied social segments in the community and five functionaries involved in women's welfare activities at village level such as the Adult Education Instructor, Anganwari Worker, Primary School Teacher, Mahila Mukhya Sevika and the Dai. Auxiliary Nurse Midwife (ANM) is the Member-Convener. A major new initiative undertaken during 1991-92 was the *Chid Survival and Safe Motherhood Project*, an integration of Universal Immunization Programme with expanded/intensified MCH activities in high IMR states/districts of the country.

VIII Five Year Plan

To impart new dynamics to the Family Welfare Programme, several new initiatives were introduced and ongoing schemes were revamped in the Eighth Plan (1992-97). The broad features of these initiatives are as under :

World bank assisted area projects which seek to upgrade infrastructure and development of trained manpower have been continued during the 8th Five Year Plan. Two new area projects namely *India Population Project (IPP)*-VIII and IX have been initiated during the 8th plan. The IPP-VIII project aims at improving health & family welfare services in the urban slums in the cities of Delhi, Calcutta, Hyderabad and Bangalore. IPP-IX will operate in the States of Rajasthan, Assam and Karnataka.

An US aid assisted project named *"Innovations in Family Planning Services"* has been taken up in Uttar Pradesh with specific objective of reducing TFR from 5.4 to 4 and increasing CPR from 35% to 50% over the 10 years project period.

Recognising the fact that demographic and health profile of the country is not uniform, 90 districts which have CBR of over 39 per thousand (1991 census) were identified for differential programming. Enhanced allocation of financial resources, amounting to Rs. 50 lakhs per year per district, was made for upgradation of health infrastructure in these districts from 1992-93 to 1995-96. This amount is being used for providing well equipped operation theatres, labour room, a six-bedded observation ward and residential quarters for paramedical workers in 5 PHCs of each district per year. All the block level PHCs of these 90 districts have been covered.

Realising that government efforts alone in propagating and motivating the people for adaptation of small family norm would not be sufficient, greater stress has been laid on the involvement of NGOs to supplement and complement the government efforts. Four new schemes for increasing the involvement of NGOs have been evolved by the department of family welfare.

The *Universal Immunisation Programme (UIP)* was launched in 1985 to provide universal coverage of infants and pregnant women with immunisation against identified vaccine preventable diseases. From the year 1992-93, the UIP has been strengthened and expanded into the *Child Survival and Safe Motherhood (CSSM) Project.* It involves sustaining the high immunisation coverage level under UIP, and augmenting activities under Oral Rehydration Therapy, prophylaxis for control of blindness in children and control of acute respiratory infections. Under the Safe Motherhood component, training of traditional birth attendants, provision of aseptic delivery kits and strengthening of first referral units to deal with high risk and obstetric emergencies are being taken up.

The targets fixed for the 8th plan of a National level birth rate of 26 was achieved by all States except the States of Assam, Bihar, Haryana, Madhya Pradesh, Orissa, Rajasthan and Uttar Pradesh.

IX Five Year Plan (1997-2002)

Reduction in the population growth rate has been recognised as one of the priority objectives during the Ninth Plan period.

The *objectives* during the Ninth Plan were :

i) to meet all the felt-needs for contraception
ii) to reduce the infant and maternal morbidity and mortality so that there is a reduction in the desired level of fertility.

The *strategies* during the Ninth Plan were :

i) to assess the needs for reproductive and child health at PHC level and undertake area-specific micro planning.
ii) to provide need-based, demand-driven, high quality, integrated reproductive and child health care.

The expected levels of achievement by the terminal year of Ninth Plan (2002) are given below :

Indicator	If current trend continues	If acceleration envisaged in Approach Paper to the Ninth Five Year Plan is achieved
CBR	24/1000	23/1000
IMR	56/1000	50/1000
TFR	2.9	2.6
CPR	51%	60%
NNMR	35/1000	
MMR	3/1000	

Community Needs Assessment Approach (CNAA) in Family Welfare Programme

1. The International Conference on Population and Development, Cairo, Egypt held on 5-13 September, 1994 recommended that the aim of

family planning programme must be to enable couples and individuals to decide freely and responsibly the number and spacing of their children and to have the information and means to do so and to ensure informed choices and make available a full range of safe and effective methods. The success of population education and family planning programme in a variety of settings demonstrates that informed individuals everywhere can and will act responsibly in the light of their own needs and those of their families and communities. The principle of informed free choice is essential to the long-term success of family planning programmes.

2. Under the Target Oriented approach, the national level targets in respect of different family planning methods were used to be fixed in consultation with the states/union territories, keeping in view the long-term demographic goals and past performance levels of the states/union territories. These targets, however, became an end in itself and not the means to bring about the expected decline in the birth rates. The target based system followed up to 31st March, 1996, suffered from negligence of the quality of services provided to the people under family welfare programme. The needs of the individual client were not properly met. Thus, the numerical method-specific targets provided such type of demographic planning which is against the democratic ethos of the country. Thus, a need arose to introduce decentralised, participatory approach with emphasis on clients' satisfaction and quality of services under target free approach doing away the target oriented approach.

3. The approach of determining targets was given up after extensive consultation with the states and after making pilot studies in one district of each of the 18 states in 1995-96. In the 4th conference of the Central Council of Health & Family Welfare, the council placed on record its appreciation of the efforts made by all the state governments to implement the family welfare programmes on the basis of target free approach with effect from 1996-97. In its 5th conference held in January, 97, the council urged all states & UTs and voluntary organisations to secure the full involvement of the community in the implementation of family welfare programme under target free approach.

4. On the basis of the experience gained during the experimental approach and in pursuance of the decision taken in conference of state secretaries (Family Welfare) held on 2nd February, 1996, the target free approach for the family welfare programme was extended all over the country from 1st April, 1996, which necessitates the decentralised participatory planning renamed as **Community Needs Assessment Approach (CNAA)** in 1997-98. Under this approach, planning of family welfare services will be formulated in consultation with the community at the grass root level and it is expected to lead to improvement in quality of services and client satisfaction. Besides, monitoring and evaluation of the performance also require a fresh look at the issues of quality of care at different levels of the primary health care system. Decentalised planning implicates close association of the community and its leading lights and opinion leaders such as village pradhans, mahila swasthya sanghs, primary school teachers, etc. in formulation of the PHC based family welfare and health care plan. In this connection, a manual of CNAA on family welfare programme has already been circulated to all the states and UTs to provide guidance in decentralized planning at the level of SC/PHC.

5. Forms :

   5.1 A total of 9 forms are prescribed in the CNAA manual in which the reports are to be made by the ANM for the sub-center, by in-charge medical officer for the PHC/FRU/sub-district hospital/district hospital to the district family welfare officer and by the District FW Officer to the state government and to the govt. of India (Department of FW).

   5.2 These 9 forms are of two types – forms 1 to 5 are action plan forms which have to be prepared once in every year prior to the beginning of the financial year by the ANM, In-charge MO PHC/FRU/Sub-district hospital/district hospital, district medical officer and the state action plan by the state FW officers.

   5.3 Form No. 6 to 9 of the CNAA manual are the monthly report forms to be submitted by 15th–25th of the following month by ANM/MPW(Male) for sub-center/urban health post/revamping center to the PHC, by medical officer in-charge FRU/CHC/sub divisional hospital/PPC district hospital to the district FW officer and the consolidated monthly report by the district FW officer to the state FW department and the department of FW (Ministry of Health & FW, New Delhi).

NATIONAL HEALTH POLICY

Policy

A system which provides the logical framework & nationality of decision making for the achievement of intended objectives :

Utilities of Policy

- A guide to action to change.
- Policy sets priorities & guides resource allocation.
- Vital for development of nation.
- Health policy aims at the improvement of the condition that make people feel secure, safe, adequate & sustainable livelihoods, life-styles & healthy environment housing.
- Every 6th person on the globle today is an Indian.
- India adds about 10 lakh persons to its population every fortnight.
- 49% including in India's population is from 4 states – BIMARU states.

Role of Media

The communication media have played an important role in promoting the family welfare programme. Following the pattern of the successful agricultural extension services, during the third Five Year Plan, a strategy shift from 'clinic approach' to 'extension approach' was adopted and family planning workers were required to visit people in their homes to inform and educate them about various aspects of the family planning programmes.

Family planning communication received a new impetus with the creation of the *Mass Education Media (MEM)* division within the department of family welfare during the inter plan period of 1966-69. Simultaneously, the media units of information and broadcasting ministry were strengthened for family planning communication. The objective was to evolve a differential communication strategy. Simple messages with simple pictures were selected for wider dissemination and through media which were easily visible and audible.

Demography and Family Planning

Red Triangle

It was during the Fourth Five year Plan that communication efforts began to be much more meaningful. The famous *Red Triangle* symbol for family planning was conceived during this period and a national campaign was launched for advocating " two or three children- enough". The campaign for male contraception-the condom under the brand name 'Nirodh' as the first social marketing effort which carried professional communication orientation was also initiated about this time. Films were seen as a major vehicle of communication and the district units of the MEM division were equipped with audio-visual vans for exhibiting a series of motivational films. The Satellite Instructional Television Experiments (SITE) programme helped to assess the impact of TV programmes about family planning on the beliefs and practices of the rural communities.

KNOWLEDGE OF CONTRACEPTIVE METHODS IN STATES/UTS

States/Uts	Any Method	Any Modern Method
Delhi	99.7	99.7
Haryana	99.9	99.8
Himachal Pradesh	100.0	100.0
Jammu Region	98.8	98.8
Punjab	100.0	100.0
Rajasthan	98.8	98.7
Madhya Pradesh	97.8	97.8
Uttar Pradesh	98.4	98.3
Bihar	99.2	99.2
Orissa	98.6	98.3
West Bengal	99.6	99.4
Assam	98.4	98.3
Gujarat	98.5	98.3
Maharashtra	99.4	99.4
Andhra Pradesh	98.9	98.9
Karnataka	99.4	99.3
Kerala	99.7	99.7
Tamil Nadu	99.9	99.9
India	**99.0**	**98.9**

Source : National Family Health Survey, India 1998-99.

Landmark Strategy

During the fifth five year plan, the government of INDIA executed an agreement with the advertising agency association of India to design a communication strategy for the states of Uttar Pradesh, Andhra Pradesh and West Bengal and this agreement is still considered a landmark in evolving communication strategies in family planning programme. The objectives of the strategy were to provide appropriate knowledge about methods of contraception, allay fears among the people, provide accurate information as to where one can have family planning services, and finally to stimulate inter-personal contacts. Finally the strategy was required to motivate people for increasing the practice of family planning.

The gains of such strategies were fairly obvious as during this time multi-media approach was put into practice, different messages were evolved for different audience and in almost all cases, local languages received due importance. Around 400 prototype materials were prepared and sent to Uttar Pradesh, Andhra Pradesh and West Bengal for use. The strategy also envisaged covering all media of mass communication such as radio, press, song and drama, exhibition, group discussion through extension educators and field workers. Eminent lyricists like Prem Dhawan and singers like Lata Mangeshkar and Asha Bhonsle were utilised. The involvement of voluntary organisations was much wider and special campaigns were organised to ensure greater acceptance of family planning by minorities. Considerable efforts to involve scholars, writers, journalists, doctors, opinion leaders for promoting Family Planning programme were also initiated.

New Initiatives

As part of the new IEC strategy in tune with the **Reproductive & Child Health Programme**, it has been decided by the centre to utilise private professional agencies for creating audio-visual and advertising campaigns for the mass media. For effective communication and optimal impact, it has been decided to utilise the services of eminent filmmakers for producing full length feature films with sensitive depiction of messages on reproductive health and population issues.

In the new strategy, the centre has chosen a few specific channels of communication viz. television, radio, the song and drama division, directorate of field publicity and the print media for promoting the reproductive health and population issues.

Television

Beside utilising the services of eminent filmmakers for production of films, the department utilises the services of creative producers in the making of video spots, arranging interactive panel discussions with opinion leaders of district and region and audiences and panel discussions on important RCH issues with subject specialists.

Radio

Apart from revamping of old programmes, a new folk song programme has been launched on AIR's vivid bharti channel from August 1999. Audio spots are produced and broadcast by the All India Radio and inserted in the popular sponsored programmes. To maximise the audience only the channels like vividh bharati and national channel are used.

Song and Drama Shows

Song and drama division of the ministry of information & broadcasting (MIB), whose troops perform live shows in the villages have been asked to intensify coverage by assigning one troupe the responsibility of covering 2-3 districts in a phased manner with their live shows on reproductive health and population issues.

Field Publicity

The directorate of field publicity, another media unit of the MIB, which have been organising a variety of programmes such as film shows, song and drama shows, special plays, photo exhibitions, seminars, symposia, debates, baby shows and other contests through its field units at the district level, have been asked to involve women, students and youth in a big way.

Print Media

Advertisement campaigns on reproductive health issues are being designed from time to time and released to all major news papers in 13 languages viz. English, Hindi, Assamese, Oriya, Bengali, Marathi, Gujarati, Urdu, Punjabi, Kannada, Malayalam, Telugu and Tamil. Recently, the RCH newsletter has been started in Assamese, Oriya, Hindi and English. The copies of this newsletter being sent to health functionaries in the district on a regular basis.

At the state level, similar activities are being undertaken by the states governments. Funds for maintenance of Mahila Swasthya Sangh-women's groups are being provided by the centre. States are being encouraged to open separate IEC (Information, Education and Communication) bureaus for better planning and evolve local specific media strategies.

Decentralised Strategy

An important initiative of the new IEC (Information, Education and Communication) strategy is to decentralised IEC efforts to the level of district, so that every district is able to plan and implement local specific IEC keeping in view the cultural, ethnic, linguistic requirements. IEC through *Zila Saksharta Samitis*, ZSS, (part of the national literacy mission) are new thrust areas aimed at for integrating education with family welfare by utilising the already existing network. Under the ZSS scheme, the concerned districts are to plan and implement their IEC plans, with a thrust on the folk media, design and display of posters, wall writing and paintings and specific cultural medium in their resoective areas. Decentralisation of IEC campaign is giving the district much more flexibility to work with freedom and creativity. When compared with the top-down approach from either the centre or the state governments, the decentralised efforts have the potential of opening up unlimited, region specific possibilities in the sphere of inter-personal and group communication as well.

Three-tier Approach

While the IEC division of the ministry of health and family welfare, department of family welfare, government of India has the overall responsibility for planning major IEC activities and national campaigns, the implementation is being largely carried out by the states and union territories, various media units of ministry of information and broadcasting (MIB) and professional agencies. District becomes focal point for local IEC campaigns as well as a sub-centre of activities in the surrounding rural areas.

IEC at State Level

Each state/UT has state directorate of information and publicity, which plays the same role as the MIB at the central level. The responsibility of planning and conducting IEC activities rests with the state IEC division headed by the state media officer.

IEC at District Level

At the district level, there is a district extension & media officer. There is a block extension education officer, and at the sub centre level IEC is combined with clinical service delivery and is carried out by multipurpose workers. Community workers/health functionaries used for IEC and advocacy activities in most states include auxiliary nurse cum midwives (ANMs), multipurpose workers, male health workers and mahila swasthya sanghs. Rajasthan and a few other states have developed special networks such as the Jan Mangal and Swasthya Karmi. Unfortunately, the understaffed IEC structure in the field has often been found overworked and used for other activities and projects. It is assumed with the introduction of independent district IEC efforts, these personnel will not be used for other activities any more.

Non Government IEC Efforts

In addition to the government initiatives, a large number of NGOs at the national, state and district levels carry out IEC activities independently. Prominent NGOs who have contributed significantly to the IEC campaigns include the Family Planning Association of India, Bombay; Voluntary Health Association of India, New Delhi; Society for Services to Voluntary Agencies, Pune and Gandhigram Institute of Rural Health and Family Welfare Trust who cover vast areas independently.

Population Education

Population education programmes are implemented through cells in the centre and the states at the primary, secondary, post-literacy, higher education and vocational training programme levels. Presently, four national projects on population and development with the assistance of UNFPA are in progress.

Project on School education is being implemented with the help of the National Council of Education Research and Training (NCERT) in 30 out of a total of 32 States/U.T. In this project, over 2.2 million teachers and educational functionaries have been oriented in Population education. Over 540 titles on various themes have been published in 17 Indian languages. Introduction of adolescence education in school curricula, which already includes Population related messages, have been introduced.

Project on post-literacy & continuing Education is being implemented by department of adult education (National literacy mission) through state/regional resource centres in 430 districts of 26 States/UTs. Major activities under this project includes training of Project functionaries, preparation, production and distribution of training and education material including integrated primers, supplementary readers, follow-up materials and reading materials for continuing education, outreach activities like exhibitions and fairs, street plays, awareness camps for mothers-in law and research and evaluation. Motivational material for electronic media was also produced.

Project on Higher Education is being implemented since 1986 through 17 Population Education Research Centres (PERCs), set up in various University campuses all over India, to disseminate information regarding Reproductive Health and Population issues to the university and college students. Thirty-five Universities have introduced special paper on population education. Over 1400 population education clubs have been set up under the project to organise various education activities with the cooperation of the community and the NGOs.

Project on Vocational Training is being implemented through Directorate General of Employment and Training (DGET), Ministry of labour in 600 Industrial Technical Institutes (ITI) all over the country in its second phase. The first phase covered about 1000 ITIs. The component of population education have been integrated in the social studies curriculum in all the ITIs which runs a number of vocational courses for the adolescents and youth.

Project for Involvement of Elected Representatives

The Project titled "Involvement of elected representatives" for advocacy on population, RCH, HIV/AIDS, Reproductive rights and women's involvement' is being implemented by Indian Association of Parliamentarians on Population and Development, New Delhi. Launched in November 1999, it is initially sanctioned for a period of two years. The project will cover the entire states of Madhya Pradesh and Rajasthan and 20 more districts of Maharashtra, Gujarat, Orissa and Kerala where UNFPA funded integrated population and development projects are under implementation.

The goal of the project is to sensitize, mobilise and involve elected representatives (including Panchayat Raj representatives) in effective population stabilisation, reproductive health programmes including awareness of HIV/AIDS.

Cause of Population Growth

- Widening gap between birth rate & death rate.
- Low age at marriage.

- High illiteracy (mainly of women).
- Religious attitude towards family planning.
- Status of female – no decision power.
- Desire for male child.
- Joint family system – less responsibility of couple to bring up their children.
- Lack of information.
- Lack of choice of contraceptives.
- Side effects of contraceptives.
- Poor services of family planning.
- Poverty – poor parents need more children to earn bread & butter consequently child labour.

NPP (1983)
- Average size of family 1 to 2.3.
- Birth Rate/1000 population 1 to 21.
- Death Rate 1 to 9.
- Infant mortality rate, IMR < 60.
- Effective couple protection rate > 60%.

NPP, 1986
Evolved & promoted the slogan "movement of the people, by the people, for the people".

Failure due to
- Lack of political commitment.
- Lack of people participation.
- Lack of quality of health services.
- Lack of education.
- Lack of overall development.
- Lack of appropriate technology.

NPP 2000
Immediate Objectives
- To meet the unmet need of contraception.
- Strengthening health infrastructure.
- Strengthening of health personnel.
- Health services should be integrated services to RCH.

Medium Objective
- Bring the TFR (2-1) to replacement level by 2010.

Long term Objective
- Stable population by 2045.

National Socio-demographic goals for 2010

1. Address the unmet needs for basic reproductive and child health services, supplies and infrastructure.
2. Make school education upto age 14 free and compulsory and reduce drop cuts at primary and secondary school levels to below 20 per cent for both boys and girls.
3. Reduce infant mortality rate to below 30 per 1000 live births.
4. Reduce maternal mortality rate to below 100 per 100,000 live births.
5. Achieve universal immunization of children against all vaccine preventable diseases.
6. Promote delayed marriage for girls not earlier than age 18 and preferably after 20 years of age.
7. Achieve 80 per cent institutional deliveries and 100 per cent deliveries by trained persons.
8. Achieve universal access to information/counselling and services for fertility regulation and contraception with a wide basket of choices.
9. Achieve 100 per cent registration of births, deaths, marriage and pregnancy.
10. Contain the spread of Acquired Immunodeficiency Syndrome (AIDS) and promote greater integration between the management of reproductive tract infections (RTI) and sexually transmitted infections (STI) and the National AIDS Control Organisation.
11. Prevent and control communicable diseases.
12. Integrate Indian Systems of Medicine and Homoeopathy (ISM & H) in the provision of reproductive and child health services and in reaching out to households.
13. Promote vigorously the small family norm in achieve replacement levels of TFR.
14. Bring about convergence in implementation of related social sector programms so that family welfare becomes a people centered programme.

Demography and Family Planning 201

Strategies
- Decentralization.
- Empowerment of women.
- Child survival & child health.
- Meeting family need for FID services.
- Greater emphasis for understated population growth – slums, tribals.
- Village level services – Gram panchayat.
- Diverse health care providers.
- Collaboration with private agencies & NGOs.
- Integration of Indian system of medicine in delivery of MCH services.
- Contraceptive technology & research in RCH.
- Providing for older population.
- IEC.

National Levels
National population policy suggested a commission on population with prime minister as chairman & all chief ministers & senior officials of FW as members.

State Levels
State level commission for intersectoral coordination.
- Technology mission should be constituted in FW development.
- 42 constitutional amendment – LS seats frozen to 2007 further extended till 2026.
- Ensuring adequate funds for the policies.
- Containment of AIDS and greater interaction between AIDS & STD.
- Prevention & control of communed diseases.
- Integration of Indian system of medicine in provision of RCH services.
- Promote small family norm to achieve replacement level of TFR.
- Bring about conversions in implementation of related, social sector programmes so that FW become people centered programme.
- Achieve 100% registration of births, deaths, marriage & population.

Small Family Motivation and Promotional Measures

- Panchayat and Zila parishad rewards.
- Balika Samridhi Yojana – Girl child reward by department of women and child development Rs. 50/-.
- Maternity benefit scheme – Rs. 500/-.
- Health insurance – sterilization Rs. 5000/-.
- Below poverty line couple rewarded.
- Village-level self help group.
- Creches and child care centre.
- Wide choice of contraceptives.
- Safe abortion facilities.
- Social marketing.
- Ambulance services – soft loans.
- Vocational training for girls.
- Enforcement of child marriage restraint act.
- Soft loans for ANMs for their vehicle.
- 42nd constitutional amendment – Freezing of seats. For giving power to panchayat and reservation for females in it.

CHAPTER-10

MATERNAL AND CHILD HEALTH

MATERNAL & CHILD HEALTH (MCH)

It refers to the promotive, preventive, curative and rehabilitative health care for mothers and children.

The package for mother :

(1) Antenatal care.
(2) Intranatal care.
(3) Postnatal care.

Antenatal Care

The objective is to ensure a normal pregnancy with safe delivery of a healthy baby from a healthy mother.

AIMS

1. To protect and promote the health of the mother during pregnancy.
2. To prevent or to detect at the earliest and to treat the complications that may arise out of pregnancy.
3. To identify "High Risk" cases and provide them special attention.
4. To remove the fear and anxiety associated with pregnancy from the mind of the mother.
5. To educate the mother about child care, nutrition, personal hygiene, etc.
6. To provide the mother with information regarding family planning services.
7. To reduce the maternal and infant mortality and morbidity.

Antenatal care comprises of following elements :

(i) Antenatal visits.
(ii) Prenatal advice.

(iii) Specific health protection.
(iv) Family planning services.

Antenatal Visits

Ideally there should be atleast one visit during first 7 months of pregnancy followed by twice a month in next 2 months, then weekly visits. Therefore in India, the ministry of health and family welfare recommends at least 3 antenatal visits.

First visit

Objectives :

(1) To obtain the information about the health status of mother and foetus.
(2) Screening of 'high risk' cases and formulation of subsequent plan of action.
(3) To obtain the information important in determining the gestational age.

Components

History taking and examinations :

(I) History taking – includes information about the vital statistics, history of present pregnancy, obstetrical history, menstrual history, family history, etc.
(II) General physical examination
(III) Obstetrical examination.
(IV) Routine investigations – includes
  (i) Blood examination – Hb estimation, ABO grouping, Rh typing, VDRL test, etc.
  (ii) Urine examination for albumin, sugar and pus cells.
  (iii) Pap smear.
  (iv) G.C. culture test for gonorrhoea.
  (v) Stool examination.

Risk Approach

It is a management technique which is now in use for improvement of MCH services. Here the purpose is to provide essential services to all but 'special attention' to those who are in high risk category. By the use of these methods – the range of MCH services can be extended to include the mothers who need it the most. The criteria for selection of high risk cases are :

1. Primi gravidae above the age of 30 years.

Maternal & Child Health

2. Grand multiparas.
3. Pre-eclampsia.
4. Ante partum haemorrhage.
5. Anaemia.
6. Short statured primi (below 145 cm).
7. History of two or more previous abortions.
8. Previous still birth or neonatal death.
9. Previous medical diseases or operations.
10. Previous caesarean section or hysterotomy.
11. Hypertensive primi.
12. Abnormal presentation and position.
13. Multiple pregnancy.

Home visits is an important part of MCH services. At least one home visit should be made by either female health worker or public health nurse. They help in gaining confidence of the mother and also in providing proper antenatal advice keeping in mind the environmental and socio economic conditions at home.

Subsequent visits
Objectives :
(a) To identify at the earliest the signs and symptoms of retarted foetal growth, pre edampsia, hydramnios, anaemias, toxaemia, etc.
(b) To decide the time for amniocentesis.
(d) To detect any mal-presentation, if present.

Components
(I) History — for new complaints.
(II) General examination as weight, pallor, odema, B.P., etc.
(III) Obstetrical examination.
(IV) Laboratory examinations
   (i) Urine examination.
   (ii) Blood examination — Hb estimation.

Antenatal Advice
Principles :
(1) To make the mother realise the importance of regular antenatal checkups.
(2) To protect and maintain the health of the mother by giving advice regarding diet, drugs and personal hygiene.
(3) To give information about the working signs of pregnancy.

(a) Diet – The diet during pregnancy should be providing adequate nutrients for the maintenance of maternal health and growth of the foetus. It should also be adequate for successful lactation. During pregnancy there is increased calorie requirement. This needs increased intake of energy rich foods. The diet should be *light, nutritious* i.e. rich in proteins, minerals, vitamins and carbohydrates and *easy to digest*.

(b) Personal Hygiene – It includes personal cleanliness, regular bowel movements, dental care rest and sleep.

Specific Health Protection

(a) Tetanus Toxoid, Vaccination

In India, an important cause of death in infancy is neonatal tetanus, which is caused by infection of newborn infants by tetanus organisms, usually at the umbilical stump. Neonatal tetanus is most common among children who are delivered in unhygienic environments and when unsterilized instruments are used to cut the umbilical cord. Tetanus typically develops during the first or second week of life and is fatal in 70-90 per cent of cases (Foster, 1984). If neonatal tetanus infection occurs where expert medical help is not available, as in many rural areas in India, death is almost certain. Neonatal tetanus, however, is a preventable disease. Two doses of tetanus toxoid vaccine given one month apart during early pregnancy are nearly 100 per cent effective in preventing tetanus among both newborn infants and their mothers, Immunity against tetanus is transferred to the foetus through the placenta when the mother is vaccinated.

In India, the tetanus toxoid immunization programme for expectant mothers was initiated in 1975-76 and was integrated with the Expanded Programme on Immunization (EPI) in 1978 (Ministry of Health and Family Welfare, 1991). To step up the pace of the immunization programme, the government of India initiated the Universal Immunization Programme (UIP) in 1985-86. An important objective of the UIP was to vaccinate all pregnant women against tetanus by 1990. In 1992-93, the UIP was integrated into the Child Survival and Safe Motherhood Programme, which in turn has been integrated into the Reproductive and Child Health Programme. According to the National Immunization Schedule, a pregnant woman should receive two doses of tetanus toxoid injection, the first when she is 16 weeks pregnant and the second when she is 20 weeks pregnant (Central Bureau of Health Intelligence, 1991). Reinoculation is recommended every three years. If two doses were received less than three years earlier, a single booster injection is recommended.

(b) Iron and Folic Acid Supplementation

Nutritional deficiencies in women are often exacerbated during pregnancy because of the additional nutrient requirements of foetal growth. Iron deficiency anaemia is the most common micronutrient deficiency in the world. It is a major threat to safe motherhood and to the health and survival of infants because it contributes to low birth weight, lowered resistance to infection, impaired cognitive development, and decreased work capacity.

Studies in different parts of India have estimated that the proportion of births with a low birth weight (less than 2,500 grams) ranges from 15 per cent to 46 per cent (Nutrition Foundation of India, 1993). Overall, about one-third of newborn children in India are of low birth weight, indicating that many pregnant women in India suffer from nutritional deficiencies. Improvement in a woman's nutritional status, coupled with proper health care during pregnancy, can substantially increase her child's birth weight. To this end, the provision of iron and folic acid (IFA) tablets to pregnant women to prevent nutritional anaemia forms an integral part of the safe-motherhood services offered as part of the MCH activities of the Family Welfare Programme (Ministry of Health and Family Welfare, 1991), and now offered as part of the Reproductive and Child Health Programme. The programme recommendation is that pregnant women consume 100 tablets of iron and folic acid during pregnancy.

Nutritional Anaemia

- More than 50% pregnant females suffer from anaemia : 1/3 crore.
- It is one of the cause among 5 death.
- 60-70% children below 6 years suffers from anaemia.
- More than 50% are adolescent girls.
- It is not due to specific cause.

Factor :

- Lack of sufficient absorption of iron.
- Presence of disease, diarrhoea, worms.
- Increased demands, chronic disease.

Anaemia in Pregnancy
- More prone as increased requirement.
- Increased requirements interfere with maternal Hb formation.

Pregnant female seldom develops anemia, if :
- Eats a diet containing ample supply of essential material.
- Free from parasite.
- Increased demand is satisfied readily.

Causative factors :
1. Pre-pregnant state of female.
2. Intake of food during pregnancy.
3. Absorption & demand of food during pregnancy.
4. Iron requirement increased for foetus, placenta, enlarged uterus, increased blood volume.
5. During parturition – increased blood loss. (especially PPH) & this demand increases with each pregnancy.
6. Social values prevailing in community is also important.
7. Woman trends to eat last especially in conservative families.
8. Total calories required is met but diet suffers the quality.
9. Fasting during pregnancy.
10. Smoking & drinking.
11. Social belief & tabooes require 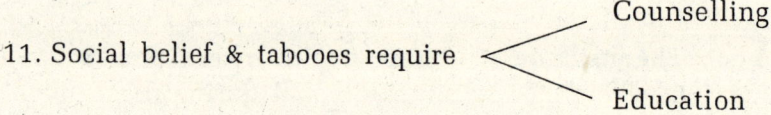 Counselling / Education
12. Lack of availability of food.
13. Lack of education and knowledge of food stuff.

Weight gain & outcome :
1. 10 kg. of weight is gained during pregnancy.
2. If women do not eat enough & do hard physical work the weight gain is less.
3. Baby born < 2.5 kg. prone to disease & death.
   [< 2 kg (India)].
4. Emergency health care is provided for pregnant female.

Family Planning Services

Educational and motivational efforts for family planning during antenatal period. If the mother has had 2 or more children, she should be motivated for puerperal sterilization.

Natal Care

Natal period starts from the onset of labour till the delivery is complete.
- Places with appropriate medical facility.
- Institutional delivery
  - Early seeking.
  - No delay.
  - Good services.
  - Care of mother & new born.
  - Management of complication.

If institutional delivery not possible, 2nd option is to conduct the delivery by a trained person.

Intranatal Care

Objectives :
1. Safe delivery – hands thoroughly clean till elbow.
2. Clean hands to – handie the sterilized things.
3. Clean surface.
4. Clean cord.
5. Clean tie.
6. Clean blads.
7. Minimum injury to infant and mother.

Home delivery

The following clean practices must be ensured.
- Female must lie on clean cort.
- Clean hand.
- Cut nails, remove rings & bangles.
- New blade, etc.

Assistance Required :
- Encourage frequent emptying of bowel & bladder.
- Soap & water as enema or plain water as enema.
- Emergency care – Give sweet warm drinks during 1st stage and soft food (100k for hydration state).

- Let her walk between labour pain.
- After membrane rupture – Don't let her move.
   – Don't leave her alone.
- 2nd stage : Dilatation of cervix to delivery – Encourage pushing in between pain & relaxation.
- Provide perineal support to prevents prolapse.
- Don't leave the cotton gauge inside the pelvic area as it increases maternal mortality rates.
- As hand comes out ask the mother to relax because afterwards baby comes out on its own. Tie cord 2.5 cm or less from patient.

Complications during delivery

Timely identification of danger signs :
1. Excessive bleeding.
2. Female in labour > 12 hrs.
3. Placenta not delivered during 30 min.
4. Child not cried.
5. Yellow colour skin of the child.
   (Action – transfer child to an appropriate health centre)

Post Natal Care

Signs :

1. Fresh uterine contractions.	Takes 15-20 min.
2. Extravalviular part of cord lengthens. Put two artery forceps.	
3. Gush of blood.	

- Post natal period starts from delivery of placenta to 42 day.
- Mother and baby are vulnerable to death.
- They are physically weak and need rest and proper nutrition to recover from the process of delivery (to prevent hypothermia and hyperthemia – Breast fed the baby).
- Support is necessary for proper and complete restoration of mother's health and newborn's care.

Wait and watch method should be applied.

Neonatal Care

Objectives :
- Prevent morbidity and mortality.

Maternal & Child Health

- Maintaining vital parameters.
- Early diagnosis of congenital disease.

Immediate Care

1. Cleaning the air ways.
2. Cleaning of mucus.
3. Head low position.
4. Suction
5. Resuscitation if natural breathing fails to establish.

Apgar Score

It is a quantitative method for assessing the infant's respiratory, circulatory and neurological status. A five minute score is to be taken.

Observe the
- Heart Rate
- Resp. Rate
- Pulse.
- Muscle tone.
- Reflexes.
- Colour.

Sign	0	1	2
Heart rate min.	Absent	Low < 100	Over 100
Respiratory effort	Absent	Slow, irregular	Good crying
Muscle tone	Flaccid	Some flexion	Active movements
Reflex response	Absent	Present	Cry
Colour	Blue coloured	Body pink, extremities blue	Pink
Total 10.	Severe depression 0-3	Mild depression 4-7	No depression 7-10

Care of Cord

- Cut the umbilical cordafter pulsation stop.
- Care to prevent tetanus.
- Cord must be ept dry.
- Falls off after 7-8 days.
- Takes long time in winter season & caesoaian baby.

Care of Eyes

- Application of topical neomycin may be helpful.
- Ophthalmia neonatorum/Red eye.
- Clean with a cotton swab from medial to lateral side.

Care of Skin
- Maintain the body temp. (36.5 - 37.5° C).
- 70% heat lost from head so cover the head.
- Gently wash the skin. Cover with soft cotton cloth.

Initiation of Breast Feeding
- Within 1 hour.
- Helps in starting milk secretion reflex.
- Colostrum is most suitable, as contains high% of vitamins and antibodies.

Examination

1st Examination :
In 24 hours — To detect injuries soon after birth Cony.
— Congential anomalies.
— Assess the maturity.

2nd Examination :
After 24 hrs. — Head to toe examination.
— Neonatal tetanus & syphilis.
— HIV, HBV, HEV.

Advise Given
Risk
- 90% of transmission if mother is HBsAg positive.
- 30% of transmission if HIV infected through breast feeding.
- Malnutrition play important role in death of Baby.

Baby Measurements
- Baby placed on clean towel in scale pan, spring balance, sling bag & salter, weight scale.
- Length should be recorded within 3 days using infantometer to nearest of 0.1 cm.
- Head circumference — Changes slightly due to moulding. Note the change before discharge.

Neonatal Screening
It should be done for congenital anomalies. At risk infants are to be identified.
- < 2.5 kg.
- Twins.

- Birth order 5 or more.
- Artificial feeding.
- Birth weight < 70% of expected.
- Failure to grow within 3 successive month.

Supportive Care of PHC Includes
- Nutrition.
- Mother should eat more than her usual diet.
- She should be given fruits, vegetables & milk in her diet.
- She should drink plenty of water and other fluids.
- Addition nutrients like iron and vitamins (x100 days) and folic acid.
- Demand feeding – (not the clock feeding) in day as well as night.
- Feed every 2-3 hourly or at least 7 times/day.
- Do not stop feeding if the baby or mother is sick.

Breast Feeding

Breast feeding is the ideal form of feeding in the neonate. It is the nature's device to ensure the survival of young ones and promotes close physical and emotional bonds between the mother and baby.

Major Practical Considerations

Avoid the followings :
- Discarding or minimum feeding of colostrum by 80% of mothers.
- Non-exclusive breast feeding by 85-95% in first 4 months of life.
- Unnecessary utilization of commercial infant milk food and animal milk.
- Pre-time or delayed feeding.

Advantages of Breast Milk

Nutritional Superiority

Breast milk contains all the nutrients a baby needs for normal growth and development, in a proper proportion and in a form that is easily digested and absorbed.

Carbohydrates :
- High concentration of lactose (6-7 g/dl).
- Lactose helps in absorption of calcium and enhances the growth of lactobacilli in the intestine.

Proteins :
- Low protein content (0.9-1.1 g/dl) so as to lactalbumin in more than caseinogen.
- Cause lower solute load on the kidneys.

Fats :
- Rich in polyunsaturated fatty acids (PUFA) promotes brain growth.
  Active lipase promotes digestion of fats and provides free fatty acids.
- Omega 3 and omega 6 fatty acids helps in formation of prostaglandins, cholesterol, necessary for steroid hormones.

Vitamins & Minerals :
- Sufficient for the needs of the baby in the first 4-6 months of life.

Water & Electrolyte :
- 88% water content sufficient enough to excrete low mineral and sodium content.

Convenient
- Breast milk can be given at any time.
- Easy availability at room temperature and can be stored for 10 hours at room temperature.
- No fuel consumption, thus breast feeding is eco-friendly.
- Time saving.

Maternal Benefits
- Exclusive breast feeding serves as an effective contraceptive as lactation suppresses ovulation.
- Lowers the risk of ovarian and breast cancers.
- Helps to stop maternal bleeding after delivery along with uterine involution.
- Improves the figure of the mother bymobilising the extra fat of the body.

Protection against Infection
- Secretory IgA, IgM, lysozyme, antistaphylococcal factor and specific inhibitory substances protect against viral infections.
- Lactoferrin and iron protects against enterobacteria.

- High level of bifidus factor protects the baby from the infection with Escherichia coli.
- Colostrum has viable phagocytic macrophages and lymphoid cells, which provide non-specific gastro intestinal host defenses and offer protection against diarrhoea.
- Para-amino-benzoic acid (PABA) provides protection against malaria.

Protects from Allergy
- Secretory IgA protects from milk allergy in exclusively breast fed infants.

Specific Protection
- Protects against neonatal hypocalcaemia and tetany nectrotizing enterocolitis, deficiencies of vitamin E and zinc, celiac disease, ear infections and orthodontic problems.

Economic Factors
- The cost of human milk is negligible as compared to the fresh milk or commercially obtained powder milk for artificial feeding including the costly feeding bottles and rubber teats.

Emotional Bonding
- Breast feeding pronotes close physical and emotional bonds between the mother and the baby.

Saves Life
- Effective breast feeding for first 4-6 months of life and then weaning in addition to breast feeding for first year of life is very helpful as it has been documented that it prevents death of additional 1.3 million infant per year.
- Child with effetive breast feed is 14 times less likely to die from diarrhoea and 4 times less likely to die from acute respiratory infections.

Varying Types of Breast Milk

1. Colostrum

The milk secreted during the first three days after delivery. It is yellow and thick and thick and contains more antibodies and cells and increased amounts of vitamins A, D, E and K. It should not be discarded.

2. Transitional Milk

It is secreted during the following two weeks. The immunoglobulin and protein content decreases while the fat and sugar content increases.

3. Mature Milk

It follows the transitional milk. It is thinner and watery but contains all the nutrients essential for optimal growth of the body.

4. Preterm Milk

The milk of a mother who delivers prematurely contains more energy, protein, fat, sodium, zinc, anti-infective factors and macrophages and has lower content of lactose, calcium and phosphorus to meet the requirement of a preterm baby.

5. Fore Milk

It is secreted at the start of a feed. It is watery and rich in proteins, sugar, vitamins, minerals and water to satisfy the baby's thirst.

Proper Feeding Technique

- Breast feeding should be initiated as soon as possible after birth (within half an hour after normal delivery and four hours of caesarean section).
- Do not give prelacteal feeds like sugar water, gripe water, honey, breast milk substitutes or formula before initiation of breast feeding.
- The baby should be given only breast milk and nothing else (not even water) for first 4 months of life.
- Breast feeding should be given, whenever baby feels hungry (demand feeding).
- Mother should sit down preferably with her back, well supported.
- The baby's head and neck should be supported, in a straight line with his body, and should face the breast.
- Head of the infant should be slightly elevated while feeding and feed the child with a alternate breast during each feed.
- When the mother's breast touches the baby's upper lip, cheek or the side of the mouth, the baby opens up the mouth & searches for the nipple with an open mouth. This is called the rooting reflex.

Maternal & Child Health

- Insert whole of the nipple and most of areola in child's mouth for drawing milk from the lactiferous sinuses and effective suckling through suckling reflex.
- The child's mouth is filled with milk by one to three suckles, the baby swallows the milk through swallowing reflex and then breathes.
- When the baby does not get sufficient feed, he sucks more vigorously resulting in sore nipple.
- During first few days babies should be aroused by gentle tickling behind the ears or soles but it should not be unpleasant.
- Most of the babies take 15-20 minutes for total feed.
- Contented baby is playful, sleeps well, gain weight regularly and passes urine at least 6 or more times per day.
- Act of burping must be explained to safegaurd against regurgitation.
- Colostrum should always be fed to the baby for the initial 2-3 days.
- Exclusive breast feeding is the natural normal nutrition of the baby for 4-6 months.

Baby Friendly Hospital Initiative

- Baby Friendly Hospital Initiative (BFHI) was launched in 1992 as part of the Innocenti Declaration on promotion, protection and support of breast feeding by WHO and UNICEF.
- Bottle feeding is the biggest killer in developing countries.
- Steps are taken to improve knowledge, attitude and practice of health care workers by providing information and scientific methods to proote exclusive breast feeding during 4-6 months.
- Mother baby bondage at birth, avoidance of prelacteal feed, early breast feeding, practice of keeping the mother and baby together in 'rooming in' the ward is encouraged.
- Representatives of infant food manufacturers are strictly forbidden to contact mother or health care staff for distribution of low cost or free infant feed formula.
- Advertisement of breast milk substitutes in media and distribution of pamphlets, calenders, growth chart is against "The Infant Milk Substitutes, Feeding Bottles and Infant Foods Acts 1992" and can lead to fine or imprisonment.

- Medical and nursing graduates, family physician and all personnel should be provided information for breast-feeding.

Recommendations for Successful Breast Feed

- Education and advice must be given to every mother in antenatal clinic. Retracted and cracked nipples to be managed before delivery.
- The first feed should be exclusively breast feed.
- Baby should be held in correct position.
- Mother can feed in any position that is comfortable for both.
- Allow 'rooming in'.
- Feeding must be on demand and not by clock.
- Bottle feeding should not be introduced.
- No supplementation with water.
- Frequent suckling, complete emptying of breast, correct position and supportive care are corner stones of successful breast feeding.

Ten Steps to Successful Breast Feeding

Step 1 : Have a written breast-feeding policy that is routinely communicated to all health care staff.

The policy guidelines should be prominently displayed in ANC, delivery room, special care baby unit and maternity ward to act as repeated reminders to mother and health care staff.

The hospital authorities should clearly state their commitment of not accepting any full or low cost sample of infant formula or any promotional material. Policy statement should be available both in English and in local language. It should be readily understood by mother and health care staff.

Step 2 : Train all health care staff in skills necessary to implement this policy.

Staff should be trained in science and art of breast feeding. They should be taught 10 steps to successful breast feeding. Practical skills should be imparted to mother for breast feeding like position, etc.

Step 3 : Inform all pregnant women about the benefits and management of breast feeding.

During antenatal period mother should be informed regarding nutritional, biological and emotional advantage of breast feeding. They should be motivated and assisted for promotion of breast feeding even if nipples are cracked, retracted or small as they should be managed during antenatal period.

Principles known to promote lactation should be explained. She should be made aware of danger of bottle feeding.

Step 4 : Help mothers initiate breast feeding within a half-hour of birth.

Establish mother baby bonding soon after the delivery & avoid prelacteal feeds.

Step 5 : Show mothers how to breast-feed and how to maintain lactation even if they should be separated from their infants.

In small & sick infants, exclusive breast milk and correct technique is to be taught to express manually or with breast pump.

Step 6 : Give newborn infants no food or drink other than breast milk, unless medically indicated.

Step 7 : Practice rooming-in. Allow mothers and infants to remain together 24 hours a day.

Practice of keeping babies alone or babies born by caesarian section in a nursery is strongly condemned because it is detrimental against successful breast feeding.

Step 8 : Encourage breast-feeding on demand.

Step 9 : Give no artificial teats or pacifiers (also called dummies or soothers) to breast feeding infants.

Expressed breast milk should be administered either through an orogastric tube or spoon depending upon vigour and maturity of infant.

Step 10 : Foster the establishment of breast-feeding support groups and refer mothers to them on discharge from the hospital or clinic.

Support group within community for breast feeding promotive and effective system of follow up.

Key family members are to be senstized and motivated to support breast feeding.

Nursing mother should be encouraged to take nutritious diet to sustain her health and to ensure good milk output.

Recognition of Baby Friendly Hospitals

Baby Friendly Hospital Initiative (BFHI) movement is active in India under National task force comprising of government of India, UNICEF, WHO, promotional bodies and voluntary organisations.

Steps for the hospitals to be recognised as baby friendly are :

1. Hospital conducts minimum 250 deliveries per year can seek recognition. After implementation of 10 global steps for breast feeding promotion, aduly completed self assessment form and registration form are sent to BHFI secretary.
2. The hospitals or nursing homes meeting 10 criteria is visited by assessor for on the spot checkings, to interview mothers and health care staff. The assessors sends their report to BFHI secretriate to be reviewed by reviewed committee.
3. The hospitals fulfilling the national BHFI criterias are recognised as baby friendly. The national task force organise a public ceremony for presentation of BFHI recognition certificate and a logo plaque. The hospitals unable to fulfil the required criteria for certification are informed regarding short coming.

Contraindication of Breast Milk

- Cialactosemia.
- Phenylketonuria.
- Temporarily during maternal's acute febrile illness.
- Development of breastinflammation or mastitis.
- Mother taking, anti thyroid drug, anti cancerous drugs or radio pharmaceuticals.

Weaning

Weaning refers to accustoming the infant to nourishment other than the mother's milk. It is a gradual process which is implemented for the infant after the age of 4 months when the mother's milk is no longer sufficient for the baby.

Desirable Qualities of Weaning Foods

- Adequate energy, protein, vitamins and minerals content.
- Easy to digest and nourishing.
- Semi-solid in consistency.
- Low in bulk & viscosity (Not too thick).
- Fresh & clean.

- Affordable and easy to prepare.
- Culturally acceptable, in consonance with the traditional feeding practices.
- Locally available and inexpensive.
- Easily prepared at home, with the existing facilities.
- Clean & hygienic, so that it should not become a source of infection.

Principally give one food item at a time without enforcing the child with clean hands.

Groups of Weaning Food

Group I : Protein, e.g. meat, milk, egg, pulses, beans, etc.

Group II : Oil/Fats, e.g. butter, nut.

Group III : Vegetables and fruits.

Various preparation of Weaning food :

1. Sprouting to increase the nutrients.
2. Fermentation to increase the digestibility, e.g. curd, idli, khmiri roti, dhokla, etc.
3. Malting : Here the grain is dampened, allowed to germinate, dried, husked and milled. Malted products have riboflavin, vitamin C and Iron. Gruel (khichri, kanji) prepared from rice (3 parts), legume (1 part), green leafy vegetable and some milk curd is a satisfactory weaning food.
4. Drying : Dried fish is rich in protein and calcium.
5. Milling : It improves digestibility but nutrients are lost.
6. Parboilng.
7. Amylase rich food (ARF) are germinated food which directly address the twin problum of dietary bulk and poor energy density of most weaning gruel. It is low in viscosity and dietary bulk. So, mothers can add then in weaning food.

Growth and Development

Growth : It denotes a net increase in the size or mass of tissues. It is largely attributed to multiplication of cells and increase in the intracellular substance.

Development : It specifies maturation of function. It is related to the maturation and myclination of the nervous system and indicates acquisition of a variety of skills for optimal functioning of the individual.

Growth Chart : It is used for monitoring the child's growth and development.

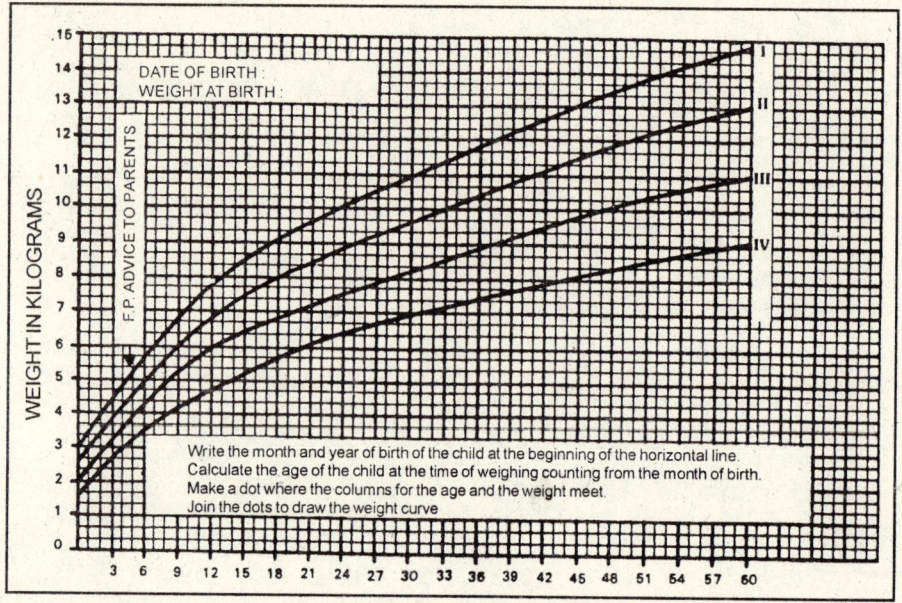

Growth chart in use in India, showing use of several reference curves to indicate the nutritional status of the child

Weights of average well-fed healthy children should be above the uppermost line I.
Children whose weight falls between lines I and III are under-nourished and require supplementary feeding at home.
Children whose weight falls below the line III are severely malnourished. Consult the doctor and follow his advice.
Children whose weight falls below line IV will have to be hospitalized for treatment.

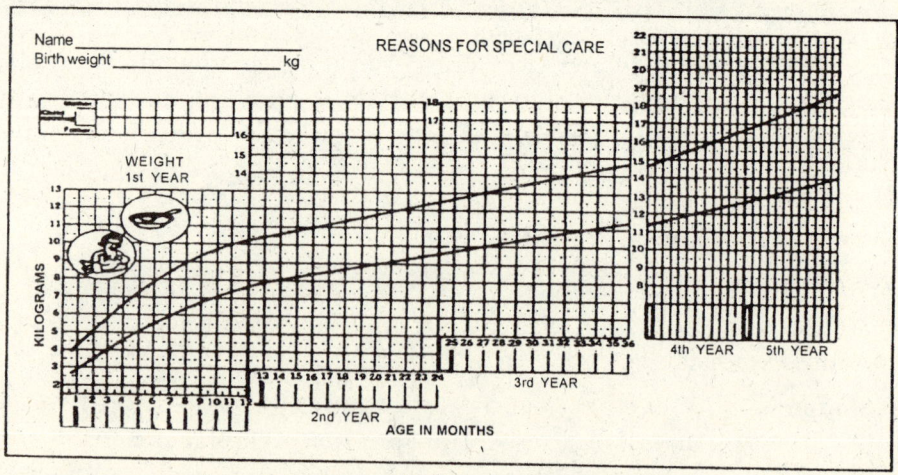

A prototype growth chart developed by WHO

National Immunisation Schedule

1. At birth : BCG + OPV – 'O' Dose
(For institutional deliveries)
   - 6 weeks : BCG (if not given at birth), DPT-1, OPV-1
   - 10 weeks : DPT-2, OPV-2
   - 14 weeks : DPT-3, OPV-3
   - 9 months : Measles
2. 16-24 months : DPT + OPV (Booster)
3. 5-6 years : DT. second dose of DT should be given at an interval of one month if there is no clear history or documental evidence of previous immunization with DPT, TT or DT.
4. Pregnant female : Early in Pregnancy – TT-1 or booster (16-20 weeks).

If second pregnancy occurs within 3 years of first, only 1 dose is required.

Note : Interval between 2 doses of vaccine should not be less than one month.

Minor cough, cold or mild fever are not contraindications to vaccinations.

Indicators of MCH Care

Maternal and child health status is assessed through measurement of mortality, morbility and growth and development. The commonly used mortality indicators of MCH care are :

1. Maternal mortality rate.
2. Mortality in infancy and childhood.

Maternal Mortality Rate

As per WHO, a maternal death is defined as "the death of a woman while pregnant or within 42 days of termination of pregnancy, irrespective of the duration and site of pregnancy, from any cause related to or aggravated by the pregnancy or its management but not from accidental or incidental causes."

$$M.M.R. = \frac{\text{Total number of female death due to complications of pregnancy, child birth or within 42 days of delivery from "puerperal causes" in an area during a given year}}{\text{Total number of live births in the same area and year}} \times 1000$$

Maternal in Infancy and Childhood

- They generally reflect the status of survival of children.
- As per experience gained within country and outside, it is established that the health of women in reproductive age group and below 5 years is of crucial importance.
- The more effective way of ensuring good health of the child is to ensure health of the mother.
- Estimation of infant and child mortality rate of an area or state is important as they reflect the impact of various interventions currently implicated under RCH program.

Infant Mortality Rate

It is defined as "the ratio of infant deaths registered in a given year to the total number of live births registered in the same year; usually expressed as a rate per 1000 live births."

$$IMR = \frac{\text{Number of deaths of children less than 1 year of age in a year}}{\text{Number of live births in the same year}} \times 1000$$

- It has been difficult to bring down the rate below 15 even after very good awareness in the community.
- However it is the indicator of the program for –
  i) Immunisation.
  ii) Diarrhoea management.
  iii) ARI management.
  iv) Adequate newborn care.
  v) Malnutrition.

Neonatal Mortality Rate

Neonatal period is from birth to first 28 day of life. Neonatal mortality rate is defined as "the ratio of neonatal deaths in a given year to the total number of live births in the same year"; usually expressed as a rate per 1000

$$N.M.R = \frac{\text{Number of deaths of children under 28 days of age in a year}}{\text{Total live births in the same year}} \times 1000$$

- It constitutes 2/3 of all deaths during infancy.
- In 1995, N.M.R. was 48/1000
- It can be reduced by institutional deliveries.

Major causes of deaths peculiar to infancy reported by RCH (1994) act are :

- Prematurity.
- Respiratory infection.
- Diarrhoea of newborn.
- Cord infection.
- Birth injuries.
- Congenital malformation.
- Non-detectable causes.

Strategies for improving child survival are :

- Appropriate management of diarrhoea.
- Appropriate management of A.R.I.
- Strengthen essential newborn care.
- Sustain high level of immunization.
- Vitamin A prophylaxis.
- Improving maternal care.
- Proper birth spacing.

Under Five Mortality Rate (child death rate)

It is estimated as :

$$\frac{\text{Number of deaths of children aged 1-4 years during a year}}{\text{Total number of children aged 1-4 years at the middle of the year}} \times 1000$$

- Child death rate is a more refined indicator of the social situation in a country than I.M.R.
- 2nd year of life is more susceptible to infection.
- It reflects the adverse enviornmental health hazards e.g. malnutrition, poor hygiene, infections, accidents, even economic, educational and cultural characteristics of the family.

School Health

School health is an important branch of community health.

Enrolment, attendance in school, preformance and learning are adversely affected by :

- Poverty.
- Poor school.

- Sexual behaviour.
- Physical and mental disability.
- Risk, crime behaviour.
- Religion.
- Parasitic infection.
- Acute respiratory infection.

The health bebefits through education (esp. girls) are :
- Benefits to themselves (physical, social and mental).
- Their future children.
- Their society.
- Population control.
- Enviornment protection.

School cannot affect health through curriculum alone, it needs the support of :
- Enviornment.
- Prevention programmes.
- Psychological health services.
- Nutritional and food safety service.
- Social service.

School Health Programme

This is a program to promote health through school & it involves all health activities.

Benefits :
- It is most efficient investment and a cost effective way to improve students' health and their academic performance along with that of school teachers and other staff.
- Schools generate higher income and healthier work force.
- 1-3 years of schooling to mother decreases mortality by 15%.
- Marked effect on attendance and performance.
- It can reach 1 billion students world wide every day.
- comprehensive health education curriculum can prevent certain adverse behaviours like :
  * Tobacco use.
  * Illicit drug use.
  * Dietary practice.
  * Unsafe sexual behaviour
  * Physical inactivity.

- Reduces school absenteism.
- Decreases injuries.
- Improve cognitive behaviour.
- Increases self esteem.
- Improves life skills, decision making, communications, understing emotions, etc.

Areas which needs emphasis are :
- Improvement, prevention and treatment of :
  * Malnutrition.
  * Infection.
  * HIV/AIDS, STDs.
  * Violence, injuries, crimes.
  * Uninfended pregnancy.
  * Poor reproductive health care.
- Handling conflicting message.
- Changing roles.
- Resources.

Components of School Health Programmes

1. School health services
   - Preventive, curative and referral services focussing not only students but school staff, too.
   - Health appraisal.
     * Regular periodic medical examination.
     * Daily inspection by trained teachers.
     * Make the check list and follow it.
   - Health record card
     * To be maintained by teacher or health worker.
   - Special clinical/health centre for 500 students in urban and less than 500 students in rural area.
   - Provision of beds in general hospital.
   - Focus on common endemic diseases.
   - First aid box/emergency care.
   - In-service training of teachers and other staff.
   - Special emphasis on dental health, eye care, mental health and E.N.T. care.
   - Dental hygienists.

2. School health education.

   It provides :
   - Academic skills and knowledge.
   - Health and nutritional education.
   - Inservice training.
   - Personal hygiene.
   - Mental hygiene.
   - Learning, correct :
     * Sitting posture.
     * Reading style.
     * Standing posture.
   - Extra curricular activity.
   - Community work and interaction.
   - Vaccination program.
   - Enviornmental pollution control.
   - Construction of latrines, sanitary wells, chlorination of water, etc.
   - Prevention of high risk and injuries by following traffic rules.
   - First aid.
   - Sex education.

3. School health enviornment
   - Physical, social psychological & cultural development.
   - Safe water supply.
   - Safe sanitation service.
   - Proper location.
   - Appropriate structure.
   - Surroundings free of diseases, injuries or pollution.
   - 10 square feet space for each student.
   - Maximum 40 students in a class.
   - Sufficient cross ventilation.
   - Sufficient lighting.
   - Furniture with safety designs.
   - Separate room for mid-day meals.
   - Proper lavatory facilities for boys and girls.

4. Health promotion for school personal.
   - Teachers should be the role model.
   - School staff presents the best social, physical & mental health

5. School community projects to out reach the difficult terrains and hilly areas.
    - Involvement of NGOs and private practitioners.
    - Involvement of community for better planning and delivery.
6. Nutritional and food safety.
    - Midday meal program containing ½ protein and $1/3$ calories which is to be free of cost.
    - Safe and nutritional lunch or meal on no profit no loss.
    - Applied nutition program for cultivating vegetables and other food items.
7. Physical education.
8. Mental health, social support and counselling.

Psychiatric Disorders of Children

1. Behaviour problems.
    - Anti social in nature – Lying, stealing, gambling, etc.
    - Habit disorders – Nail biting, thumb sucking, etc.
    - Personality problems – Timidity, jealously, fear, etc.
    e.g. Role of over protection in schizoid personality can be depicted as –

    Overprotection
    ↓
    Overdependent
    Obedient   } Submissive traits
    Authority acceptancy
    ↓
    Difficult development
    ↓
    Increased withdrawl
    ↓
    Schizoid personality

    - Educational problem – School phobia, school failure, etc.
2. Organic disorders.
3. Psychosomatic disorders – Asthma, skin diseases, obesity.
4. Psychoneurosis – Anxiety, hysteria, obsessive compulsive neurosis.

5. Psychosis – Schizophrenia, Maniac depressive psychosis.
6. Mental deficiency :
    (i) Hyperkinetic reaction.
    (ii) Over anxious reaction.
    (iii) Withdrawal reaction.
    (iv) Run away reaction.
    (v) Unsocialised aggressive reaction.
    (vi) Group deliquent reaction.

Causes of Behaviour Disorders

1. Heredity : Child's outburt of temper, etc. not directly attributed to any factor except predisposition.
2. Physical & Organic factor : Imbalanced endocrinology plays important role.
3. Cultural & social factors : Mainly concerned with feelings and attitudes.
4. Factors of intelligence
    - It is not related to success.
    - Dull children are easily persuaded into anti-social behaviour.
5. Emotional factors
    - Guilt about masturbation.
    - Ambivalent feeligns towards parents.
    - Hostility.
    - Jealousy, esp. towards siblings.
    - It can cause neurosis, psychosis, psychosomatic disease, etc.
6. Enviornmental factors :
    - Commonest cause of behaviour disorders.
      e.g. unhealthy parent child relationship is the most important factor.
    - Poverty.
    - Step mother situation.

Child Placement

1. Orphanages
2. Foster homes.
3. Adoption.
4. Borstals.
5. Remand homes.

Child Guidance Clinic

It was firstly started in chicago in 1909. Its objective is to prevent children from the possibility of becoming neurotics and psychotics in later life.

Juvenile Justice Act, 1986

It come into force on 2nd October, 1987. Its objectives are –
- Uniform legal frame work.
- Specialized approach.
- Establishes norms and standards of administration of juvenile justice.
- Linkage and co-ordination.

UN Declaration of the Right of Child

- Right to enjoy the benefits of social security including housing, nutrition and medical care.
- Right to develop in an atmosphere of affection and security and wherever possible, in the care and under the responsibility of his/her parents.
- Right to free education.
- Right to full opportunity for play and recreation.
- Right to special care, if handicapped.
- Right to a name and nationality.
- Right to be among the first to receive protection and relief during disaster.
- Right to learn to be a useful member of society and to develop in a healthy and normal manner and in conditions of freedom and dignity.
- Right to enjoy these rights, regardless of race, colour, sex, religion, national or social origin.
- Right to be brought up in a spirit of understanding, tolerance, friendship among people, peace and universal brotherhood.

Integrated Child Development Services Scheme

ICDS scheme was launched on 2nd October, 1975 in persuance of the national policy for children in 33 blocks.

Beneficiaries :

1. Children below 6 years.
2. Pregnant and lactating women (upto 6 months).

3. Women in age group of 15-44 years.
4. Adolescent girls in 507 blocks (3.5 lacs girls in age group 11-18 years).

Objectives :
1. To improve nutritional and health status of children 0-6 years old.
2. To lay the foundation for proper psychological, physical and social development of the child.
3. To reduce the incidence of mortality, morbidity, malnutrition and school drop out.
4. Achieve effective co-ordination of policy and implementation among the various departments to promote child development.
5. To enhance the mother's capability of looking after the health and nutrition needs through proper nutrition and health education.

To achieve these objectives a package of services is being rendered through 'Anganwadi Workers' at the village centre called 'Anganwadi'.

Supportive supervision by functionaries of nodal and health departments is being done regularly

ICDS Package include :
1. Supplementary nutrition, vitamin A, iron and folic acid.
2. Immunization.
3. Health check up.
4. Referral services.
5. Treatment of minor illness.
6. Nutrition and health education to women.
7. Preschool education of children 3-6 years.
8. Convergence of other supportive services like water supply, sanitation, etc.

Other features :
- Stepwise distribution of ICDS project is maximum in U.P., Bihar, M.P. and West Bengal.
- 1 Anganwadi for 1,000 population.
- 25 Anganwadi under 1 Mukhya sevika/Supervision.
- 1 Sector consists of 25 Anganwadi.
- 1 Block consists of 1 lakh population.
- It is headed by child development project officer (CDPO) under Social Welfare Department.

Functioning of Anganwadi Workers

Organisation and forward flow of monthly monetary reports.

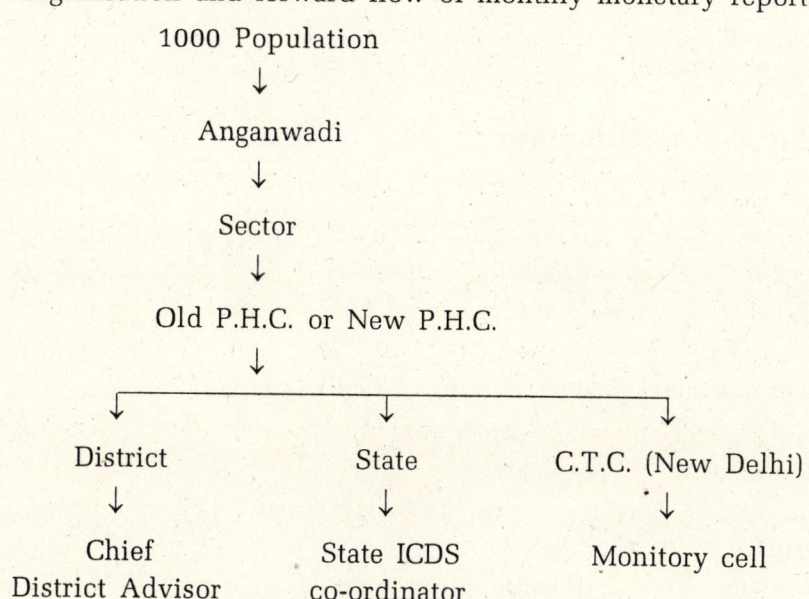

Features of Anganwadi Workers

It is a part time work for which the person receives an honorarium. She is assisted by helped who is also locally chosen and paid an honorarium.

Functions

1. Organising non-formal, pre school education for children 3-6 years.
2. Organising supplementary nutrition feeding for children under 6 years of age, pregnant and lactating mothers.
3. Giving health and nutrition education to mothers.
4. Making home visits for education of mothers.
5. Eliciting community support and participation in running the programme.
6. Assisting P.H.C. staff in implementing the health component of ICDS programme.
7. Maintaining liasons with other institutions in village and other village functionaries.
8. Maintain records on the village survey and submiting monthly progress reports.

REPRODUCTIVE HEALTH

It is a state of complete physical, mental and social well being and not merely the absence of a discase or infirmity in all matters related to reproductive system and its function and process.

Reproductive Health Care

It encompasses :
- All aspects of human sexuality and reproductive health needs during various stages of life cycle.
- Enable clients to make informed choices, receive screening and counselling services.
- Education for responsible and healthy sex.
- Access services for the prevention and management of reproductive morbidity.
- Envisage a situation where the people have the right to reproduce and regulate their fertility.
- Women are able to undergo pregnancy and abortion safely.
- The outcome of pregnancy are successful in terms of maternal and infant survival and well being.
- Couples are able to maintain healthy sexual relationship without fear of pregnancy or STDs.

Reproductive Health Components

- Encompasses terms like reproduction, obstetrical morbidity, reproductive tract infection, STDs, etc.
- Safe motherhood.
- Modes of delivery.
- Abortion practices.
- Family planning practices.
- Sexual life, etc.

There are three categories of reproductive morbidity viz. –

i) Obstetric – Direct, indirect, psychological.

ii) Gynaecological – Direct, indirect, psychological.

iii) Contraceptive morbidity.

CHAPTER-11

NUTRITION AND HEALTH

As we have already read in previous chapters that nutrition plays an important role in protection, promotion and maintenance of health.

CLASSIFICATION OF FOODS

(i) On the basis of chemical composition
- (a) Protein
- (b) Fats
- (c) Carbohydrate
- (d) Vitamins
- (e) Minerals
- (f) Roughage

(ii) By origin
- (a) Food of animal origin like egg, fish, meat.
- (b) Food of plant origin like fruits, wheat, etc.

NUTRIENTS

Nutrients is a substance which is essential for body in order to maintain proper health, growth and development.

Macronutrients — Protein, fats, carbohydrates.
Micronutrients — Vitamins, minerals.

Carbohydrates

They are made up of three elements : carbon, hydrogen and oxygen. They are the main source of energy. The major carbohydrates in the diet are starch, glucose, sucrose, etc.

They provide energy when oxidised in the body. 1 gram of carbohydrate produces about 17 KJ of energy or **4 kcal/gram**.

Functions

Cellulose acts as a roughage and adds bulk to our food. They also helps in maintaining the healthy digestive system. Glucose gets converted to glycogen in our body and provides necessary energy when required.

Sources

Major sources of carbohydrates are potatoes, wheat, rice, etc.

Daily Requirements

Commonly active females between age of 19-22 years requires 1500-2500 kcal per day while males of the same age group requires 2500-3300 kcal per day.

Deficiency of carbohydrates can lead to many diseases like Kwashiorkar and Marasmus.

Kwashiorkar

It is a malnutrition disease which occurs due to the deficiency of proteins as well as carbohydrates. It mainly occurs in children of age group between 1 to 5 years. Children having this disease have stunted growth, swelling of feet along with oedema, enlarged liver and anaemia as well. Mental development is also retarded.

Marasmus

It occurs due to deficiency of proteins, fats and carbohydrates mainly in infants upto 1 year of age. Infants suffering from marasmus shows wasting of muscles, loosely folded skin ribs becomes prominent along with loss in body weight. Their intestinal digestion is also impaired.

Differences between Kwashiorkar and Marasmus

	Kwashiorkar	Marasmus
1.	It occurs mainly due to the deficiency of proteins and amounts of carbohydrates.	It occurs due to the deficiency of proteins as well as carbohydrates and fats also.
2.	Child suffers from the oedema.	Child does not suffers from oedema.
3.	It occurs in children of age group 1-5 years.	It occurs in infants of 1 year.
4.	Skin becomes dark and scaly.	Skin colour does not change and no scales appear.
5.	There is no wasting of muscles and ribs do not become prominent.	Ribs become prominent due to wasting or degeneration of muscles.

Proteins

They are made up of 20 types of different amino acids . Apart from oxygen, hydrogen and carbon, they also contains sulphur and phosphorus.

Among the 20 amino acids only eight are essentially. They are leucine, isoleucine, valine, methionine, lysine, phenylalanine, threonine and tryptophan.

Functions

They occurs in many different forms and serves many important functions in the form of enzymes, hormones, transport proteins, etc. Pepsin and Trypsin acts as enzyme. Myosin and Actin serves as contractile proteins. Collagen is an important structural proteins.

Sources

Main sources of proteins are eggs, milk, meat, pulses, etc. The plant proteins due to their less protein content as compared to the animal proteins like, pulses are called as 'rich man's meat'.

Daily Requirement

Proteins on oxidation inside our body gives **4 kcal per gram**.

An average adults weighing 75 kg. should take 75 grams of proteins per day. Growing children and nursing mothers should take rich protein diet.

Fats

They are the esters of fatty acids. They can be saturated due to the presence of single bond or unsaturated due to the presence of multiple bonds. Unsaturated fatty acids are important and essential for us as they can not be synthesised inside our body e.g. – linoleic, linolenic, oleic and arachidonic acids.

They can provide twice as much energy as that can be provided by the same amount of carbohydrate.

1 gram of fats on oxidation can provide **9 Kcal or 37 Kilojoules**.

Functions

They are used as reserve food source. Though they are expensive but can provide twice as much energy can be provided by the carbohydrates and proteins. In body they mainly supports the visceral organs.

Sources

Their main sources are butter, ghee, vanaspati, groundnut, meat, egg, yolk, cheese, etc.

Daily Requirements

An average adult should take 75 grams of fats per day in his diet. Unsaturated fatty acids should be taken more than the saturated ones.

Types of Fats

- *Saturated* – They are single bonded, e.g. – animal fats like butter.
- *Mono unsaturated* – They have single double bond in the fatty acid chains.
  E.g. – olive, peanut, etc.
- *Poly unsaturated* – They have two or more double bonds.
  E.g. – safflower oil, cottonseed oil, etc.
- *Trans-fat* – They have been partially hydrogenated producing fever double bonds and the remaining are converted from a cis to trans configuration.
- *Omega-3-fat* – They have at least one double bond three carbon atoms in from the end of the fatty acid molecule.
  E.g. – Linolenic acid.

Minerals

The metals, non-metals and their salts are called minerals. They are also equally important as the proteins, carbohydrates and fats are. They include calcium, potassium, sodium phosphorus, sulphur, copper, zinc chlorine, fluorine and magnesium.

However they do not supply any energy to our body, but they are essential for metabolic activities.

Most of the minerals are obtained from plants.

Calcium

It gives strength and rigidity to bones and teeth along with phosphate. It is required for making bones, teeth, etc. It also helps in blood clotting. Calcium also plays a role in altering the permeability of nerve fibers during impulse transmission. Children needs more calcium than adults as they are growing. It is also necessary for the development of foetus. Its main sources are whole gram, cereals, meat, fish, ragi, etc.

A 15 years old child needs at least 1 gram of calcium in his diet every day.

It is also a component of hormone calcitonin, vitamin D and parathyroid hormone. (PTH).

Sodium and Potassium

Mainly the salts of sodium and potassium are needed for the maintenance of the osmotic pressure of the body. In muscle and nerve cells, a high order of difference exists between intracellular K^+ and extra cellular Na^+. This results in the formation of potential difference in the nerve cells. Sodium ions are necessary to initiate and maintain the contraction of heart. Nacl also helps in the formation of hydrochloric acid of gastric juice present in the stomach for digestion of food.

It is mainly obtained by the common salt, some vegetables, etc.

Iron

It is one of the most important mineral require by our body. It is a main constituent of protein haemoglobin which helps in transporting oxygen from lungs to the body cells. It also occurs in oxygen storing pigment – myoglobin. Electron transport chain enzymes cytochromes oxidases are also made up of iron.

Its deficiency can cause anaemia. Its main sources are spinach, ground nuts, eggs, bajra, ragi and other green leafy vegetables.

Phosphorus

Like calcium it is also require for the formation of bones and teeth. It is a component of energy releasing ATP and also others like nucleic acid, NAD and NADP. It also acts as buffers by forming diabasic phosphate (HPO_3^{2-}) and mono basic phosphate ($H_2PO_4^-$) and thus neutralizes strong acids and bases.

It mainly occurs in milk, green leafy vegetables, bajra, ragi and nuts.

Iodine

It forms the important constituent of the horame thyroxine (T_4) and triiodothyronine (T_3) produced from the thyroid glands which plays an important role in controlling the mental, physical and sexual development of the body.

Its deficiency can lead to 'goitre' which can be prevent by used iodized salt.

Vitamins

They are complex organic compounds necessary for the well being of our entire body. Like minerals they also do not provide any energy, but are important.

They can be water soluble like vitamin B complex and vitamin C or they can be fat soluble e.g. – vitamin A, D, E and K.

They are found in vegetable, milk, meat, etc. in sufficient amounts.

(1) Vitamin A (Retinol)

It is the precursor to retinal, the prosthetic group of all four of the light absorbing pigment in the eye.

Sources

Cream, fish liver oils, butter, eggs, carrots and some vegetables. Mainly in green leafy vegetables.

Excess of vitamin A in diet can be harmful. It is stored in the liver, and can be toxic, especially in children.

Deficiency

Its deficiency leads to xerophthlmia.

(2) Vitamin B_1 (Thiamine)

It is essential for growth, carbohydrate metabolism, functioning of heart, nerves and muscles. It is also a coenzyme in cellular respiration.

Sources

Meat, yeast, unpolished cereals grains, soyabean, sea food, green vegetables.

Deficiency

It's deficiency can cause beriberi. Rarely found in developed countries except among alcoholics.

As it is a water soluble vitamin and can be easily excreted if present in excess amount.

(3) Vitamin B_2 (Riboflavin)

It is mainly necessary to keep skin and mouth healthy. It also helps in normal functioning of the eyes. It is a prosthetic group of flavin protein enzymes used in the cellular respiration.

Sources

Milk, peas, beans, whole grain cereals, eggs, green leafy vegetables, yeast and cheese.

Deficiency

It's deficiency can cause damage to eyes, mouth and genitals.

(4) Vitamin B_4 (Niacin)

It is mainly essential for maintaining healthy skin. It is a precursor of NAD and NADP. It is also necessary for a good digestive tract.

Sources

Meat, fish, potato, whole grain, tomato, ground nut and green vegetables.

Deficiency

Its deficiency causes pellagra (producing skin lesions) a risk where corn is the staple carbohydrate.

(5) Folic acid (Folacin)

Its main function is to synthesis purines and pyrimidines. It is also necessary for the formation and maturation of red blood cells (RBC) in human body.

Sources

Green leafy vegetables, sprouted pulses, cauliflower, meat, liver, kidney and grams.

Deficiency

Its deficiency can cause anaemia, birth defects. Pregnant woman should take an adequate amount of 400 mg/day.

(6) Vitamin B_{12} (Cyano-cobalamin)

It is mainly required for DNA synthesis and also for proper growth and functioning of body.

Sources

Liver, eggs, milk (needs intrinsic factors to be absorbed) and meat.

Deficiency

Its deficiency can cause pernicious anaemia which is caused by lack of intrinsic factor.

(7) Vitamin C (Ascorbic acid)

It is necessary for keeping teeth, gums and joints healthy. It acts as coenzyme in the synthesis of collagen. It increases the body resistance to infection and helps fight diseases.

Sources

Citrus fruits especially Amla, Lime, lemon, orange, gooseberry, guava and tomatoes.

Deficiency

Deficiency of Vitamin C can cause scurvy.

Excess

Its excess generally do not causes major harms.

(8) Vitamin D (Calciferol)

It is a fat soluble vitamin. It is necessary for normal growth of bones and teeth by the absorption of calcium from the intestine and bone formation.

Sources

It is synthesised when the ultraviolet rays strikes the skin. It is present in fish, milk, cod liver oil, eggs and butter.

Deficiency

Deficiency of vitamin D can cause rickets in children and osteomalacia (softening of bones) in adults.

Excess

Excess of vitamin D can cause excess of calcium deposits and mental retardation especially in infants.

(9) Vitamin E (Tocopherol)

It is necessary for the normal reproduction, normal functioning of muscles and also for protection of liver. It acts as a reducing agents in the cells.

Sources

Egg yolk, salad, greens tomatoes, milk, wheat germ oil and vegetable oils.

Deficiency

It's deficiency can cause anaemia and damage to retina.

Excess

High doses of Vitamin E can be toxic in infants.

(10) Vitamin K (Phylloquinone)

It is necessary for the normal blood clotting and prevents haemorrhage. It is synthesized by intestinal bacteria.

Sources

Spinach, green leafy vegetables, cabbage, soyabean, tomatoes.

Deficiency

Deficiency of vitamin K causes delay in blood clotting and haemorrhage.

Excess

Excess of this vitamin can prove toxic in infants.

NUTRITIONAL PROFILES OF PRINCIPAL FOODS

MILK – It is a complete food.

Table-1
Nutritive value of milks compared
(Value per 100 grams)

		Buffalo	Cow	Goat	Human
Fat	(g)	6.5	4.1	4.5	3.4
Protein	(g)	4.3	3.2	3.3	1.1
Lactose	(g)	5.1	4.4	4.6	7.4
Calcium	(mg)	210	120	170	28
Iron	(mg)	0.2	0.2	0.3	–
Vitamin C	(mg)	1	2	1	3
Minerals	(g)	0.8	0.8	0.8	0.1
Water	(g)	81.0	87	86.8	88
Energy	(kcal)	117	67	72	65

Source : (157)

FRUITS – See the table 2.
CEREALS – See the table 2.
PULSES – See the table 2.
VEGETABLES – See the table 2.
EGG – See the table 2.
MEAT – See the table 2.
FISH – See the table 2.

Table-2
Nutritive Value of Different Food Stuffs

Food stuffs (per 100 gm)	Calories	Protein (grams)	Calcium (mg)	Iron	Vit. A (mg)	Vit. B$_1$ (Iu)	Vit. B$_2$ (mg)	Niacin (mg)	Vit. C (mg)
1	2	3	4	5	6	7	8	9	10
CEREALS :									
Wheat	346	11.5	41	4.9	103	0.45	0.17	5.0	0
Jowar	349	10.4	25	5.8	79	3.37	0.13	2.8	0
Rice (parboiled)	345	6.4	9	4.0	0	0.23	0.05	3.1	0
Rice (hand pounded)	346	7.5	15	3.2	4	0.21	0.04	3.2	0
Rice (Milled)	345	6.8	10	3.1	000	0.85	0.04	1.9	0
Maize	125	4.7	9	4.1	54	0.11	0.13	0.6	6
Wheat flour (refined)	348	11.0	10	2.5	43	0.12	0.08	0.9	0
Ragi	325	7.3	344	17.4	70	0.42	0.19	1.1	0
Bajra	361	11.6	42	3.2	200	0.33	0.25	3.2	0
PULSES :									
Red gram dal (Arhar)	355	22.3	73	5.8	220	0.45	0.15	2.6	0
Green gram dal	348	24.5	75	8.5	83	0.72	0.21	2.4	0
Peas (dry)	315	19.7	75	5.1	66	0.47	0.19	1.9	0
Lentil	343	25.1	69	4.8	450	0.45	0.20	1.5	0
Black gram dal	347	24.0	154	9.1	64	0.42	0.20	1.5	0

Food stuffs (per 100 gm)	Calories	Protein (grams)	Calcium (mg)	Iron	Vit. A (mg)	Vit. B_1 (Iu)	Vit. B_2 (mg)	Niacin (mg)	Vit. C (mg)
1	2	3	4	5	6	7	8	9	10
Bengal gram, whole	360	17.0	202	10.2	316	0.30	0.15	2.1	0
Bengal gram, dhal	372	20.8	56	9.1	216	0.48	0.16	2.4	1
Bengal gram, roasted	369	22.5	58	9.5	189	0.20	0.16	1.3	0
Khesari dal (Lathyrus sativus)	345	28.2	90	6.3	120	0.39	0.17	2.3	0
Soyabean	432	43.2	340	11.5	436	0.73	0.39	3.3	0
LEAFY VEGETABLES :									
Onion tops	61	4.7	71	—	—	—	—	—	—
Curry leaves	108	6.1	830	7.0	2600	0.08	0.21	2.3	4
Cauliflower leaves	66	5.9	626	4.0	—	—	—	—	—
Cabbage	27	1.8	39	0.3	2000	0.06	0.09	0.4	170
Gogu	56	1.7	172	5.0	4830	0.07	0.39	1.5	20
Tamarind leaves tender	115	5.8	101	5.2	418	0.24	0.17	4.1	3
Ambat chuka	15	1.6	63	8.7	6102	0.03	0.06	1.0	12
Amaranth	46	4.0	332	25.5	8200	0.03	0.03	1.0	99
Mint	48	4.8	302	15.6	2700	0.05	0.26	1.4	27
Pon	73	5.0	513	16.7	3210	—	0.14	1.2	17
Spinach	26	2.0	73	10.9	3900	0.03	0.26	0.5	28
Drumstick leaves	92	6.7	443	7.0	14300	0.06	0.05	0.82	20
Fenugreek leaves	49	4.2	395	16.5	3900	3.04	0.31	0.3	53
Bathua leaves	30	3.7	190	4.2	1740	0.01	0.14	0.6	61

Food stuffs (per 100 gm)	Calories	Protein (grams)	Calcium (mg)	Iron	Vit. A (mg)	Vit. B_1 (Iu)	Vit. B_2 (mg)	Niacin (mg)	Vit. C (mg)
1	2	3	4	5	6	7	8	9	10
Bengal gram leaves	97	7.0	380	23.8	978	0.09	0.10	0.6	135
Coriander leaves	44	3.3	134	13.5	6911	0.05	0.06	0.8	135
Mustard leaves	34	4.0	155	16.3	2622	0.03	–	–	33
Radish leaves	28	3.8	265	3.6	5295	0.28	0.47	0.8	81
ROOTS AND TUBORS :									
Onion	49	1.4	180	0.7	0	0.08	0.01	0.4	11
Tomato	221	1.4	60	1.3	130	0.07	–	0.7	–
Caroler	48	0.9	80	2.7	3150	0.04	0.02	0.6	3
Sweet Potato	223	1.2	20	0.8	10	0.03	0.04	0.7	21
Colacasia	84	3.0	40	1.7	40	0.09	0.03	0.4	0
Maci Khol	92	1.1	70	1.4	–	–	0.01	0.4	11
Potato	97	1.6	10	0.7	40	0.10	0.01	1.2	17
Beet root	53	1.7	200	1.8	0	0.04	0.09	0.4	83
Radish	17	0.7	50	0.4	5	0.06	0.02	0.5	15
Turnip	23	0.5	30	0.4	0	0.04	0.04	0.5	43
Taricca	117	0.7	50	0.9	–	0.05	0.10	0.3	25
OTHER VEGETABLES :									
Plantain, raw	64	1.4	10	0.6	50	0.05	0.02	0.3	24
Platain flower	34	1.7	32	1.6	46	0.05	0.04	0.3	16
Plantain stem	42	0.5	10	1.1	0	0.02	0.01	0.2	7

Food stuffs (per 100 gm)	Calories	Protein (grams)	Calcium (mg)	Iron	Vit. A (mg)	Vit. B$_1$ (Iu)	Vit. B$_2$ (mg)	Niacin (mg)	Vit. C (mg)
1	2	3	4	5	6	7	8	9	10
Indian goosberry (Amla)	53	0.5	50	1.2	15	0.03	0.01	0.2	600
Bittergourd	25	1.6	20	1.8	210	0.07	0.09	0.5	83
Cauliflower	30	2.6	33	1.5	51	0.04	0.10	1.0	56
Cluster beans	50	3.2	130	4.5	330	0.09	0.03	0.6	49
Pumpkin	25	1.4	10	0.7	84	0.06	0.04	0.5	2
Field beans	158	7.4	50	2.6	57	0.34	0.19	0.0	27
Amarnath stalks	19	0.9	260	1.8	425	0.01	0.18	0	10
Cucumber	13	0.4	10	1.5	0	0.03	0.01	0.2	7
Jack fruit, raw	51	2.6	30	1.7	0	0.05	0.04	0.2	14
Snake-gourd	18	0.5	50	1.1	160	0.04	0.06	0.3	0
French beans	48	3.8	50	1.7	221	0.08	0.06	0.3	14
Ridge-gourd	17	0.5	40	1.6	56	0.07	0.01	0.2	5
Ladies fingers	35	1.9	65	1.5	88	0.07	0.10	0.6	13
Mango raw	44	0.7	10	5.5	150	0.04	0.01	0.2	6
Chillies, green	29	2.9	30	1.2	292	0.09	0.39	0.9	111
Chillies, giant	25	1.3	10	1.2	712	0.05	0.55	0	137
Drumstick	26	2.5	30	5.3	184	0.05	3.07	0.2	120
Brinjal	24	1.4	18	0.9	124	0.24	0.11	0.9	12
Calabash cucumber	12	0.2	20	0.7	0	0.30	0.01	0.2	6
Papaya green	27	0.7	28	0.9	0	0.01	0.01	0.1	12
Tomato green	23	1.9	20	1.8	192	0.07	0.01	0.4	31

Food stuffs (per 100 gm)	Calories	Protein (grams)	Calcium (mg)	Iron	Vit. A (mg)	Vit. B$_1$ (Iu)	Vit. B$_2$ (mg)	Niacin (mg)	Vit. C (mg)
1	2	3	4	5	6	7	8	9	10
NUTS AND OILSEEDS :									
Coconut, dry	652	6.8	400	2.7	0	0.03	0.01	2.6	7
Cashew nut	596	21.2	50	5.0	100	0.63	0.16	2.1	0
Gingells seeds	563	18.3	1450	10.3	100	1.01	0.34	4.5	0
Ground nut	549	26.7	50	1.6	63	0.90	0.13	14.1	0
FRUITS :									
Apple	55	0.3	9	1.0	0	0.12	0.08	0.2	2
Orange	53	0.9	50	0.1	326	0.12	0.06	0.3	68
Guava, Country	51	0.9	10	1.4	0	0.03	0.03	0.4	212
Cashew fruit	53	0.8	10	0.2	39	0.02	0.05	0.4	180
Tomato, ripe	20	0.9	48	0.4	585	0.12	0.06	0.4	27
Pomegranate	65	1.6	10	0.3	0	0.06	0.10	0.3	14
Lime	59	1.5	90	0.8	26	—	—	—	—
Jack fruit	83	1.9	20	0.5	292	0.03	0.13	0.4	7
Watermelon	16	0.2	11	7.9	0	0.02	0.04	0.1	1
Papaya, ripe	32	0.6	17	0.5	1110	0.04	0.25	0.2	57
Mango, ripe	51	0.6	10	0.3	4800	0.04	0.05	0.3	13
Wood apple	134	7.1	130	0.6	102	0.04	0.17	0.8	3
Sapota	110	0.8	31	0.1	117	—	—	0.1	6
Custard apple	114	0.6	398	0.3	0	0.33	0.17	1.3	16

Nutrition and Health

Food stuffs (per 100 gm)	Calories	Protein (grams)	Calcium (mg)	Iron	Vit. A (mg)	Vit. B_1 (Iu)	Vit. B_2 (mg)	Niacin (mg)	Vit. C (mg)
1	2	3	4	5	6	7	8	9	10
Apricot (Fresh)	53	1.0	20	2.0	2160	0.04	0.18	0.6	6
Dates (Fresh)	144	1.2	22	—	—	—	—	—	—
Figs	37	1.3	80	1.0	162	0.06	0.05	0.6	5
Grapes (blue variety)	58	0.6	20	0.5	3.0	0.04	0.03	0.2	1
Lemon (citrus)	57	1.0	70	2.3	00	0.02	0.01	0.1	39
Lichi	61	1.1	10	0.7	0	0.02	0.06	0.4	31
Lime sweet (musambi)	43	0.8	40	0.7	00	—	—	0.0	50
Plums	52	0.7	10	0.6	166	0.04	0.1	0.3	5
Rasians	323	1.8	87	7.7	2.4	0.07	0.19	0.7	1
Seethaphal	104	1.6	17	1.5	00	0.33	0.44	1.3	37
MILK AND MILK PRODUCTS :									
Cow's milk	67	3.2	120	0.2	174	0.05	0.19	0.1	2
Buffalo milk	117	4.3	210	0.2	160	0.04	0.10	0.1	1
Breast milk	65	1.1	28	0.1	137	0.02	0.02	—	3
Cheese	348	24.1	790	3.1	273	—	—	—	—
Curds	60	3.1	149	0.5	102	0.05	0.06	0.1	1
Goat's milk	72	3.2	70	0.3	182	0.05	0.04	0.3	1
OTHER FRESH FOODS :									
Egg hen	173	13.5	60	2.1	1200	0.10	0.18	0.1	0
Beef muscle	114	22.6	10	0.8	60	0.15	0.04	6.4	2

F - 17A

Food stuffs (per 100 gm)	Calories	Protein (grams)	Calcium (mg)	Iron	Vit. A (mg)	Vit. B$_1$ (Iu)	Vit. B$_2$ (mg)	Niacin (mg)	Vit. C (mg)
1	2	3	4	5	6	7	8	9	10
Liver, sheep	150	19.3	10	6.8	22300	0.36	1.70	17.6	17
Mutton	194	18.5	150	2.5	31	0.18	0.27	6.8	—
Pork, muscle	114	18.7	30	2.2	0	0.54	0.69	2.8	2
Egg, duck	181	13.5	70	3.0	1200	0.18	0.28	0.2	—
Goat meat muscle	118	21.4	12	—	—	—	—	—	—
Liver, goat	197	20.7	17	—	—	—	—	—	—
MISCELLANEOUS FOODSTUFFS:									
Betel leaves	44	3.1	109	—	9600	0.07	0.03	0.75	5
Bread	245	7.8	11	1.1	—	0.02	—	0.7	—
Sago	351	0.2	10	1.3	0	0.01	—	0.2	—
Jaggery	383	0.4	80	11.4	0	0.02	—	1.0	0
Sugar	393	0.1	13	—	—	—	—	—	—
Oil or ghee	900	—	—	—	—	—	—	—	—

NUTRITIONAL REQUIREMENTS

RDA – Recommended daily allowance definition – the amount of nutrient sufficient for the maintenance of health in needy all people, the due given in table 3 is given by ICMR.

Table-3
Recommended Dietary Allowances for Indians

Group	Particulars	Body Wt kg	Net energy kcal/d	Protein* g/d	Fat mg/d	Calcium mg/d	Iron** mg/d	Vit. A μg/d Retinol-βcarotene		Thiamin mg/d	Riboflavin mg/d	Nicotinic acid mg/d	Phyridoxin mg/d	Ascorbic acid	Folic acid μg/d	Vit. B₁₂ μg/d
Man	Sedentary work	60	2425	60	20	400	28	600	2400	1.2	1.4	16	2.0	40	100	1
	Moderate work		2875							1.4	1.6	18				
	Heavy work		3800							1.6	1.9	21				
Woman	Sedentary work	50	1875	50	20	400	30	600	2400	0.9	1.1	12	2.0	40	100	1
	Moderate work		2225							1.1	1.3	14				
	Heavy work		2925							1.2	1.5	16				
	Pregnant woman	50	+300	+15	30	1000	38	600	2400	+0.2	+0.2	+2	2.5	40	400	1
	Lactation				45	1000	30	950	3800				2.5	80	150	1.5
	0-6 months		+550	+25						+0.3	+0.3	+4				
	6-12 months		+400	+18						+0.2	+0.2	+3				
Infants	0-6 months	5.4	108/Kg	2.05/Kg		500		350	1200	55μg/Kg	65μg/Kg	710μg/Kg	0.1	25	25	0.2
	6-12 months	8.6	98/Kg	1.65/Kg						50μg/Kg	60μg/Kg	650μg	0.4			

Group	Particulars	Body Wt kg	Net energy kcal/d	Protein* g/d	Fat mg/d	Calcium mg/d	Iron** mg/d	Vit. A µg/d Retinol-βcarotene		Thiamin mg/d	Ribo-flavin mg/d	Nicoti-nic acid mg/d	Phyri-doxin mg/d	Ascorbic acid	Folic acid µg/d	Vit. B$_{12}$ µg/d
Children	1-3 year	12.2	1240	22	25	400	12	400	1600	0.6	0.7	8	0.9	40	30	0.2-1.0
	4-6 years	19.0	1690	30			18	400	2400	0.9	1.0	11	0.9		40	
	7-9 years	26.9	1950	41			26	600	2400	1.0	1.2	13	1.6		60	
Boys	10-12 years	35.4	2190	54	22	600	34	600	2400	1.1	1.3	15	1.6		70	
Girls	10-12 years	31.5	1970	57			19			1.0	1.2	13	1.6		70	0.2-1.0
Boys	13-15 years	47.8	2450	70	22	600	41	600	2400	1.2	1.5	16			100	
Girls	13-15 years	46.7	2060	65			28			1.0	1.2	14			100	0.2-1.0
Boys	16-18 years	57.1	2640	78	22	500	50	600	2400	1.3	1.6	17	2.0		100	
Girls	16-18 years	49.9	2060	63	22		30			1.0	1.2	14			100	0.2-1.0

Source:

* Mixed vegetable protein with NPU 65% relative to egg. Human milk protein in case of infants[5]
** On mixed cereal diet with absorption of 3% in man, 5% in woman 8% in pregnant woman.

Nutrition and Health

DIETARY GOALS – WHO

(a) Dietary fat should not be more than 20-30 per cent of total daily protein.
(b) There should be no excessive consumption of any component of food.
(c) Salt protein should be reduced to an average of not more than 5g/day.
(d) Protein should be around 18-20% of the total daily protein.
(e) No junk foods.

BALANCED DIET

It is a diet contain by all essential nutrients in proper and adequate quantities for maintenance of health, vitality and general well being.

NUTRITIONAL PROBLEMS

There are at present a large number of nutritional problems affecting a large portion of population. Some of the major problems are as follows :

Protein Energy Malnutrition (PEM)

It is one of the most prevalent nutritional problems. The age group affected mainly are the children. PEM is responsible for childhood mortality and morbidity.

Classification of PEM

PEM can be classified on the basis of :
(I) Weight for age (Gomez Classification)
(II) Weight for height
(III) Height for age
(IV) Midarm circumference

(I) Weight for age – Gomez's classification is based on the criteria of weight retardation in comparison to 'reference weight for age. The 'normal reference weight' corresponds to 50th percentile of Boston standards.

$$\text{Weight for age} = \frac{\text{Weight of child at present}}{\text{Weight of reference child at same age}} \times 100$$

Grade	Weight as % of reference
Normal	90-110%
1st degree, mild malnutrition	75-89%
2nd degree moderate malnutrition	60-74%
3rd degree severe malnutrition	below 60%

According to Indian academy of pediatrics 80% is taken as cutoff point. It correspond to approximately 2 standard deviation or the 3rd percentile. So, the children between 89 and 80 per cent are not labelled malnourished as happens in Gomez classification.

(II) Weight for height

It follows the same principle as weight for age. Here the comparison is made with reference weight for height.

$$\text{Weight for height \%} = \frac{\text{Weight of child}}{\text{Weight as \% of reference}} \times 100$$

Grade	Weight as % of reference
Normal	80% or above
I	70-79%
II	60-69%
III	below 60%

(III) Weight for age

It is a indicative of chronic condition of malnutrition. Here the **growth is retarded**.

$$\text{Height for Age \%} = \frac{\text{Height of child}}{\text{Height of normal child at same age}} \times 100$$

Grade	% of height for age
Normal	95% or above
I	87.5-95%
II	80-87.5%
III	below 80%

(IV) Midarm circumference

It estimates the body muscle mass. It can be used if facilities for weighing are not present and also it is quite simple to measure. It is not used before the age of one year. The cut off value is 13.5 cm.

Grade	Midarm circumference
Normal	13.5 cm or more
Mild-moderate malnutrition	12.5-13.5 cm
Severe malnutrition	below 12.5 cm

PEM manifests itself in two clinical forms
  (i) KWASHIORKOR
  (ii) MARASMUS

Epidemiology of PEM

- *Agent factors* – Due to deficiency of protein and energy.
- *Host factors*
  (i) Age – Children are affected most commonly.
  (ii) Sex – Female children are affected more.
  (iii) Low birth weight.
  (iv) Delayed weaning or absence of weaning altogether.
- *Environment factors*
  (i) Socio economic factors – poverty.
  (ii) Cultural practises – late start of breast feeding, food fad, less attention to female child, improper weaning.
  (iii) Over-crowding.
  (iv) Poor sanitation.
  (v) Infectious conditions like ARI, diarrhoeal diseases, etc.

Principles of Prevention

(1) Primary Prevention

(a) Health Promotion – it includes :
- Proper feeding of pregnant, women.
- Promote breast feeding.
- Nutritional education to family.
- Measures directed to improve diet of the family.
- Family planning, birth spacing.
- Better economics application.
- Improved sanitation.
- Environment betterment.

(b) Health Promotion for child includes :
- Proper balanced diet to child.
- Immunization against common disease BCG, DPT, MMR, TT, OPV.
- Food participation.

(2) Secondary Prevention

(a) Early diagnosis and treatment
- Growth monitoring.
- Early diagnosis and treatment of infection and diarrhoeal diseases.
- Supplementary feeding programmes.

- De-worming.
- Hospital treatment, follow up.

(3) Tertiary Prevention

(a) Nutritional rehabilitation.

Nutritional Anaemia

Anaemia is a major nutritional deficiency disorder in India and other developing countries. The prevalence is around 38 to 72 per cent. The most vulnerable group is compound of pregnant women and children.

Epidemiology – The main etiological factor is inadequate iron intake in food. Indians usually are vegetarian and take iron lacking diet. Also other inhibitors of iron absorption like phytic acid, etc are present suppressing the bio availability of iron.

Requirements – The Dietary Iron Requirements (RDA) is given in table-4.

Table-4
Dietary Iron Requirements (RDA) Expressed as mg/1,000 kcal*

Group	Recommended Energy Intake kcal/d	Dietary Iron Requirement mg/d	mg/1000 kcal
Children			
1-3 years	1240	11.5	9.3
4-6 years	1690	18.4	10.9
7-9 years	1950	26.0	13.3
Adolescent boys			
10-12 years	2190	34.2	15.6
13-15 years	2450	41.4	16.9
16-18 years	2640	49.5	18.8
Adolescent girls			
10-12 years	1970	18.9	9.6
13-15 years	2060	28.0	13.6
16-18 years	2060	29.9	14.5
Adults**			
Men	2875	28.0	9.7
Women	2225	30.0	13.5
Pregnant women	2525	37.5	14.9
Lactating women	2775	30.0	10.8

* ICMR, Recommended Dietary Allowance for Indians; Report of an Expert Group, 1990.
** Reference person with moderate activity.

Energy and iron intakes in Indian diets are highly correlated (r=0.769), presumably because a major proportion of both dietary iron and energy are derived from cereals. Apart from inadequate content of iron, reduced intake of energy (food) which is widely seen among the poors in the country, further reduces daily iron intake. This is particularly so among young children, women and pregnant women. This is evident from Table-5 where dietary iron intakes (corrected for contaminant iron) are compared with RDA. It is, therefore, not surprising that there is widespread dietary iron deficiency in India, particularly among the vulnerable groups who suffer from varying degrees of energy (food) deficiency.

Table-5
Dietary Iron Intake by Indians and its Adequacy

Age (years)	Sex	RDA for iron mg/d	Average* dietary iron intake	percent adequacy
1-3	M+F	12	7.7	64
4-6	M+F	18	11.0	61
Adult	M	28	22.5	89
	F	30	19.7	63
Pregnant Women		38	17.1	45
Lactating women		30	23.7	79

*Corrected for contaminant iron (30 per cent).

Iron absorption from diets. Men and Children 3 per cent, Women 5 per cent, Pregnant women 8 per cent.

Decrease Iron content of circulating haemoglobin and tissue iron contents, is known to lead to several functional abnormalities with health consequences. The consequence of a mild form of anaemia is not yet clearly recognised. Although mild anaemia with haemoglobin levels above 10 g/dl is not known to result in any serious impairment of function, moderate to severe anaemia is known to have several functional consequences. They included the following : impaired maximal work capacity; decreased immunological competence; behavioural abnormalities and reduced learning ability among children; poor pregnancy outcome.

Although a moderate degree of anaemia may not seriously affect day-to-day work, most of which corresponds to sedentary to moderate levels of activity. Impaired work capacity is seen only in those engaged in hard physical labour with moderate to severe anaemia. Iron deficienc·

anaemia with haemoglobin level below 10 g/dl is known to reduce cell mediated immunity. Anaemia of pregnancy is known to cause increased maternal morbidity and mortality; increased foetal morbidity and mortality; and, increased risk of low birth-weight.

The Control of Anaemia in India

Iron fortification programme : The two obvious approaches to the control of anaemia are :

- Increasing the iron content of the diet by including iron-rich foods such as green leafy vegetables (GLVs) and/or enhancing iron bio-availability in the existing diets by including foods rich in absorption promoters such as ascorbic acid and animal foods such as fish and meat. This important approach is a long-range effort which may not yield results in the immediate future.
- The alternative approach is to increase iron intake through fortification of a universally consumed food item with iron. Iron fortification has been attempted in several countries, and in India a highly successful technology for the fortification of common salt with iron has been developed.

Iron fortified salt has been extensively tested in the community and its effectiveness in improving iron status and reducing the prevalence of anaemia has been clearly demonstrated. The merit of this technology is that the vehicle used for fortification, namely salt, is universally consumed by all segments including the poor among whom anaemia is much more prevalent.

Although the technology for the fortification of salt has been available for the past one decade, it has not been introduced on a large scale to combat iron deficiency anaemia in India, despite being strongly recommended.

Iron-fortified salt is currently being produced on a small scale only by a few private manufacturers and by the Food and Nutrition board of the ministry of food and agriculture. Large-scale introduction of iron-fortified salt is currently being organised only in Tamil Nadu by the Tamil Nadu government with support from the UNICEF, the food and nutrition board and the Tamil Nadu State industrial corporation.

A possible reason for the hesitation to introduce the fortification programme on a countrywide scale may be the apprehension that it might impede and complicate the important ongoing salt iodation programme to combat iodine deficiency.

In view of this, a new technology for the double fortification of salt with iron and iodine has been recently developed; this is currently undergoing field evaluation. The double fortified salt could be introduced in areas of the country where both anaemia and goitre are prevalent and iron-fortified salt could be introduced in the rest of the country where only anaemia is prevalent. The same formula developed for the double fortified salt can be used for the manufacture of iron-fortified salt also by omitting the addition of iodine. If the iron balance in the total population is improved through iron-fortified salt, the anaemia prophylaxis programme among pregnant women through distribution of folifer tablets will have better success. Iron fortification of salt is being suggested as an adjunct and not as an alternative to the present anaemia prophylaxis programme.

Anaemia prophylaxis through supplementation of medicinal iron (tablets) : The most vulnerable groups with regard to anaemia prevalence are women, pregnant women and pre-school children. In the background of widespread prevalence of anaemia among women, the stress of pregnancy with its increased demand for iron further aggravates anaemia. Dietary iron requirement during the second and third trimesters of pregnancy is 25 mg/1,000 kcal. A normal diet with 10 mg/1,000 kcal can hardly meet the iron requirement during pregnancy. Therefore, additional iron supplementation is needed in the form of medicinal iron. This widely recognised therapeutic iron supplementation is recommended during pregnancy even for women who start their pregnancy with normal haemoglobin levels. If a woman starts her pregnancy not with a normal level of haemoglobin but with various degrees of anaemia as it happens with the majority of pregnant women in our country, therapeutic supplementation to such women should cover both her requirements of iron during pregnancy plus the amount needed to correct the existing anaemia.

The Current Anaemia Prophylaxis Programme in India

A study group on nutritional anaemia of the nutrition society of India recommended in 1968 an anaemia prophylaxis programme for the eradication of anaemia of pregnancy and childhood. According to this expert group, the most practical and expeditious way is to give supplements of iron and folate to anaemic pregnant women during the last 100 days of pregnancy. Based on the results of controlled supplementary trials then available and theoretical computations, the group recommended 60 mg of elemental iron in the form of ferrous compound and 500 µg of folic acid. They recommended at least 50 per cent of all pregnant women to be covered during the first five years. They suggested the use of public health centres (PHCs), sub-centres and mother and child health (MCH) centres as outlets for the distribution of tablets. They also gave a plan for the distribution of tablets and their quality control. Besides, they emphasised the educational component to motivate the women, and periodic evaluation of the impact of the programme.

In pursuance of the above recommendations, the government of India had set up the National Anaemia Prophylaxis Programme (NAPP) in 1970 in all states of the country. The target population under this programme comprises pregnant women, lactating women, family planning acceptor women (of terminal methods and IUDs) and children of both sexes between one and 11 years (both years inclusive). The supplementation provided under this programme consists of tablets of iron folate containing 60 mg of elemental iron (ferrous sulphate) and 500 µmg folic acid for all adult woman beneficiaries. For children, smaller tablets containing 20 mg of elemental iron ($FeSO_4$) and 100 mg of folate are provided. For children who cannot swallow tablets, iron and folic acid in the same dose as in a single tablet is given in 2 ml of syrupy liquid.

Each beneficiary is given one tablet daily for a period of 100 days once a year for every year of his/her beneficiary status.

Although the programme has been in operation for more than 15 years, no improvement in anaemia prevalence was discernible, as several studies conducted during this period indicated. There were many speculations as to the cause behind the lack of impact of the programme. One reason that was strongly advanced was that the dose of iron given to pregnant women was insufficient and their were proposals to increase the dose to 120 or 240 mg/day based on a study in India. A multicentric field study to test different doses of iron, namely 60, 120, 180 and 240 mg, was organised by ICMR; though the study is reported to have been completed, the results are not yet available. However, an evaluation of the programme in 11 states of the country, conducted by the ICMR during 1985-86, yielded the following depressing conclusions :

- The programme has not made any significant impact on the prevalence of anaemia.
- The important drawback of the programme was that a large proportion of the women did not receive the tablets due to poor supply of tablets to PHCs.

- The monitoring of supply of tablets and their distribution as well as compliance were far below the desired levels.
- There were also the problems of poor quality of the tablets.

Apparently the programme has remained all these years as a 'low priority' programme! An aspect of the programme which has not been highlighted is adequacy of production of folifer tablets and the availability of chemicals.

Arising from the evaluation, certain recommendations for the improvement of the programme have been made (Table 6). Another important point that has not been mentioned in the recommendation is the question of dosage of iron. **Iron dosage to anaemic pregnant women should be 120 mg/day**. It could be delivered as a single tablet or two tablets of 60 mg each by which side effects can be reduced. There is also a need to improve the appearance of the tablet – that is the change from brown to red colour. Hopefully, the implementation of these guidelines will improve the programme.

Table-6

Recommendations of the ICMR Task Force on Evaluation of NAAP

1. All the pregnant women to be covered, since there are no simple methods of identifying anaemics.
2. Education of the health functionaries involved in implementation of the programme at all levels.
3. Periodic checking of the quality of tablets.
4. Pilot study to find out the best strategy for delivery of the supplement.
5. Ensuring adequate and regular supply of the supplement at the PHC level.
6. Insuring the quality of tablets with regard to its contents as well as the coating.
7. A rationalised fixing of targets in different states based on population statistics.
8. To consider alternate strategies as additional measures to control.

It is clear that present efforts towards prevention and control of anaemia in the country are wholly inadequate. To a considerable extent, this could be a reflection of the general inadequacies of our health system with respect to the delivery of health care. With improved outreach, and greater motivation of health workers and of the community, it should be possible to promote better implementation. Better linkages between the ICDS and the health system could facilitate wider coverage.

While medicinal iron supplementation to selected groups at risk is important, the need to augment dietary intake of iron must be recognised as this is the obvious logical approach.

Iodine Deficiency Disorders

There is a whole spectrum of Iodine deficiency disorder which, include goitre, hypothyroidism, endemic cretinism, etc.

Goitre is the most common and visible ill-effect of iodine deficiency. Less obvious but more serious condition affecting millions of iodine deficient children includes impaired mental function, poor intellectual performance, lowered IQ, muscular disorders, impaired coordination and sluggishness. In pregnancy, iodine deficiency causes spontaneous abortions, still births and infant deaths.

Iodine deficiency disorders (IDD) constitute a major public health problem in India. Accumulating evidence suggests that no state in India may be completely free from iodine deficiency. Goitre surveys conducted in 239 districts of 25 states and four Union territories (UTs) have identified 197 districts as endemic for IDD (Table)[1]. This is based on estimates of population at the risk of IDD with a cut-off point of 10 per cent for total goitre rate (TGR). The prevalence of goitre is, in fact, if the current proposed criteria for cut-off for population at risk is taken as 5 per cent TGR, and not 10 per cent TGR. It is estimated that nearly million people are exposed to the risk of IDD, of which 54 million have goitre, 2.2 million have cretinism and 6.6 million have mild neurological disorders. With continuous depletion of iodine from natural resources situation could worsen in the coming years unless control measures are taken.

Prevention, control and eventual elimination of IDD requires the establishment of an iodised salt programme in which all salt for human and animal consumption is fortified with iodine. The technology is low in cost and well established. Daily iodine supplementation, through iodine fortified salt, has been successfully applied in several developed countries resulting in total eradication of goitre several decades ago. Salt is the commonly accepted vehicle for iodine for a number of reasons. It is universally consumed in fairly uniform quantities almost daily by a large populations, and the production of salt is limited to a few regions, which makes it feasible to undertake centralised processing. Moreover iodisation does not impart any colour, taste or odour to the salt.

The strategy being adopted by the government of India for prevention IDD is the fortification of common salt with iodine.

Goitre control

(i) Iodized salt – < 1 ppm of iodine and consumes level is the requirement under PFA.

National Goitre Control Programme, 1984

Objectives

- Identify IDD endemic areas;
- Supply iodised salt in place of common salt to the entire country:
- Active private sector participation;
- Resurvey to assess the impact of supply of iodised salt.

The review also resulted in modification in organisation and management of the NGCP. Goitre Cells (IDD Cells) were recommended to be seen with central government funds in each state.

Multi-sectorial Approach

A major effort in this direction is the multi-sectorial IDD project launched by the government of India. This includes :

- Intensification of the IDD programme in 106 moderate and several districts of 13 states;
- Creating demand for iodised salt;
- Establishing a monitoring information system;
- Ensuring supply of iodised salt to selected states;
- Sensitisation meetings with potassium iodate manufacturers, salt manufacturers, wholesalers and traders for creating awareness of the problem;
- Providing support to accelerated production of iodised salt by strengthening activities for the establishment of iodised salt plants;
- Development and supply of low capacity and low cost iodisation for small salt manufacturers;
- Establishment of crusher plants and packaging units is also among the plan of action.

ASSESSMENT OF NUTRITIONAL STATUS

It has several components :

(1) General screening for nutritional problems.
(2) Anthropometry.
(3) Biochemical studies.
(4) Functional assessment.
(5) Dietary assessment.
(6) Vital statistics.
(7) Ecological studies.

General Screening for Nutritional Problems

Note the presence of the following :

- Usual body weight that is 20% above or below the ideal.
- Recent significant weight gain or loss.
- Any conditions that might increase metabolic needs, such as fever, trauma, burns, infection, or hyperthyroidism.
- Increased losses of nutrients through draining fistulas, open wounds, or chronic blood loss.
- Chronic diseases, such as diabetes, hypertension, coronary artery disease, or carcinoma.
- Recent major surgery or illness.
- GI tract diseases.
- Social history : Inadequate income, inability to buy own food, lives alone, eats meals alone, handicapped, drug addiction, alcoholism, inadequate refrigeration or cooking facilities, smoking.
- Diet history : Meals inadequate as per needs, poor appetite, ill-fitting dentures, limited diet, lack of meal appeal, impaired sense of taste, impaired sense of smell, anorexia, problems chewing or swallowing, cultural or religious limitations on diet, frequent meals away from home.

Symptoms That May Be Related to Nutritional Disease :

- Loss of appetite.
- Loss of taste or smell.
- Loss of or gain in weight.
- Pain or discomfort when eating or swallowing.

- Sore lips, tongue, or throat.
- Vomiting or regurgitation of food.
- Burning, pricking, pins and needles, or cramps in the legs.
- Swelling of the legs.
- Change in bowel habits.
- Diarrhoea.
- Blood in the stools; bulky, foul-smelling stools.
- "Rash" (dermatitis) not responding to topical medication.
- Slow healing of wound, sore, or ulcer.
- Bleeding into the skin or easy bruising.
- Changes in skin colour.
- Depression; confusion; loss of memory.
- Loss of balance.
- Light sensitivity.
- Hair loss.
- Breathlessness on exertion or at rest.

Anthropometry

Measurement of height, weight, skin bold thickness, midterm circumference are used per assessment.

Biochemical Studies

- Hb estimation
- RBC indices
- Serum proteins
- Albumin
- Prealbumin
- Transferrin
- Retinol-binding protein
- Creatinine-height index
- Immune status
- Total lymphocyte count (TLC). Delayed cutaneous hypersensitivity.

Other Biochemical Tests :

- Serum retinal
- Prothrombin time, etc.

Functional Assessment

Dietary Assessment

The purpose of the dietary assessment is to identify a person's eating habits and to estimate the average daily nutrient intake. Through a variety of methods, information should be obtained on the amount and type of food eaten.

The validity of the information obtained is affected by the person's ability to communicate, hear, and remember the recent past. Therefore, information obtained from the person should be corroborated by talking with family members and friends and by checking the pantry and refrigerator to see what food is on hand, how it is being stored, and whether it is being used. The best place to do a dietary assessment is in the person's home.

One method of assessing diet is to ask the adult to keep a record of daily dietary intake. However, the food record may not be accurate because it relies on the person's memory. Calories intake may be underestimated as a result. Because intake may vary from day to day, a 3-day food record may be more accurate than a 24-hour diet recall. However, both the 24-hour recall and 3-day food record reflect the person's current diet, not eating habits established over a long period of time. In addition, individuals keeping food records tend to be better educated and of higher socioeconomic status than the general population and thus may not be representative of the elderly.

Another way to obtain accurate information on dietary intake is to show a food model to the person so he or she could guess the approximate portion size eaten. Food models should be as realistic as possible.

Vital Statistics

Like IMR, MMR, NMR, etc.

Ecological Studies

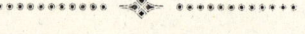

CHAPTER-12

ENVIRONMENT AND HEALTH

ENVIRONMENT AND HEALTH

Environment

Living and non living objects surrounding the man. It is divided into three components :

(a) Physical : Water, air, soil, etc.

(b) Biological : All living organisms.

(c) Socio-economical : Customs, income, religion, caste, etc.

Sanitation

As per national sanitation foundation, USA "Sanitation is a way of life. It is the quality of living that is expressed in the clean home, the clean farm, the clean business, the clean neighbourhood and the clean community. Being a way of life it must come from within the people; it is nourished by knowledge and grows as an obligation and an ideal in human relations".

WHO defines 'environmental sanitation' as 'the control of all those factors in man's physical environment which exercise or may exercise a deleterious effect on his physical development, health and survival'.

Now, the term 'environmental health' is in use instead of 'environmental sanitation'. The very aim of 'environmental health' is to promote health by providing safe water, sanitation safe housing etc.

ENVIRONMENTAL HEALTH SERVICES

These services include :

(1) Providing safe and wholesome water.
(2) Efficient sanitation facilities, safe disposal of excreta and waste products arising out of human activities includes both solid and liquid.

(3) Control of water pollution.
(4) Management of air quality.
(5) Control of noise pollution.
(6) Control of vectors like mosquitoes, rodents, flies.
(7) Maintenance of quality of consumer products.
(8) Control of adulteration of food items.
(9) Safe housing facilities.

WATER

Most of diseases in the developing world are caused by polluted water. Lack of safe and wholesome water is one of the major problems that developing countries like India faces today. Safe drinking water has been one of the basic components of 'Primary Health Care'.

SAFE AND WHOLESOME WATER by definition is the water which is free from pathogenic agents, harmful chemical substances, pleasant to taste, free from colour and odour and fit for human consumption.

Requirements

It is expressed as litres per capita per day. For physiological purposes the drinking water requirement is about 2 litres per capita per day.

For domestic purposes it is about 150-200 litres per capita per day. In India 40 litres per capita per day is the target to be achieved.

Uses of Water

(i) Domestic – Drinking, cooking, bathing.
(ii) Public – Markets, fire control, swimming pools etc.
(iii) Sanitary – Sewerage system, toilets etc.
(iv) Industrial – In various industries like chemical, steel.
(v) Agricultural – For irrigation.
(vi) For producing electricity i.e. hydroelectricity.
(vii) Commercial – Ice, cold drinks, etc.

Sources of Water

Water is a natural resource available in vast quantity but not all of the water present in the world is usable. Only a limited number of water sources are there for providing usable water. The three main sources are :

(1) Rain.

(2) Surface water
- Impounding reservoirs.
- Rivers.
- Tanks, ponds, lakes.

(3) Ground water
- Shallow Well.
- Deep Well.

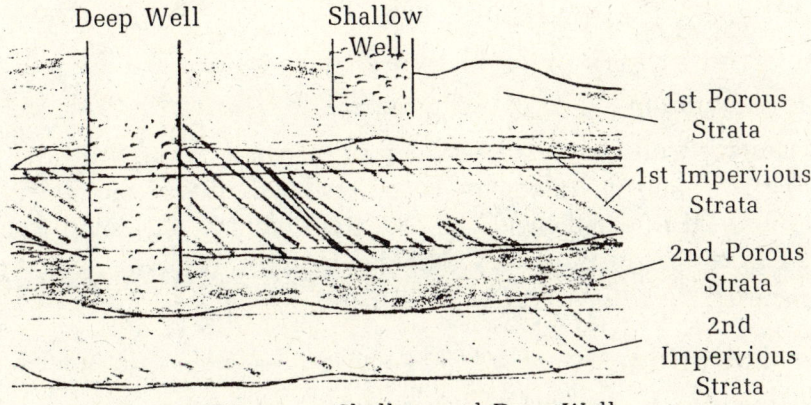

Diagram : Shallow and Deep Well

Difference between shallow and deep well :

Shallow Well	Deep Well
(i) Draws water from 1st porous strata situated above 1st impervious layer.	(i) Draws water from 2nd porous strata situated below 1st impervious layer.
(ii) Yield of water is less.	(ii) More yield.
(iii) May dry in summer.	(iii) Supplies throughout the year.
(iv) Water is hard.	(iv) Much harder water.
(v) Water obtained is likely to be contaminated.	(v) Free from contamination.

Sanitary Well

It is a well which is properly located, well constructed and protected against the danger of contamination.

It should not possess steps and should be located at least 15 m (50 feet) from likely sources of contamination. But it should be within 100 m distance from residential area to facilitate use. Various important parts of a sanitary well are :

(i) *Lining* – It should be made up of bricks or stones and cement. The lining of the well should go upto a depth of at least 6 m.

The lining should be above the ground for a distance of 100 cms.

(ii) *Parapet* – It is situated around the mouth of well and should be made up of cement. It height should be 70-75 cms.

(iii) *Platform* – It is made up of cement and extends at least 1 m in all directions around the well. It should have a slope away from the well.

(iv) *Drain* – It carries spilled water to a public drainage system.

(v) *Covering* – To closev the top of the well.

(vi) *Handpump* – For drawing the water from well.

A sanitary well is a very useful source of water mainly in rural area. Its proper care and maintenance is the responsibility of the consumers. It should be disinfected regularly. Washing, bathing, etc. should not be allowed in the vicinity of well. Regular monitoring of water quality is also essential *Health Education* should be given to all the users.

Water Pollution

It is the presence of any foreign matter in water. Most of the pollution is man made. The sources of pollution are :

(i) Sewage – Includes organic matter, microbes, etc.

(ii) Industrial waste – Toxic chemical substances.

(iii) Agricultural pollutants – Night soil, fertilizers.

(iv) Physical pollutants – Radioactive substances, heat.

The water contamination results in more than 50 million illnesses every year in India with more than 5 million deaths. Various water borne disease are :

(i) *Viral* – Include hepatitis A, E, polio, etc.

(ii) *Bacterial* – Typhoid, salmonellosis, cholera, diarrhoeas.

(iii) *Protozoal* – Amoebiasis, giardiasis.

(iv) *Helminthic* – Round worm, thread worm.

Water Quality

It is usually assessed from acceptability, chemical, microbiological and radiological parameters.

The quality of water from microbiological point of view is very important. Presence of E. coli and other coli forms are indicative of sewage contamination of water.

Acceptability Aspects
Physical Parameters
Taste and odours

Taste and odour originate from natural and biological sources of processes from contamination by chemicals water treatment (chlorination).

Taste and odour in drinking water may be indicative of some form of pollution or of malfunction during water treatment or distribution. The cause of tastes and odours should be investigated and the appropriate health authorities should be consulted. No health based guideline value is proposed for taste and odour.

Temperature

Cool water is generally more potable than warm water. High water temperature enhances the growth of micro organisms and may increase, taste, odour and colour and corrosion problems.

Colour

It is due to coloured organic matter and humus concentration of soil, iron and other metals. The source of colour should be always investigated. Colours above 15 to 0 (true colour units) are detectable with naked eye.

Turbidity

Turbidity in drinking water is due to particulate late matter. High levels of turbidity can protect micro organisms from the effects of disinfection and can stimulate bacterial growth. The turbidity must be low so that disinfection can be effective. The appearance of water with a turbidity of less than 5 nephelometric turbidity units is usually acceptable to consumers. No health based guideline for turbidity has been proposed.

Inorganic Constituents
Aluminium

The presence of aluminium at concentrations in excess of 0.2 mg/litre often leads to consumer complaints as hydroxide floc in distribution system occurs.

Ammonia

The threshold odour concentration of ammonia at alkaline pH is approximately 1.5 mg/litre and a taste threshold of 35 mg/litre has been proposed for the ammonium cation.

Chloride

High concentrations of chloride give an undesirable taste to water and beverages. Taste thresholds for the chloride anion are in the range of 200-300 mg/litre for sodium, potassium and calcium chloride. No health based guideline value is proposed for chloride in drinking water.

Copper

Copper in public water supplies increases the corrosion of galvanised iron and steel fittings. At levels above 5 mg/litre, it also imparts colour and an undesirable bitter taste to water.

Hardness

Public acceptability of the degrees of hardness of water varies. The taste threshold for the calcium ion is in the range of 100-300 mg/litre.

Hard water on heating forms deposits calcium carbonate scale. Soft water, with hardness of less than 100 mg/litre may on the other hand, have a low buffer capacity and so be more corrosive for water pipes. No health based guideline value has been proposed for hardness.

Hydrogen Sulphide

The taste and odour thresholds of hydrogen sulphide in water are estimated to be between 0.05 and 0.1 mg/litre. The "rotten eggs" odour of hydrogen is particularly noticeable in some ground waters and in stagnant drinking water.

Iron

Iron promotes the growth of "iron bacteria". At levels about 0.3 mg/litre iron stains laundry and plumbing fixtures. There is usually no noticeable taste at iron concentrations below 0.3 mg/litre although turbidity and colour may develop. No health-based guideline value is proposed for iron.

Manganese

Although manganese concentrations below 0.1 mg/litre are usually acceptable to consumers. If it exceeds 0.1 mg/litre in water supplies, it stains sanitary ware and laundry and causes an undesirable taste. It is considered that taste impairment is minimal at levels below 250 mg/litre. As sulphate is one of the least toxic anions, no health-based guideline value has been derived.

Zinc

Zinc imparts an undesirable astringent taste to water. Tests indicates a taste threshold concentration of 4 mg/litre. Although drinking water seldom contains zinc at concentrations above 0.1 mg/litre levels in tap water can be considerably higher because of the zinc used in the plumbing materials.

Total dissolved solids

Total dissolved solids (TDS) can have an important effect on the taste of drinking water. The palatability of water with a TDS level of less than 600 mg/litre is generally considered to be good.

No health – based guideline value for TDS has been proposed.

Organic Constituents

Toluene

Toluene has a sweet, pungent, benzene like odour. The reported taste threshold ranges from 40 to 120 mg/lire. The reported odour threshold for toluene in water ranges from 24 to 170 mg/litre.

Xylenes

Xylene concentrations in the range 300 µg/litre produce a detectable taste and odour. The odour threshold for xylene isomers in water has been reported to range from 20 to 1800 µg/litre.

Others :
- Ethyl benzene.
- Styrene.
- Mono chlorobenzene.
- Dischloro benzene.
- Tri chlorobenzene.
- Synthetic detergents.

Disinfectants and their by-products

Chlorine

The taste and odour thresholds for chlorine in distilled water are 5 and 2 mg/litre respectively. The taste threshold for 5 mg/litre is at the health based guideline concentration.

Chlorophenols

Chlorophenols have very low organoleptic thresholds.

Micro Biological Aspects

Infectious diseases caused by pathogenic bacteria, viruses and protozoa or by parasites are the most common and widespread health risk associated with drinking water. They are transmitted generally through water infected with human or animal excreta.

Some of the important orally transmitted waterborne pathogens and their significance are given in Table-1.

Microbial indicators of water quality

(i) E. coli and other coliforms

They are the members of family *Entero bacteriaceae*. Their presence is an indicative of recent faecal pollution. They serve as quite useful indicators of water pollution as they are present abundantly in faeces, can be detected easily by various tests and are more resistant than other pathogens present in water.

Coliform Test is still useful for monitoring the microbial quality of treated piped water supplies.

(ii) Faecal streptococci

The term refers to those streptococci present in faeces of humans and animals. They belong to germs Entero coleus and streptococci. In children commonly found organisms are species E. avium, E. faecalis E. faecium, E. mundtii, E. celorum etc.

They are regarded as specific indicators of human faecal pollution under certain circumstances.

They are more resistant than E.coli and they also serve as additional indicators of treatment efficiency.

(iii) Sulphite – reducing clostridia

Anaerobic sporing bacilli of clostridium perfringum (Cl. welchii) is normally seen in faeces, but fewer in comparison to E.coli. They can survive much longer and their resistance is very high to disinfectant. Their presence in disinfected water may thus indicate deficiencies in treatment.

They thus have as phial value but are not included in routine monitoring of distribution systems.

(iv) Coli phages and other alternative indicaters includes bacteriophages, Bacteroides fragilis.

Table-1
Orally transmitted waterborne pathogens and their significance in water supplies

Pathogen	Health significance	Persistence in water supplies[a]	Resistance to chlorine[b]	Relative infective dose[c]	Important animal reservoir
BACTERIA					
Campylobacter jejuni, C. coli	High	Moderate	Low	Moderate	Yes
Pathogenic Escherichia coli	High	Moderate	Low	High	Yes
Salmonella typhi	High	Moderate	Low	High[d]	No
Other salmonellae	High	Long	Low	High	Yes
Shigella spp.	High	Short	Low	Moderate	No
Vibrio cholerae	High	Short	Low	High	No
Yersinia enterocolitica	High	Long	Low	High (?)	No
Pseudomonas aeruginosa	Moderate	May multiply	Moderate	High (?)	No
Aeromonas sppl	Moderate	May multiply	Low	High (?)	No
VIRUSES					
Adenoviruses	High	?	Moderate	Low	No
Enteroviruses	High	Long	Moderate	Low	No
Hepatitis A	High	?	Moderate	Low	No
Enterically transmitted non-A, non-B, hepatitis viruses, hepatitis E	High	?	?	Low	No
Norwalk virus	high	?	?	Low	No
Rotavirus	High	?	?	Moderate	No (?)
Small round viruses	Moderate	?	?	Low (?)	No
PROTOZOA					
Entamoeba histolytica	High	Moderate	High	Low	No
Giardia intestinalis	High	Moderate	High	Low	Yes
Cryptosporidium parvum	High	Long	High	Low	Yes
HELMINTHS					
Dracunculus medinensis	High	Moderate	Moderate	Low	Yes

? Not known or uncertain.

[a] Detection period for infective stage in water at 20°C : short, up to 1 week; moderate, 1 week to 1 month; long, over 1 month.

[b] When the infective stage is freely suspended in water treated at conventional doses and contact times. Resistance moderate, agent may not be completely destroyed.

[c] Dose required to cause infection in 50% of health adult volunteers; May be as little as one infective unit for some viruses.

[d] From experiments with human volunteers.

[e] Main route of infections is by skin contact, but can infect immunosuppressed or cancer patients orally.

Bacteriological quality

Water intended for drinking and household purposes must not contain waterborne pathogens. Because the most numerous and the most specific bacterial indicator of faecal pollution from humans and animals is E.coli. It follows that E.coli or thermotolerant coliform organisms must not be present in 100-ml samples of any water intended for drinking.

During distribution, the bacteriological quality of water may deteriorate. Coliform bacteria other than E.coli can occur in inadequately treated supplied, or those contaminated after leaving the treatment plant, as a result of growth in sediments and on unsuitable materials in contact with the water (washers, packing, lubricants, plastics and plasticizers, for example). They may also gain entrance from soil or natural water through leaky valves and glands, repaired mains, or back-siphonage. This type of contamination is most likely to be found when the water is untreated or undisinfected, or where there is limited or no residual disinfectant. Allowance can be made for the occasional occurrence in the distribution system of coliform organisms in up to 5% of samples taken over any 12-month period, provided E.coli is not present. It must be stressed that any regular occurrence of coliform organisms is a matter of concern and should be investigated.

Virological quality

Drinking water must essentially be free of human enteroviruses to ensure negligible risk of transmitting viral infection. Any drinking water supply subject to faecal contamination presents a risk of viral disease to consumers. Two approaches can be used to ensure that the risk of viral infection is kept to a minimum : providing drinking water from a source verified free of faecal contamination, or adequately treating faecally contaminated water to reduce enteroviruses to a negligible level. Virological studies have shown that drinking water treatment can considerably reduce the levels of viruses but may not eliminate them completely from very large volumes of water. Virological, epidemiological, and risk analyses are providing important information, although it is still insufficient for deriving quantitative and direct virological criteria. Such criteria cannot be recommended for routine use because of the cost, complexity, and lengthy nature of virological analyses, and the fact that they cannot detect the most relevant viruses.

The guideline criteria are based upon the likely viral content of source waters and the degree of treatment necessary to ensure that every very large volumes of drinking water have a negligible risk of containing viruses.

Ground water obtained from a protected source and documented to be free from faecal contamination from its zone of influence, the well, pumps, and delivery system can be assumed to be virus-free. However, when such water is distributed, it is desirable that it is disinfected, and that a residual level of disinfectant is maintained in the distribution system to guard against contamination.

The water must meet guideline criteria for turbidity and pH bacteriological quality and parasitological quality.

Chemical Aspects

Inorganic Constituents

(a) Lead – It is a toxic metal and leads to multi system disorders affecting peripheral nervous system, hemopoietic system, etc. The guideline value of lead is 0.01 mg/litre.

(b) Mercury – It affects CNS. Guideline value is 0.001 mg/litre.

(c) Arsenic – It comes into water supply through dissolution of minerals and ores, industrial effluents, etc. The provisional guideline value is 0.01 mg/litre.

(d) Cyanide – One of the must toxic substance known. Affects the enzymes of respiratory chain. The guideline value is 0.07 mg/litre.

(e) Fluoride – Causes fluorosis – skeletal and dental. The guidelines value is 1.5 mg/litre. But a number of countries have a very high fluoride content upto 5 mg/litre.

(f) Nitrate and nitrite – They are present in surface and ground waters in mg/litre concentration. At higher values than the provisional guideline nitrate causes metheamoglobinaemia.

   Nitrate – 50 mg/litre
   Nitrite – 3 mg/litre

(g) Cadmium – Guideline value is 0.003 mg/litre.

(h) Chromium – Guideline value is 0.05 mg/litre.

Organic Constituents

Given below are the guideline value for health related organic constituents :

Organic constituents	Concentration (mg/litre)
Chlorinated alkalies	
– Carbon tetra esloride	2
– Dichloromethane	20
Chlorinated ethenes	
– Vinyl chloride	55
– 1, 1 - dichloroethene	30
– 1, 2 - dichloroethene	50
Aromatic hydrocarbon	
– Benzene	10
– Toluene	700
– Xylenes	500
– Ethyl benzene	300
– Styrene	20
– Benzolalpyrene	0.7

Poly nuclear aromatic hydrocarbons – they can be carcinogenic even in small quantities.

Pesticide – live DDT, Aldrin, Lindere etc. get inside living organism.

Health Risk Assessment

Tolerable daily intake (TDI) is an estimate of the amount of a substance in fluid or drinking water, expressed on a body weight basis (mg/kg or g/kg or body weight) that can be ingested daily over a life time without health risk.

It can be derived as follows :

TDI = (NOAEL or LOAEL)/UF

Where :
- NOAEL = No-observed-adverse-effect level;
- LOAEL = Lowest-observed-adverse-effect level;
- UF = Uncertainty factor.

The guideline value (GV) is then derived from the TDI as follows:

GV = (TDI × bw × P)/C

Where :
- bw = Body weight (60 kg for adults, 10 kg for children, 5 kg for infants),

- P = Fraction of the TDI allocated to drinking water,
- C = Daily drinking water consumption (2 litres for adults, 1 litre for children, 0.75 litre for infants).

Radiological Aspects

It aims as at giving the guidelines for radioactivity in drinking water. So, as to have minimal or no effect on human health.

The provisional guidelines are :
gross alpha (α) activity – 0.1 αq/L
gross beta (β) activity – 1.0 βq/L

Homoeopathic Aspects

Some of the important rubrics with medicines from various repertories for enviornmental hazards are :

- Arsenic poisoning – Ars., Camph., Carb-v., Chin., Euph., Ferr., Iod., Phos., Tab., Verat., etc.
- Carbon gas poisoning – Acet-ac., Acorl., Am-c., Bell., Bry., Carb-v., Lach., Op.
- Carbon monoxide from – Acon., Bell., Bry., Carb-v., Op.
- Iron abuse of – Chin., Ferr., Ferr-p., etc.
- Lead poisoning – Alum., Alumin., Bell., Caust., Plat., Verat., etc.
- Mercury abuse of – Carb-v., Aur., Hep., Merc., etc.
- Mining ill effects of – Ant-c., Carb-s., Cadm-m., Nat-as., Sil., Sulph.
- Ptomaine poisoning ailments from – Cupr-act, Pyrog., Verat.
- Sewer gas poisoning – Bapt., Pyrog., Tub.
- Silica poisoning ailments – Calc., Lyco., Puls., Sil.
- Stone cutter ailments in – Calc., Lyc., Puls., Sil.
- Side effects of radiation – Cadm-s., Sol., Rad-br., X-rays.

EXCRETA DISPOSAL

It is a potent reservoir of infection, habouring a large number of pothentially dangerous microorganism. It can cause soil or water pollution, food contamination and diseases such as typhoid, cholera, salmonellosis, etc.

Methods of Excreta Disposal
Unsewered Areas
(1) Service type – Now abolished.

(2) Non service type (Sanitary latrine)
   (a) Bore hole latrine
   (b) Pit or dug well latrine
   (c) Water-seal type of latrines.
      (i) R.C.A type
      (ii) P.R.A.I type
      (iii) Sulabh Shauchalya.
   (d) Septic tank
   (e) Aqua privy.

Sewered Areas

Water carriage system and sewage treatment.
   (a) Primary treatment
      (i) Screening
      (ii) Grit removal
      (iii) Plain sedimentation.
   (b) Secondary treatment
      (i) Trickling filters
      (ii) Activated sludge process.
   (c) Others :
      (i) Oxidation ponds.
      (ii) Sea out fall.
      (iii) River out fall.
      (iv) Sewage farming.

Sanitary Latrines

(1) Bore Hole Latrine

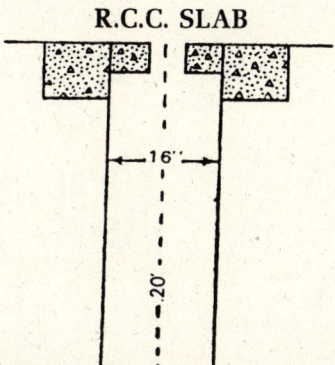

(2) Dug-Well Latrine

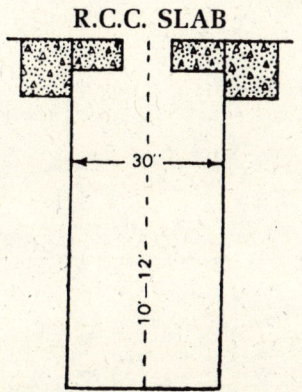

(3) Water Seal Latrine

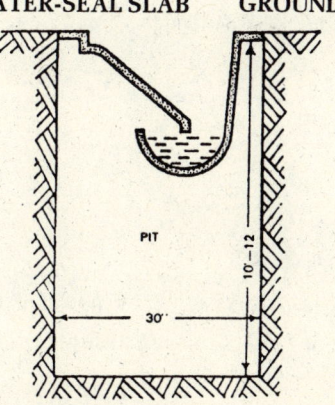

(a) R.C.A. Latrine

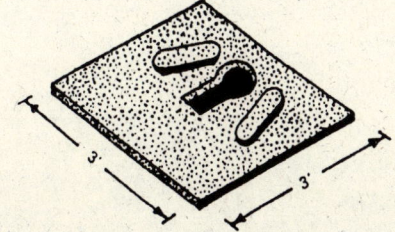

(b) Pan

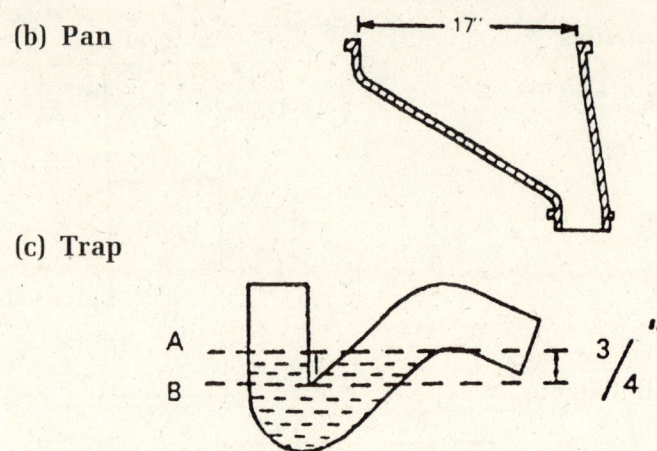

(c) Trap

(d) Connecting Pipe

(e) Dug Well

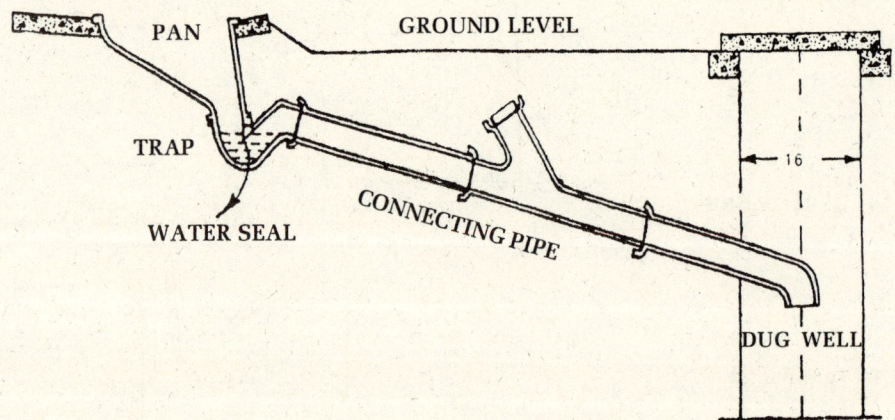

Septic Tank

It is an excellent means of excreta disposal in unsewered areas. It can be of various designs.

Main design features are :

1. Capacity – 20-30 gallon per person.
2. Dimension – length and breadth can very but length is generally twice the breadth.

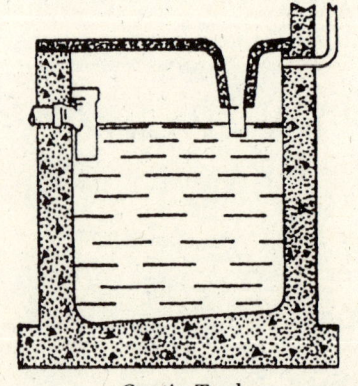

Septic Tank

F - 19B

3. Depth – 1.5-2 m.
4. Airs pole – between the liquid beside and under surface of cover. It should be around 30 cm.
5. Liquid height – 120 cms.
6. Inlet and Outlet – both are sub-merged.
7. Cover made up of concrete slab, having a man hole converted to inlet pipe.

Functioning of Septic Tanks

The solids in feaces settles down at the bottom of the tanks and forms the sludge where as the lighter parts rise to the surface forming

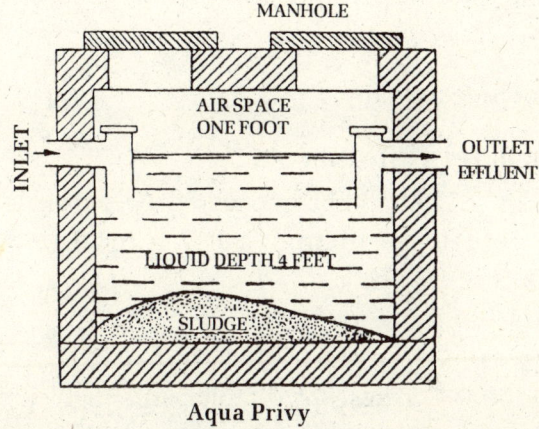

Aqua Privy

slum. The solids are attached by anaerobic bacteria and undergoes anaerobic digestion to form liquids and gases. The liquid, through outlet pipe, now called effluent pass into perforated pipes to percolate into the soil where it is affected by aerobic bacteria leading to oxidation of the effluent into simples compounds like carbon dioxide, water, etc.

An aqua privy also function on the same principle. Its capacity is about 35 cubic foot.

MEDICAL ENTOMOLOGY

Sir Patrik Manson was the first person to realise the important of insects in transmission of diseases. The role played by flies, ticks and other blood sucking arthropods in transmission of diseases is of great importance.

Diseases like malaria and plague, were responsible for worldwide epidemics. They have earned a permanent place in the history of mankind.

Classification

I Class

Insecta

Orders
- Diptera — Mosquitoes, sandflies, tsetse flies.
- Siphonaptera — Fleas
- Anoplenra — Lice
- Hemiptera — Bed-bug.

II Class

Arachnida includes ticks and mites.

III Class

Crustacea includes cyclops.

General Characters of Insects

- Body form — Their body is covered by exoskeleton and body is divided into three distinct parts — head, cephalothorax and abdomen.
- Symmetry — Symmetry is bilateral.
- Germ layers — They are triploblastic.
- Reproduction — Sexes are distinct and reproduced by eggs.
- Appendages — They have jointed appendage.
- Body wall — Made up of chitinous cuticle and single layered epidermis.

Arthropod-borne Diseases

Arthropod	Diseases
1. Mosquitoes	— Malaria, filaria, yellow fever, dengue, haemorrhagic fever, west nile.
2. Lice	— Trench fever, Indian relapsing fever, typhus fever.
3. House fly	— Typhoid fever, cholera, dysentery, trachoma, anthrax, yaws, conjunctivitis, gastroenteritis.
4. Tsetse flies	— Sleeping sickness.
5. Sand-fly	— Kala azar, oriental sore, sand-fly fever, oraya fever.
6. Rat flea	— Bubonic plague, endemic typhus, chiggerosis.
7. Ticks	— African relapsing fever, rocky mountain spotted fever, tick typhus.

8. Louse	–	Epidemic typhus, trench fever.
9. Black fly	–	Onchocerciasis.
10. Hard tick	–	Viral encephalitis, tularemia, tick paralysis, human babesiosis.
11. Soft tick	–	Relapsing fever, Q fever.
12. Cockroaches	–	Enteric pathogens.
13. Itch-mite	–	Scabies.
14. Trombiculid mite	–	Scrub typhus, Rickettsial-pox.
15. Cyclops	–	Guinea worm disease, fish tapeworm.
16. Reduviid bug	–	Chagas disease.

Transmission of Arthropod-borne Diseases

- DIRECT CONTACT – Transmitted directly from one person to other by close contacts.
  e.g. scabies and pediculosis.
- MECHANICAL TRANSMISSION – The agent of disease is transmitted mechanically.
  e.g. diarrhoea, typhoid, dysentery.
- BIOLOGICAL TRANSMISSION – The agent of disease enters the arthropod host, undergoes morphological, development of change or multiplication.
  (a) Progagative – When the agent of disease doesn't undergoes cyclic change but multiplies in the host's body.
  e.g. plague bacilli in rat fleas.
  (b) Cyclo-propergative – When the agent of disease undergoes cyclical change and multiplies in the arthropod's body.
  e.g. malaria parasite in anopheline mosquito.
  (c) Cyclo-developmental – When the agent of disease undergoes cyclic changes but doesn't multiply in the arthropod's body.
  e.g. filarial parasite in culex mosquito.

Mosquitoes

Class	–	Insecta
Order	–	Diptera
Family	–	Culicidae
Sub-family	–	Culicinae.

It deposits eggs, from each of which is produced a larvae, which afterwards becomes converted into pupa from which the adult insect emerges. The egg, larval and pupal stages are spent in water, and so, water is essential for the existence of all mosquitoes.

Species belonging to the genera Anopheles, Culex and Aedes (Stegomyia) are of importance to medical man. Various species of Anopheles transmit the malaria parasite from man to man. *Culex fatigans* is the intermediate (main) host of *Wuchereria bancrofti*. Mansonioides are the true intermediate hosts of W. malayi and spread filaria in the rural areas. Aedes or *Stegomyia* are responsible for the transmission of dengue and yellow fever. The important species responsible for spread are – Aedes aegypti and Aedes albopictus.

Mosquito Anapheles

It is about 5 mm with six legs. It has hairs, scales on wing veins. Body has three divisions. It has equal length palps and proboscis. In males palpi

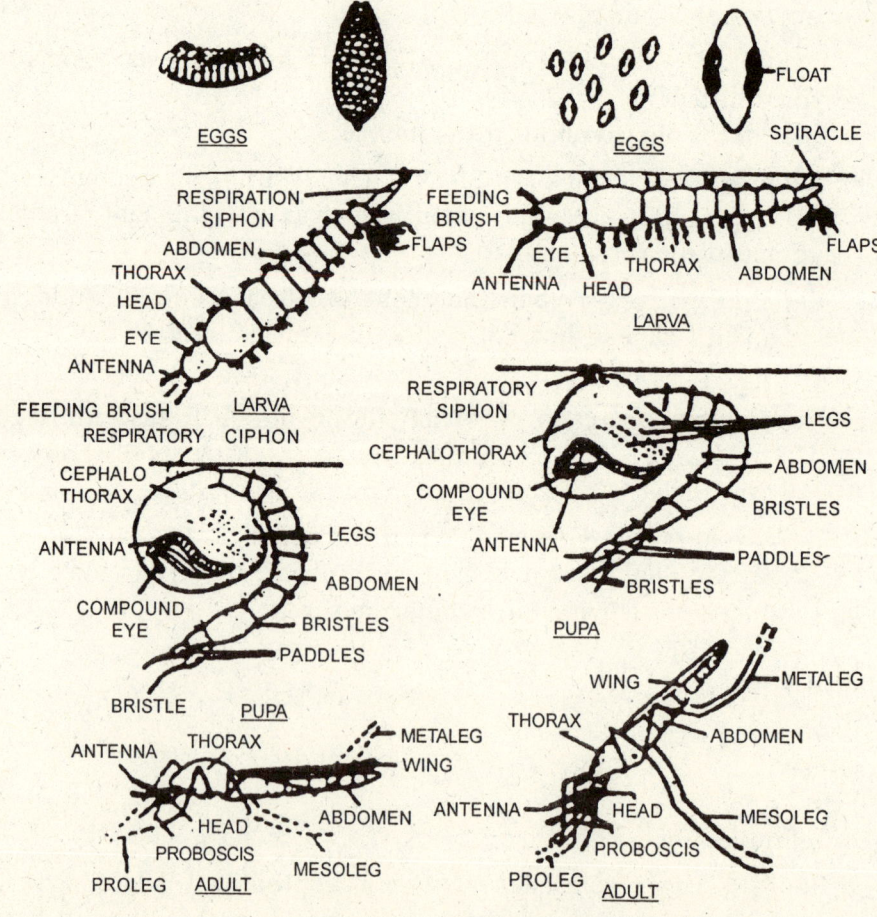

Life history of mosquito. Left (*Culex*), right (*Anopheles*).

are clubshaped while in females palpi are straight. They have complete metamorphosis. It has a life span of one to six months.

It prefers to breed in clean water or fresh water, sea water, irrigation channels, wells. Females basically feeds on the human blood while male feeds on fruit juices.

Its resting places includes dark and humid places. At rest it stands over head.

Culex Mosquito

It is about 5 mm in length. It has six legs and 2 wings. Body has three divisions and dull colour. The male has palpi that tapers at end and proboscis are shorter than palpi. In females, proboscis and palpi are short. It has life cycle of one of six months. It has complete metamorphosis. It breeds in muddy, stagnant water. Females feeds on animal or human blood, while male on fruit juices. It prefers to breed in dark and humid places. It rests parallel to the surface.

Aedes Mosquito

It is 5 mm divided into three divisions. Brown and white bands are present on abdomen, thorax and legs. It has two wings. It breeds in small water collections, pits, ditches, etc. Males depends on fruit juices and females on human blood. Resting place is near to the breeding place. Life span is about one to six months.

Mansonia Mosquito

It is 5 mm and six legs. It is divided into three divisions. It breeds in water with aquatic vegetation and pollution. Life span is about one

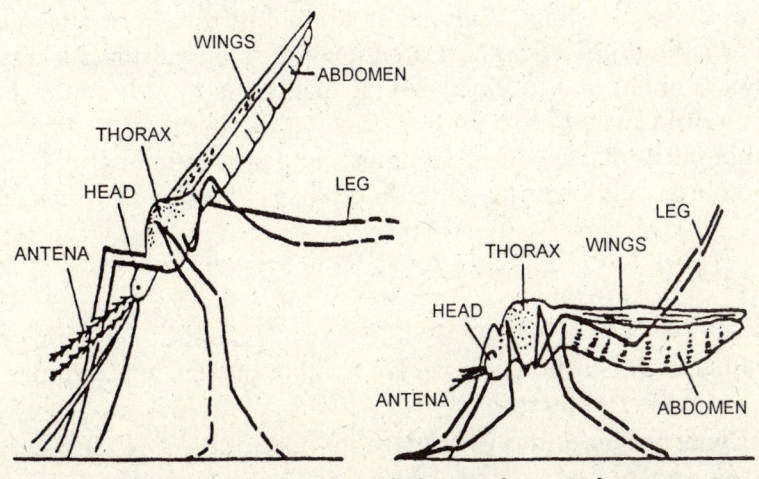

Mosquito, Left – *Anopheles*, Right – *Culex*

to six months and complete metamorphosis. Male depends on fruit juices and females on the human blood. Resting place is near the breeding place.

Anopheles mosquito	Culex mosquito
1. **Body** It has three divisions, about 5 mm and wings are spotted.	It has three divisions, dull in colour and about 5 mm. Wings are unspotted.
2. **Sex differentiation** Male palpi are clubshaped at the tip while female has straight palpi.	In male palpi tapers at end and longer than proboscis while female palpi are very short.
3. **Breeding place** Breeds in clean and fresh water tanks, streams channels, etc.	Breeds in stagnant and polluted water, muddy water.
4. **Resting position** At rest it stands over hand.	It rest more or less parallel to the surface.
5. **Eggs** Boat shaped.	Eggs are oval.
6. **Biting time** Variable.	Mainly nights.
7. **Larva** Has no siphon tube and palmate hairs.	Has conspicuous siphon tube but no palmate hairs.

Flea

It has three divisions. Body made up of chitin with bristles projecting backwards. It has six legs. There are no wings, Metamorphosis is complete. Life span is about one to four years. Females has rounded last abdominal segment while males have conical instead of rounded. It mainly breeds on animal, dirty places, deserted houses and uncleaned habitat. Its resting places includes dark, warm and humid places and also near their breeding places.

Flea Indices

Indices used in flea surveys :
1. **Specific Flea Index** – Average number of fleas of particular species, found per rodent.
2. **General Flea Index** – Average number of fleas of all species found per rodent.

3. **Percentage incidence of flea species** – Percentage of fleas of each species.
4. **Rodent Infestation Rate** – Percentage of rodents infested with various fleas indices.

Control of Fleas

1. **Insecticidal control** – Insecticides which can be used for flea control are DDT, gammatics and dieldrin. In case of resistance diazinon or malathion should be used.
2. **Repellents** – An efficient flea repellent is diethyl-toluamide. Benzyl Benzoate can also be used as an effective repellent.
3. **Rodent Control** – It can be effectively controlled by using various anti-rodent methods.

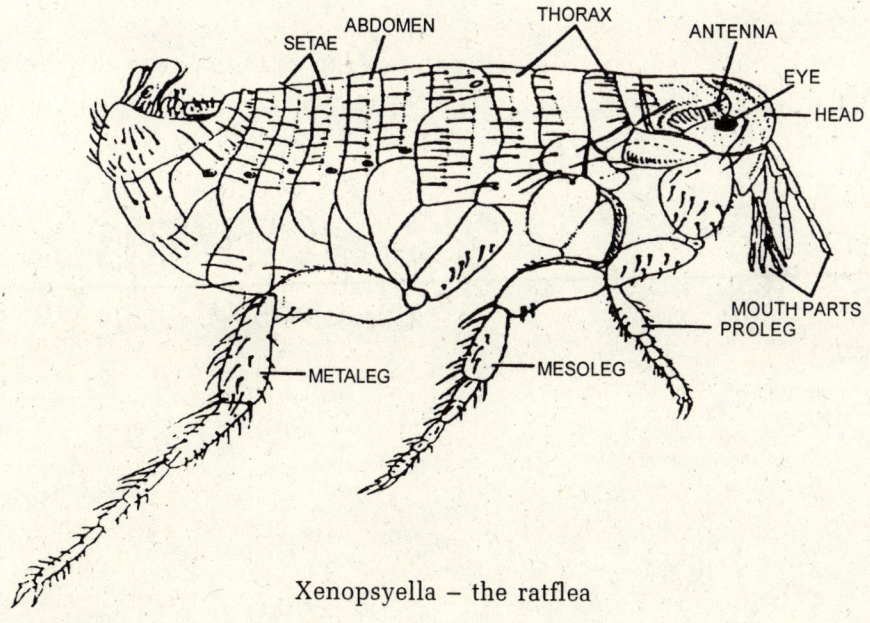

Xenopsyella – the ratflea

Housefly

It is grey in colour with narrow stripes on the thorax. The proboscis ends in a pair of fleshly lobes. It is adapted for sucking blood. It breeds freely on human excreta, garbage, etc. It can't be breed in perfectly dry materials. They are omnivorous and voracious feeder. Their life span is about two to three weeks. The resting places includes walls, kitchen, etc. There is a complete metamorphosis. It vomits frequently which consist of infectious microbes. This is called as *vomit drop*. They can be found up to 6 km from their place of origin.

Fly Control Measures

(1) *Elimination of breeding places* :
  (a) Sanitary disposal of wastes such as refuse (especially garbage), horse litter and dung, human excreta an sullage water.
  (b) Food sanitation such as keeping all foods in wire gauze or glass cupboards and containers with well fitting lids.
  (c) Tight packing of manure in trenches or pits to kill larvae by heat.
  (d) Provision of cement lined tanks or floors for stocking cowdung so that larvae cannot burrow in the soil to pupate.

(2) *Prevention of entry* : Making the houses flyproof, especially the kitchen and latrines, by putting wire gauze screens in doors and windows.

(3) *Trapping* : Using a Balfour fly trap made of wire gauge in which the flies enter through a slit to sit on the bait but cannot come out.

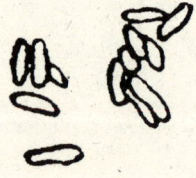
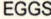

EGGS

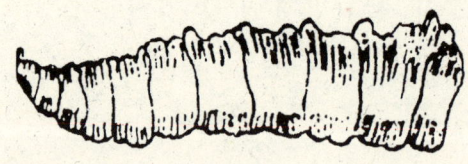

LARVA

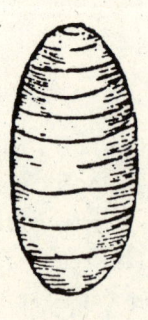

PUPA

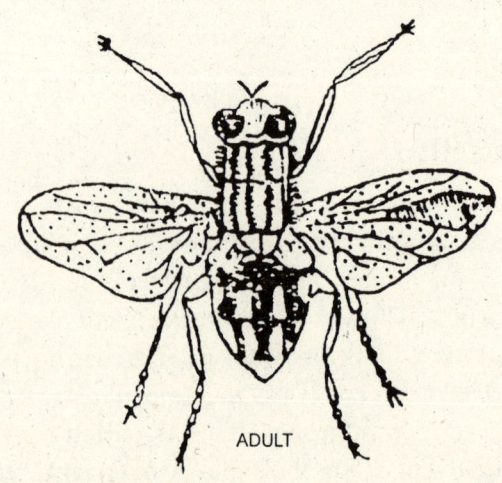

ADULT

Environment and Health

(4) *Manual killing* : Fly swatters are useful devices to kill flies.

(5) *Baiting* : Baits may be used in houses, food establishments, cattle sheds, etc. Examples are :

(i) *Adhesive fly paper* : 500 g castor oil and 800 g resin are heated together and the mixture is spread on a sheet g paper.

Sandfly

It is extremely small insects with hairs all over the body and wings. Wings at rest held up to an angle of 45° to the body. In female, abdomen is rounded at apex while in male it is narrow. Its breeding places includes cracks, holes on walls, stones or underground, damped and warm organic matter. Its life span is about 3 and ½ months like mosquitoes, its female depends on animal or human blood and male on fruit juices. Its resting place is mainly near its breeding places. It has a complete metamorphosis.

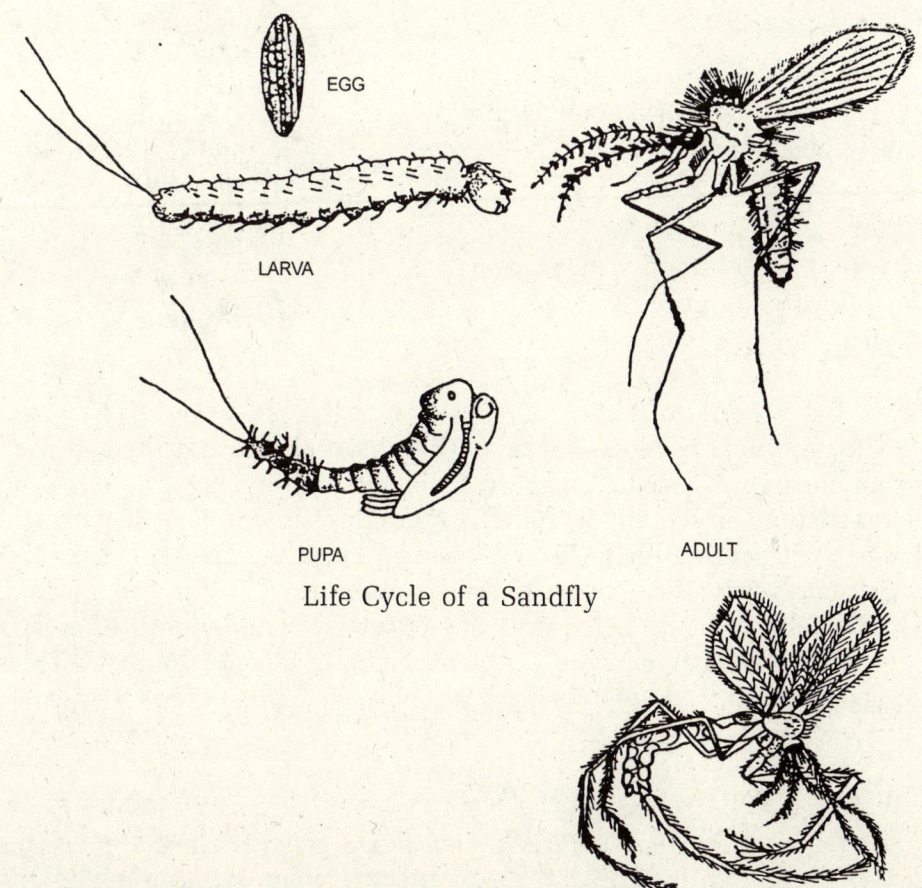

Life Cycle of a Sandfly

Control of Sandflies

1. Cleanliness – Surroundings should be kept clean. Cattle should be removed away from the living places. Cracks and Crevices should be filled up.
2. Insecticide – To kill adult fly, fumigation of sulphur or formalin, cresol or DDT should be sprayed.
3. Repellent – Repellents like Dimethyl pthalate and oils like oil of cassia or of citronella should be used.

Tsetse fly

It is nearly 10-12 mm long with 3 divisions. It has 2 wings which appears to be crossed when folded. Its breeding places includes soils near vegetation and around the water sources. Both male and female depends upon on living being for their blood as a food.

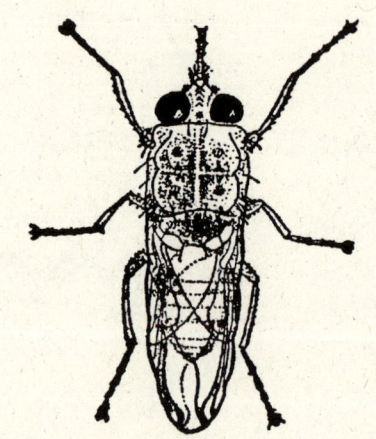

Resting places are in vegetation or it is exophilic in vegetation. Its life span is about three months.

Control

Insecticides used are organophosphorus compounds, DDT and dieldrin.

Hard Tick

They are mainly blood suckers. They have cephalothorax, abdomen but antennae ore absent. Their eyes are inflated and oval and ties on lateral margin of scutum white is a chitinous shield. They have eight legs but wings are absent. Their breeding places are cracks, crevices of walls, stones or under the stone, holes and burrows in the soil. Resting places are host's body. It requires three host for completion of their life cycles. For food they depends on blood of warm blooded animals. Their life span is about one-two years. They have incomplete metamorphosis with one nymphal stage.

Control Measures

Dimethyl phthalate (DMP) is a good tick repellant, especially against larvae. Clothes dipped in 5% DMP and 2% soap solution retain the repellant effect for 1-2 months. Infested animals may be dusted with lindane, malathion or DDT.

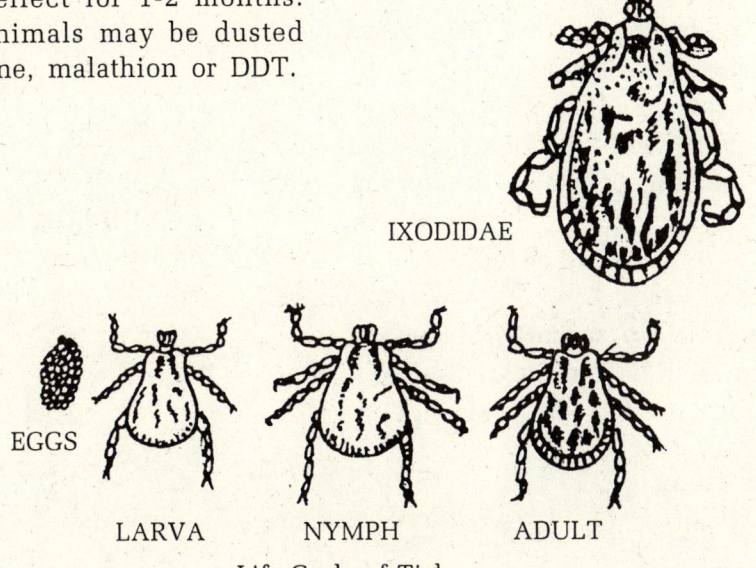

Life Cycle of Tick

Soft Tick

Mainly blood sucking insect. Their body is fused with no divisions Distinctly cuticle is leathery while scutum, the chitinous shield is absent. Their head is not visible from above. They have 8 legs but no wings. Breeding places includes cracks, holes in walls, burrows in soil, etc. same as that in hard ticks. Resting places are inside houses. For food they depends on blood of warm blooded animals but they only bite at night. Their life span is about more than an year and they show incomplete metamorphosis with 5 nymphal stages.

Control Measures

Dimethyl phthalate (DMP) is a good tick repellant, especially against larvae, clothes dipped in 5% DMP and 2% soap solution retain the repellant effect for 1-2 months. Infested animals should be dust with lindane malathion or DDT.

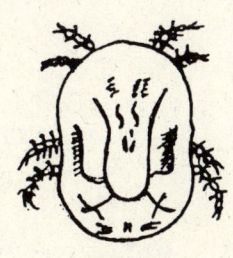

Louse

The head and body louse are extremely resembling. The other ones have conical head with constriction where it joins the thorax. They have a proboscis, a pair of jointed antennae and a compound eye lying internally. The male is smaller. They are rounded off posteriorly with a dorsal aperture for penis. The female is larger with a deep notch at the apex of last abdominal segment. Breeding places includes the hairs' root, folds of skin, seams of clothing of the host. Resting places are roots of hairs on which they are firmly attached, the combs, beddings, clothings. Depends on warm blood. Life span is about one to two months and metamorphosis is incomplete.

Rat flea

It is the carrier of plaque. They are normally nocturnal, during the day the rats remains in their nests near food. There is a seasonal migration to fields.

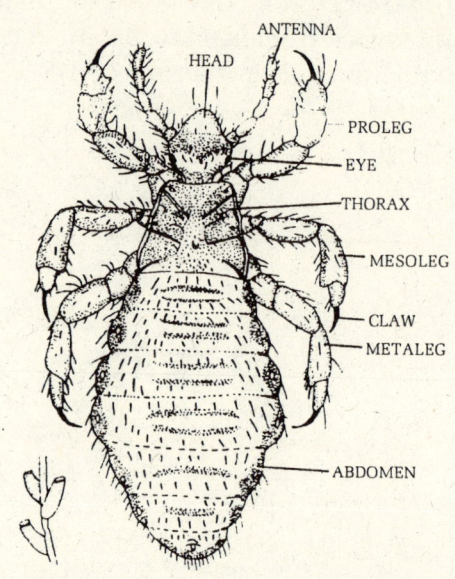

Pediculus – the human louse. Eggs glued to hair on the left.

Rats Control

Assessment of infestation should be made by special surveys by counting the dropping, runs fresh knawing and rat burrows.

Two main methods are – elimination and destruction.

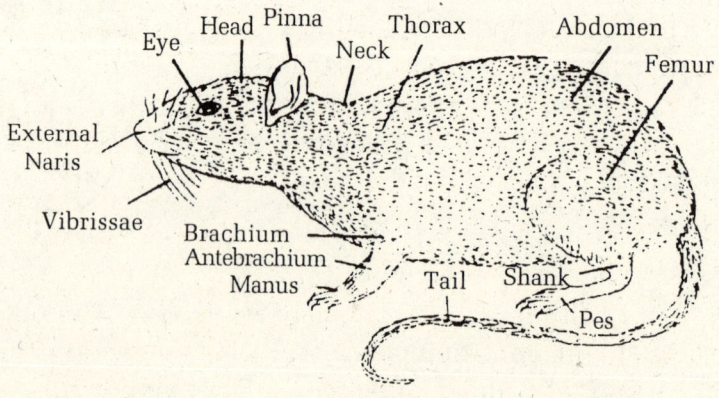

Rattus – the Rat

Environment and Health

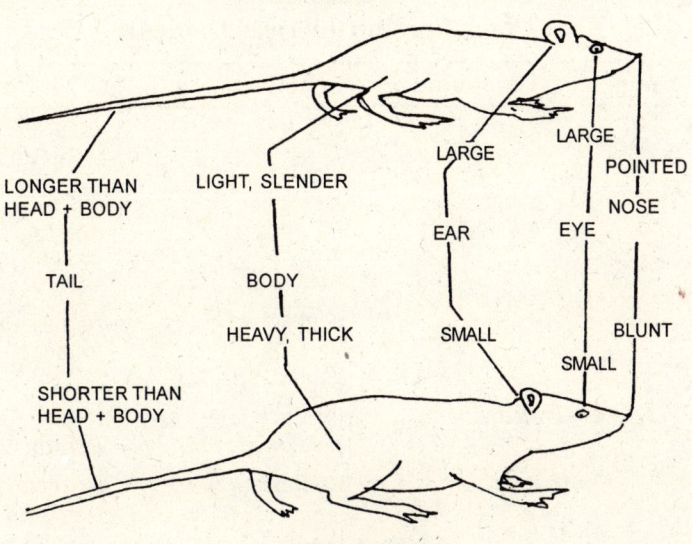

NORWAY RAT
Rattus norvegicus

YOUNG RAT

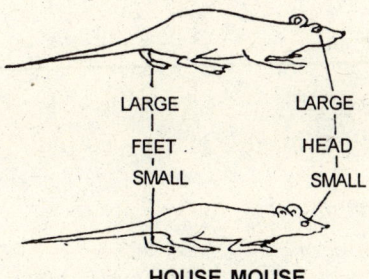

HOUSE MOUSE
Mus musculus

Pesticide

Table
Classification of Insecticides

Chemical group	Compund	Action	Notes
AMIDINES			
	Amitraz		Also ACARICIDE
BIOTANICAL			
	Azadirachtin	Insect growth regulator	Extracted from Neem
	Nicotine	Contact, non-persistent general purpose	Extracted from tobacco
	Pyrethrin	Contact, non-persistent	Extracted from *Pyrethrum*
	Rotenone	Contact	Extracted from Derris and Lonchocarpus
CARBAMATES			
	Aldicarb	Systemic	Also NEMATICIDE
	Bendiocarb	Contact & ingested	–
	Carbaryl	Contact	Also worm, killer, fruit thinner
	Carbofuran	Systemic	Also NEMATICIDE
	Methiocarb	Stomach acting	Also MOLLUSCICIDE
	Methomyl	Fly bait	–
	Pirimicarb	Contact & fumigant aphids only	–
	Propoxur	Fumigant, mainly in glasshouses	–
	Thiocarb	Pelleted bait	Also MOLLUSCICIDE
ORGANOCHLORINES			
Diphenyl aliphatic derivatives	DDT rhtohane (DDD)	– –	– –
Benzene derivatives	lindane ? gamma HCH	contact, ingested & fumigant	–
Cyclodiene derivatives	Aldrin	Persistent	UK revoked 1989
	dieldrin	Persistent	UK revoked 1989
	endosulfan	Contact & ingested	also ACARICIDE

Environment and Health

ORGANOPHOSPHATES			
	Dichlorvos	Contact, fumigant	–
Aliphatic	Dimethoate	Contact, systemic	Also ACARICIDE
derivatives	Disulfoton	Systemic, granules	–
	Malathion	Contact	Also ACARICIDE
	Phorate	Systemic	–
Phenyl	Fenitrothion	Contact, broad Spectrum	–
derivatives	Parathion	–	–
Heterocyclic	Chlorpyrifos	Contact & ingested	Also ACARICIDE
derivatives	Diazinon	Contact	–
Organotins			
	Fenbutatinoxide	–	Only ACARICIDE
Pyrethroids			
Generation 1	Allethrin	–	–
	Bioresmethrin	Contact, residual	Also ACARICIDE
Generation 2	Phenothrin	Contact & ingested	–
	Resmethrin	Contact	–
	Tetramethrin	Contact	–
Generation 3	Fenvalerate	Contact	–
	Permethrin	Contact & ingested, Broad spectrum	–
Generation 4	Bifenthrin	Contact, residual	Also ACARICIDE
	Cypermethrin	Contact & ingested	–
	Cyfluthrin	–	–
	Fenpropathrin	Contact & ingested	Also ACARICIDE

DDT

Dichlorodiphenyl trichloroethane (DDT) is a organochlorine contact insecticide that kills by acting as a nerve poison. Its insecticidal properties were discovered by the Swiss scientist Paul Muller working for J.R. Geigy (now Novartis) in 1942.

Exactly how DDT affects the nervous system is not properly understood, although a great deal of work has beer done to try and find out its precise mode of action.

DDT was originally used during World War II to control typhus which was spread by the body louse. Since then it has been used to control mosquito borne malaria, and was used extensively as a general agricultural insecticide.

Initially DDT was spectacularly successful particularly in the control of malaria, as well as against agricultural pests. But by the 1950s, resistance problems had developed and during the 1960s, a number of serious environmental problems were identified leading to wide-ranging restrictions on its use.

In recent years numerous studies on DDT have shown its environmental persistence and its ability to bioaccumulate, especially in higher animals. Of particular concern is its potential to mimic hormones and thereby disrupt endocrine systems in wildlife and possibly humans.

Classification of insecticides (based on their chemical nature)

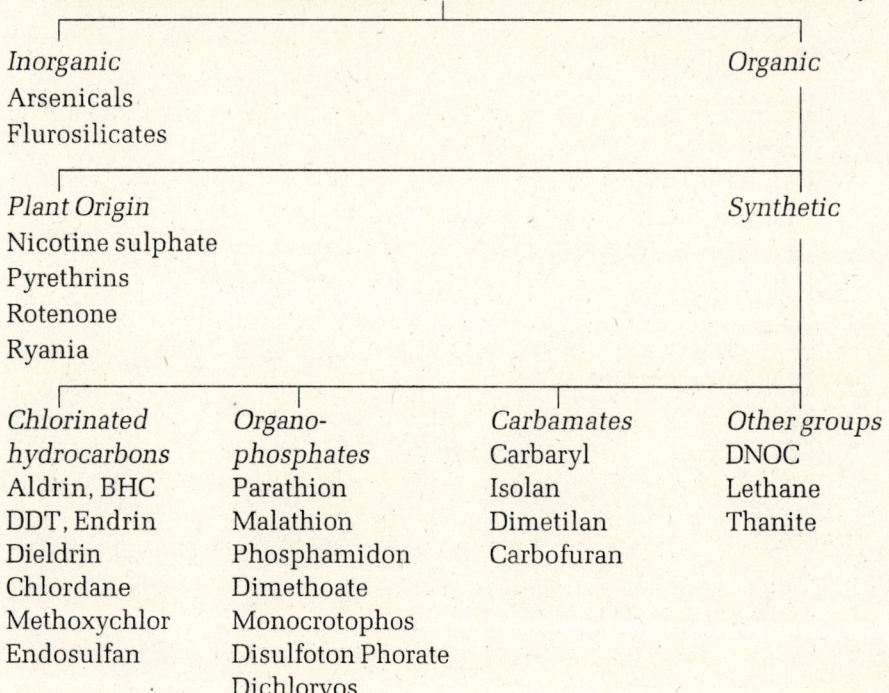

The inorganic insecticides were widely used before the synthetic organic insecticides were developed and marketed. At present, hardly any of these insecticides are being used in India. There is a feeling in some quarters that we can perhaps advantageously use arsenicals against the leaf-feeding insects, especially where some parasites or predators are known to be active against them.

Insecticides of *plant* origin have also been regulated to the background by the synthetics and at present relatively very little quantities of insecticides, like pyrethrins and nicotine sulphate, are used to control insect pests of agricultural importance. The problems of residues on insecticides on food and fodder *crops* has emphasized the necessity of using insecticides which are less toxic to mammals or breakdown into non-toxic components in a reasonable short time. Thus the insecticides of *plant* origin can be usefully employed to control a number of insect pests.

Rodenticides

- **Botanical rodenticides**
  * Scilliroside
  * Strychnine
- **Coumarin rodenticides**
  * Brodifacoum
  * Bromadiolone
  * Coumachlor
  * Coumafuryl
  * Coumatetralyl
  * Difenacoum
  * Difethialone
  * Flocoumafen
  * Warfarin
- **Indandione rodenticides**
  * Chlorophacinone
  * Diphacinone
  * Pindone
- **Inorganic rodenticides**
  * Arsenous oxide
  * Phosphorus
  * Potassium arsenite
  * Sodium arsenite
  * Thallium sulfate
  * Zinc phosphide
- **Organochlorine rodenticides**
  * Gamma-HCH
  * HCH
  * Lindane
- **Organophosphorus rodenticides**
  * Phosacetim
- **Pyrimidinamine rodenticides**
  * Crimidine
- **Thiourea rodenticides**
  * Antu
- **Urea rodenticides**
  * Pyrinuron

- **Unclassified rodenticides**
  * Bromethalin
  * Chloralose
  * Chlorohydrin
  * Ergocalciferol
  * Fluoroacetamide
  * Flupropadine
  * Hydrogen cyanide
  * Norbormide
  * Sodium fluoroacetate

Insect Repellents
Butopyronoxyl
Dibutyl phthalate
Diethyl toluamide
Dimethyl carbate
Dimethyl phthalate
Ethohexadiol
Hexamide
Methoquin-bytyl
Methylneodecanamide
Oxamate
Picaridin

CHAPTER-13

OCCUPATIONAL HEALTH

OCCUPATIONAL HEALTH

As per joint ILO/WHO "occupational health should aim at the promotion and maintenance of the highest degree of physical, mental and social well being of workers in all occupations; the prevention among workers of departures from health caused by their working conditions; protection from risks due to working conditions; the placing and maintenance of the worker in an occupational environment adapted to his physiological and psychological equipment."

Occupational health is very much based on preventive approach, with all three levels of prevention coming into play. It is very essential to provide comprehensive occupational health services to all the workers. Various different legislations are there for covering workers engaged in various occupations like *the Factories Act, Mines Act, ESI Act, Child Labour Act,* etc.

Occupational Environment

It is the sum total of all the external factors which are present at the place of work and influence the health of the worker. The environment at work place must be suitable for work because it is having a bearing on the health of the working population.

Environment essentially is composed of two components. One which deals with means for promotion, protection and maintenance of health, other is concerned with safety at work place. Environment thereby becomes a prominent feature of various legislations which lay stress on provision of safe working environment.

Three different types of interaction present in a working place are :

(i) Man and man

(ii) Man and machine
(iii) Man and material agents (physical, chemical, biological).

(i) Man to Man

Here inter personal relationships come into play. Relation with fellow workers, superiors and sub ordinates very much influence the psychosocial environment of the work place. Good interpersonal relationships not only have a positive influence over the health but also leads to increased productivity.

(ii) Man to Machine

Machines played an important role in industrial revolution. They enable mass production at low cost and are less time consuming. But they are also responsible for occupational hazards like accidents. Lack of safety measures and poor maintenance of machines, etc. are responsible for most accidents.

(iii) Man and Material Agents

- Physical Agents – Heat, cold, humidity, air movement, heat radiation, light, noise, vibrations and ionizing radiation. As well as working and breathing space, toilet, washing and bathing facilities.
- Chemical Agents – Chemicals, toxic dusts and gases.
- Biological Agents – Virus, ricketts, bacteria and parasites.

Occupational Hazards

In any occupation, occupational hazards cannot be ruled out. The hazards are mostly unique to work place and affect the health of the worker his socio economic condition, his family, the employer and the community. These are direct impacts of occupational hazards, indirect impacts include money spend for welfare and safety measures employed, cost of medical health care. Also the efforts for the rehabilitation of the affected worker are important.

Classification

They are classified into 5 types :
(a) Physical hazards.
(b) Chemical hazards.
(c) Biological hazards.
(d) Mechanical hazards.
(e) Psychosocial hazards.

Physical Hazards

(a) Heat
Direct effects – Burns, heat exhaustion, heat stroke & heat cramps.
Indirect effects – Decreased efficiency, Increased fatigue, Increased accidents.
Industries – Foundry, glass, steel, mines.
Cold – Chilblains, erythrocyanosis, emersion foot, frost bite & general hypothermia.

(b) Light
Poor illumination.
- Acute – Eye strain, headache, eye pain, lacrymation, congestion fatigue.
- Chronic – Miner's mystagmus.

Excessive brightness or glare.
- Discomfort, visual fatigue, blurring of vision, accidents.

(c) Noise
Auditory effect.
Non-auditory effect.

(d) Vibration
Frequency range – 10-500 Hz
Use of drills & hammers
Spasm of fingers.
Injuries to hands, elbow & shoulders.

(e) Ultraviolet radiation
Arc welding
Effects – conjunctivitis, keratitis.

(f) Ionizing radiations
X-rays
Radio active isotopes
Dial of watches & other instruments.
Manufacturing of radio active paints.
Effects – Genetic changes, cancer, malformation, leukaemia, depilation, ulceration, sterility & even death.

Chemical hazards
  (i) Dust
  (ii) Gases
  (iii) Metal & their compounds
  (iv) Chemicals
  (v) Solvents

Biological hazards
  Caused by :
  (i) Fungal infection
  (ii) Parasites
  (iii) Bacteria
  (iv) Virus, etc.

Mechanical hazards
  (i) Injuries.
  (ii) Accidents.

Psychosocial hazards
  Seen in form of :
  (i) Industrial neurosis.
  (ii) Hypertension
  (iii) Peptic ulcer, etc.

Occupational Diseases

Pneumoconiosis

It is the deposition and retention of inorganic dust in the lungs and the subsequent tissue reaction.

Important factors in the development of pneumoconiosis are :
  (i) Amount of dust retained in lung.
  (ii) Concentration of the substance in the air.
  (iii) Duration of exposure to the substance.
  (iv) Effectiveness of clearance mechanisms.
  (v) Size and shape of the particles (1-5 mm get to alveoli - larger particles are filtered in upper airways).
  (vi) Chemical nature and solubility of the substance.
  (vii) Individual susceptibility of the host.

Occupational Health

General clinical features
- An insidious onset.
- A long latency period between the exposure and expression of the disease.
- Irreversible and usually progressive clinical course.
- No effective treatment.

Diagnosis of Pneumoconiosis
(i) Detailed history like occupation, hobbies and nearby industries.
(ii) Light microscopy and polarised light microscopy.
(iii) Scanning electron microscopy (example silica) energy dispersive X-ray analysis elemental composition.

High temperature ashing, micro incineration, enzymatic digestion, or chemical digestion.

Silicosis

It is caused by Silica or silicon dioxide.

The crystalline forms are toxic. Different forms are :
- quartz
- cristoballite
- tridymite

It is commonly seen in :
(a) Mining or quarrying – gold, silver, nickel, tin, copper, sandstone, granite, slate, asbestos, iron, coal, uranium, mica, graphite or clay.
(b) Steel foundry work.
(c) Stone cutting, polishing and carving.
(d) Sandblasting.

Pathogenesis of Silicosis

Macrophages ingest silica particles, this the first step in the pathogenesis of silicosis. Silica particles are toxic to the macrophage and injure the macrophage releasing the silica particle as well as fibrogenic factors.

SiOH groups on the surface of the silica particles or bonds with membrane proteins and phospholipids. This leads to denaturation of membrane proteins and damage to the lipid membrane and as a result fibrosis occurs and the silica particles are re-ingested, damaging more macrophages. This results in a silicotic nodule with the most of the silica particles at the periphery of the nodule and fibrosis in the center.

Clinical Classification

1. **Simple silicosis** – Features are :
   - Fine mottling on x-ray.
   - Small nodule in lung (e.g. - show fibrosis and polarizable material in silicotic nodule).
   - Often have hilar lymph node enlargement with egg shell calcification.
2. **Complicated silicosis (progressive massive fibrosis)** – Features are :
   - Conglomerate masses > 2 cm in diameter.
   - Obliterate & contract large amounts of lung.
3. **Silicotuberculosis**
   Central cavitation with progressive massive fibrosis (PMF) occurs in it.
4. **Accelerated silicosis (Acute silicosis)**
   Here proteinaceous filling of alveoli after heavy exposure occurs.
5. **Mixed dust pneumoconiosis**
   It is stellate interstitial fibrosis with mixture of silica and another dust, usually iron oxide.

Clinical Course of Silicosis

- Asymptomatic – Usually the patients are asymptomatic and the nodules are picked up by a routine x-ray.
- Progressive massive fibrosis – Person may become breathless when this complications develops or may develop cor pulmonale (right sided heart failure).

2. **Coal Worker's Pneumoconiosis (CWP)**
   (i) Simple CWP.
   (ii) Complicated CWP (Progressive massive fibrosis).
   Diagnosis is made by X-ray changes occurring in lungs.

Pathology

The three main findings are :

(i) **Coal macule** – accumulation of coal dust with minimal fibrosis in wall or respiratory bronchiole 1-2 mm in size.

(ii) **Coal nodule** – little larger than coal macule.

(iii) **Focal emphysema** – seen around coal macule usually due to smoking, has rarely been seen in non-smokers.

Clinical features

Pulmonary symptoms of dyspnea are :
- most often due to cigarette smoking not due to simple CWP.

Importance of simple CWP
- It is the precursor of Progressive massive fibrosis (this is the lesion that causes pulmonary symptoms).

Complicated Coal Worker's pneumoconiosis (Progressive Massive Fibrosis)

Definition

A large are of fibrosis occurring in a coal miners that is by X-ray > 2 cm in diameter.

Incidence

- It occurs in 0.1% of coal miners.

Following factors are associated with an increased risk of developing complicated coal worker's pneumoconiosis (PMF).
- Tuberculosis
- Presence of silica
- High total dust content
- Immunologic factors e.g. rheumatoid arthritis.

3. Asbestosis

Asbestos is a family of crystalline hydrated silicates with fibrous geometry (length 3X > width)

Characteristics of asbestos

- Strong, flexible, resistant to acid and heat and durable.
- Small size to enter small airways and travel to subpleural areas of the lower lung fields.

Naturally occurring types

(i) Serpentine (curly and flexible) e.g. – chrysolite (most commonly used).

(ii) Amphiboles (straight and more rigid).

　　(a) Crocidolite (most fibrogenic) It is banned now.

　　(b) Amosite.

　　(c) Anthophyllite.

Exposure

Occupational exposure in :

- Asbestos cement products like sheets, corrugated, roofing, gutters, drain pipes, etc.
- Vinyl tiles.
- Insulation or fire protection in construction or shipbuilding (often sprayed).
- Textiles – especially fire resistant.
- Asbestos paper products.
- Insulation layers or pads, wall coverings, engine gaskets, roofing felts, etc.
- Brake linings and clutch facings.

Environmental exposure in :

- Proximity to mines or factories.
- Domestic exposure (to the clothings worm in mines).

Clinical types

- *Pleural plaques* – Here benign, bilateral, symmetical, fibrous thickening of parietal pleura occurs.
- *Malignant mesothelioma* – It is a lethal malignant tumor arising from pleura.
- *Asbestosis* – There is a diffuse interstitial fibrosis.
- *Lung carcinoma* – All types of lung carcinoma can occur.

Deaths due to Asbestos Exposure

- 7-12% from asbestosis.
- 11% from malignant mesothelioma up to 50% from lung cancer.

Berylliosis
- Seen in 40's.
- It is used in fluorescent light bulbs.
- Now used in nuclear and aero space industry.
- Light weight, high melting point, tensile strength, excellent alloying properties, ability to show nuclear fission.

Pathology
Pathologically it is a granulomatous disease that looks like sarcoidosis.

Clinically – Diffuse interstitial pneumonitis occurs in 50% of cases and nodular, hyaline, fibrotic lesions (40%).

Occupational Cancers
Some of the most common types of cancer seen are :
1. *Lung Cancer*

   Industries – asbestos industry, nickel and chromium manufacturing units, industries producing poly aromatic hydro carbons.
2. *Cancer Bladder*

   Industries – rubber industry, dye-industries, etc. possible carcinogens involved are benzidine, para amino diphenyl, auremine, etc.
3. *Skin Cancer*

   Industries – oil refineries, dye-industry, tar distilleries. Possible carcinogens involved are tar, X-rays, dyes etc.
4. *Leukemia*

SICKNESS ABSENTEEISM
One of the major health problems of industrial world. It provides information about the worker's state of health which includes physical, mental and social health.

The problem of sickness absenteeism is on rise, at present it is around 20-25%.

Causes
(i) *Medical* – Due to ill health the worker is unable to perform his duties. It can be due to occupational diseases, accidents, etc.

(ii) *Social* – The worker has many social and familial obligations, which he has to fulfill. e.g. – marriages, death, festivals, etc. As a result increase in the rate of sickness absenteeism.

(iii) *Economic* – As per ESI regulations each worker is entitled to cash benefits in case of sickness, in order to avail those benefits he tends to take sick leave.

(iv) *Alcoholism, Addictions* – They are an important cause of absence from work place. The worker tends to neglect his work obligations.

Prevention

1. By use of Ergonomics.
2. Improved managerial set up, practises.
3. Diagnosis and treatment of diseases.
4. Healthy working environment.

OCCUPATIONAL HEALTH

General health services

Scope : Include all type of employment.

e.g. – Mercantile and commercial enterprises, service trades, forestry and agriculture etc.

Aims –   Promotion.
            Prevention.
            Protection.

The placing and maintenance of the worker in an occ. env. adapted no his physical and psychological health. (the adaptation of work no man and of each man to his job)

Occupational Environment

1. Physical, chemical and biological agents.
2. Machines.
3. Man.

PREVENTION OF OCCUPATIONAL DISEASES

The General Conference of the International Labour Organisation 1953 gives following measures for protection of worker's health (Protection of Worker's Health Recommendation, 1953).

(I) Medical Measures

1) *Pre-placement Examination*

They are very important in prevention of occupational diseases. At the time of employment a complete *history* – past, family, occupational, personal, social. Clinical examination, lab. tests and various other investigations like X-rays, ECG, urine and blood examination, are the various components of a pre placement examination.

A very important part is looking for the qualifications the job demands in the candidate. The candidate should fulfill the requirements for the job or simple *'Right Man in the Right Job'*.

The basic principle of *Ergonomics* i.e. "To achieve best mutual adjustment of man and his work for the improvement of human efficiency and well-being" is always kept in mind. It is not desirable to employ workers suffering from some disorder which can get worsened e.g. in lead industry it is not wise to employ person having nephritis, high blood pressure, anaemia etc.

2) *Periodic Medical Examination*

They are done for detecting as early as possible signs of a particular occupational disease or of special susceptibility to that disease. It should be kept in mind what all risks and in which circumstances medical examinations should be carried out. They should be carried out by a qualified physician who should possess knowledge of occupational health. They should include investigations like chest X-rays, blood and urine examination, etc.

3) *Medical and Health Care Services*

They are provided as per the ESI regulations. At the site of work facilities for first aid and emergency treatment in case of accident, occupational disease, poisoning should be available and provided.

4) *Notification of Occupational Diseases*

Various legislations like Factories Act, 1976, Mines Act 1952 makes the notification of cases and suspected cases of occupational diseases necessary. Under Factories Act, 1976 some 22 diseases are there in the notification list Notifications are required with a view to –

(a) Initiate measures of prevention and protection and ensuring their effective application.

(b) investigation of working conditions and other circumstances which have caused or are suspected to have caused occupational diseases.

(c) Compilation of statistics of occupational diseases.

(d) Allow the initiation or development of measures designed to ensure that victims of occupation diseases receive the compensation provided for such diseases.

5) Providing Healthy Working Environment

It is done by periodic inspection of the working place, looking for various aspects of working environment like ventilation, air temperature, humidity, space available per worker, floor space, air pollution, etc. These factors are very important in determining the state of health at work place. They should be always be in such state so, as to provide healthy working environment.

6) Maintenance and analysis of Records

They are necessary for planning and development of occupation health services. All the records should be containing information about the basic health status of worker, past illnesses, sick leaves, any addictions, etc.

7) Health Education

To all the workers in order to take care of their health. Use of protective devices.

(II) TECHNICAL MEASURES

These measures should be taken by the employer to ensure that the general condition prevailing in the place of work are such to provide adequate protection of the health of the workers concerned.

(1) Proper designing of work place

(2) Providing safe working conditions

(a) Dirt and refuse should not be allowed to accumulate.

(b) The floor space and height of work rooms should be sufficient to prevent *overcrowding*.

(c) Adequate and suitable lighting should be provided.

(d) Suitable atmospheric conditions, to avoid insufficient air supply and movement, sudden temperature changes, harmful draughts, excessive humidity, cold, heat, odours, etc.

(e) Sufficient and suitable sanitary conveniences should be available like washing facilities, safe and whole some drinking water.

(f) Measures should be taken to eliminate or reduce as far as possible noise and vibrations which constitute a danger to the health of workers.

(3) Substitution

To substitute harmless or less harmful substances, processes or techniques for harmful substances, processes or techniques.

(4) Containment

Preventing the liberation of harmful substances and to shield workers from harmful radiation.

(5) Isolation

It is carrying out of hazardous processes in separate rooms or buildings.

(6) Enclosure

Hazardous processes are carried out in enclosed apparatus so as to prevent personal contact with harmful substances and escape into the air of the work room of dusts, fumes, gases fibres, mist or vapours, in quantities liable to injure health.

(7) Exhaust Ventilation

Removal, at or near their point of origin, by means of mechanical exhaust ventilation systems of harmful dusts, fumes, gases, fibres, mists or vapours.

(8) Personal Protection

Use of protective clothing, equipment and other means of personal protection. They are necessary to protect the health of the workers by shielding them from the effects of harmful agents. All the method of use should be explained to worker.

(9) Periodic Monitoring

The atmosphere of work rooms in which dangerous or obnoxious substances are manufactured, handled or used should be tested periodically at sufficiently frequent intervals to ensure that toxic or irritating dusts, fumes, gases, etc. are not present in quantities liable to damage health. i.e. following the 'permissible limits'.

(10) Newer Techniques Developments

Efforts should be made in the direction of developing newer techniques which provide protection to the health of the worker e.g. new safer machines, treatment, etc. Research should be given importance for that matter.

(III) Legislative Measures

Various laws, acts all there to safe guard the health of the worker. Some important ones are :

(1) Factories Act, 1948.
(2) ESI Act, 1948.
(3) The Mines Act.

The employees State Insurance (ASI) Act, 1948

The promulgation of Employees' State Insurance Act, 1948 envisaged an integrated need based social insurance scheme that would protect the interest of workers in contingencies such as sickness, maternity, temporary or permanent physical disablement, death due to employment injury resulting in loss of wages or earning capacity The act also guarantees reasonably good medical care to workers and their immediate dependents.

Following the promulgation of the ESI Act the central government set up the ESI corporation to administer the scheme. The Scheme, thereafter was first implemented at Kanpur and Delhi on 24th February 1952. The act further absolved the employers of their obligations under the Maternity Benefit Act, 1961 and Workmen's Compensation Act 1923. The benefit provided to the employees under the act are also in conformity with ILO conventions.

Administration

The *Employees' State Insurance Scheme* is administered by a Corporate body called the *Employees' State Insurance Corporation (ESIC)*, which has members representing employers and *employees of the Central Government, State Governments, medical profession* and *the Parliament.*

A *Standing Committee* constituted from among the members of the corporation acts as the executive body for the administration of the scheme.

There is also a *Medical Benefit Council* to advise the Corporation on matters connected with the provision of medical benefit.

The director general who is the chief executive of the corporation is also ex-officio member of the corporation and of its standing committee.

Besides the headquarters office in New Delhi, the corporation has 17 eegional offices and 5 sub-regional offices at Pune, Nagpur, Coimbatore, Madurai and Hubli and 844 local offices and cash offices all over the country for the administration of the scheme.

The medical care under the scheme is administered by state governments, who have the statutory responsibility in this regard, except in Delhi and Noida, area of U.P. Besides, the ESI Hospital, K.K. Nagar at Chennai, ESI hospital, Thakurpukur at Kolkata and ESI hospital at Nagda are also being run directly by the corporation.

The Standing Committee

The Standing Committee is the statutory executive organ of the Corporation. The members are drawn from the main body of the Corporation by nomination and election. The nominated members include three members from each of the central government and state governments. Further, three members each representing employers and employees and one each representing parliament and the medical profession are elected from amongst the members of the Corporation through a voice vote. Secretary, ministry of labour, government of India functions as the chairman of the standing committee. Director general, ESI corporation is also an ex-officio member of the standing committee.

The Standing Committee is vested with powers to administer the affairs of the corporation, exercise any of the powers and perform any functions of the corporation subject to the overall control and superintendence of the corporation. Standing committee is also empowered to constitute any non-statutory sub-committees for specific purposes as the need be.

Medical Benefit Council (MBC)

Medical benefit council is an advisory body on matters related to the administration of medical benefit under the ESI Scheme. The council is constituted by the central government for a specific term and consists of :

1. Director General, Central Health Services (ex-officio Chairman).
2. Deputy Director General/Addl. Director General, Central Health Services.
3. One member each representing respective state governments.
4. Three members each representing employees, employers and the medical profession.
5. Medical Commissioner, ESI Corporation (ex-officio member).

The ESI Act empowers the medical benefit council to advise the corporation on matters related to developments and improvements in the medical service delivery system.

Benefits under the ESI Scheme
(a) Medical Benefit.
(b) Sickness Benefit (SB).
  (i) Extended sickness Benefit (ESB).
  (ii) Enhanced sickness Benefit.
(c) Maternity Benefit (MB).
(d) Disablement Benefit.
  (i) Temporary disablement benefit (TDB).
  (ii) Permanent disablement benefit (PDB).
(e) Dependant's Benefit (DB).
(f) Funeral Expenses.
(g) Rehabilitation Benefits.
  (i) Rehabilitation allowance.
  (ii) Vocational Rehabilitation.

Existing feature of the ESI Scheme is that the contributions are related to the capacity as a fixed percentage of the workers wages, whereas, their are social security benefits according to individual needs without distinction.

Benefits are disbursed by the Corporation through its local offices LOs/mini local offices (MLOs)/sub local offices SLOs)/pay offices, subject to certain conditions.

the scheme also provides some other need based benefits to insured Includes :
  (i) Rehabilitation allowance.
  (ii) Vocational rehabilitation.

Type of Medical Benefits Provided

The Employees' State Insurance Scheme provides full medical care in the form of medical attendance, treatment, drugs and injections, specialist consultation and hospitalization to insured persons and also to members of their families where the facility for specialist consultation, hospitalization has been extended to the families.

For the families, this benefit has been divided into two categories as under :

Full Medical Care

This consists of hospitalization facilities and includes specialist services, drugs and dressings and diets as required for in-patients.

Expanded Medical Care

This consists of consultation with the specialists and supply of special medicines and drugs as may be prescribed by them in addition to the out-patient care. This also includes facilities for special laboratory tests and X-Ray examinations.

Apart from the curative services provided through hospitals and dispensaries, the corporation also provides the following facilities including family welfare services.

Immunization

The corporation has embarked upon a massive programme of immunization of young children of insured persons. Under this programme, preventive inoculation and vaccines are given against diseases like diphtheria, pertusis, polio, tetanus, measles, mumps, rubella, tuberculosis, etc.

Family Welfare Services

Along with the immunization programme, the Corporation has been undertaking provision of family welfare services to the beneficiaries of the scheme. The corporation has organized these services in 180 centres besides reserving 330 beds in hospitals for undertaking tubectomy operations. So far, 828976 sterilization operation viz. 176197 vasectomies and 652779 tubectomies have been performed upto 31.3.1999. The ESI corporation has also extended additional cash incentive to insured persons to promote acceptance of sterilization method by providing sickness cash benefit equal to full wage for a period of 7 days for vasectomy and 14 days for tubectomy. The period for which cash benefit is admissible is extended beyond the above limits in the event of any complications after family planning operations.

Supply of Special Aids

Insured persons and members of their families are provided artificial limbs, hearing aids, and artificial appliances like spinal supports, cervical collars, walking calipers, crutches, wheel chairs and cardiac pace makers as a part of medical care under the scheme.

Sickness Benefits

Sickness Benefit represents periodical cash payments made to an IP during the period of certified sickness occurring in a benefit period when IP requires medical treatment and attendance with abstention from work on medical grounds. Prescribed certificates are; Forms 8, 9, 10, 11 & ESIC-Med. 13. Sickness benefit is roughly 50% of the average daily wages and is payable for 91 days during 2 consecutive benefit periods.

Qualifying Conditions

(i) To become eligible to sickness benefit, an IP should have paid contribution for not less than 78 days during the corresponding contribution period.

(ii) A person who has entered into insurable employment for the first time has to wait for nearly 9 months before becoming eligible to sickness benefit, because his corresponding benefit period starts only after that interval.

(iii) Sickness benefit is not payable for the first two days of a spell of sickness except in case of a spell commencing within 15 days of closure of earlier spell for which sickness benefit was last paid. This period of 2 days is called "**waiting period**". This provision should be clearly understood by IMOs/IMPs as actual experience shows that such of IPs who want to avail medical leave on flimsy grounds generally come for first certificate/first & final certificate within 15 days of earlier spell, usually on unpaid holidays and/ or on each weekly off etc. to avoid loss of benefit for 2 days due to fresh waiting period.

Sickness Benefits

Extended Sickness Benefit.
Enhanced Sickness Benefit.

Extended Sickness Benefit (ESB)

IPs suffering from long diseases were experiencing great hardship on expiry of 91 days sickness benefit. Often they, though not fit for duty, pressed for a final certificate. Hence, a provision for paying sickness benefit for an extended period (Extended Sickness Benefit) of upto 2 years in a ESB period of 3 years.

1. An IP suffering from certain long term diseases is entitled to ESB, only after exhausting sickness benefit to which he may be eligible. A common list of these long term diseases for which ESB is payable, is

reviewed by the corporation from time to time. The list was last reviewed on 5.12.99 and revised provisions of ESB became effective from 1.1.2000 and at present this list includes 34 diseases which are grouped in 11 groups as per International Classification of diseases and the names of many existing diseases have been changed as under :

I. Infectious Diseases
1. Tuberculosis
2. Leprosy
3. Chronic Empyema
4. AIDS

II. Neoplasms
5. Malignant Diseases

III. Endocrine, Nutritional and Metabolic Disorders
6. Diabetes mellitus with proliferative retinopathy/diabetic foot/ nephropathy.

IV. Disorders of Nervous System
7. Monoplegia
8. Hemiplegia
9. Paraplegia
10. Hemiparesis
11. Intracranial space occupying lesion
12. Spinal cord compression
13. Parkinson's disease
14. Myasthenia gravis/Neuromuscular Dystrophies.

V. Disease of Eye
15. Immature cataract with vision 6/60 or less
16. Detachment of retina
17. Glaucoma

VI. Diseases of Cardiovascular System
18. Coronary Artery Disease :
    (a) Unstable Angina
    (b) Myocardial infraction with ejection less than 45%
1. Congestive heart failure – Left, Right
2. Cardiac valvular diseases with failure/complications

3. Cardiomyopathies
4. Heart disease with surgical intervention alongwith complications.

VII. Chest Diseases
5. Bronchiectasis
6. Interstitial lung disease
7. Chronic obstructive lung diseases (COPD) with congestive heart failure (Cor Pulmonale).

VIII. Diseases of the Digestive System
8. Cirrhosis of liver with ascites/chronic active hepatitis.

IX. Orthopaedic Diseases
9. Dislocation of vertebra/prolapse of intervertebral disc.
10. **Non-union** or **delayed-union** of fracture.
11. Post Traumatic Surgical amputation of lower expremity.
12. Compound fracture with chronic osteomyelitis.

X. Psychoses
13. Sub-group under this head are listed for clarification
    (a) Schizophrenia
    (b) Endogenous depression
    (c) Manic depressive psychosis (MDP)
    (d) Dementia

XI. Others
1. More than 20% burns with infection/complication.
2. Chronic Renal Failure
3. Reynaud's disease/Burger's disease.

1. In addition to the above list, Director General/Medical Commissioner are authorised to sanction ESB for a maximum period upto 730 in cases of rare but treatable diseases or under special circumstances, such as, adverse reaction to drugs which have not been included in the above list, depending on the merits of each case, on the recommendations of RDMC/AMO or either authorised officers running the medical scheme.

2. To be entitled to the extended sickness benefit, an insured persons should have been in continuous employment for 2 years or more at the beginning of a spell of sickness in which the disease is diagnosed and should also satisfy other contributory conditions.

3. ESB shall be payable for a period of 124 days initially and may be extended up to 309 days in chronic suitable cases by Regional Dy. Medical Commissioner/Medical Referee/Administrative Medical Officer/Chief Executive of the E.S.I. Scheme in the State or his nominee on the report of the specialist(s).

Enhanced Sickness Benefits

It was introduced w.e.f. 1.8.1976 as an incentive to IPs/IWs for undergoing Vasectomy/Tubectomy. Insured persons eligible to ordinary sickness benefit are paid enhanced sickness benefit at double the rate of sickness benefit i.e., about full average daily wage for undergoing sterilisation operations for family welfare. Duration of enhanced sickness benefits is upto 7 days in the case of vasectomy and upto 14 days in the case of the tubectomy from the date of operation or from the date of admission in the hospital as the case may be. The period is extendable in case of post operative complications.

Maternity Benefit

Maternity benefit is payable to an insured woman in the following cases subject to contributory conditions :

- Confinement-payable for a period of 12 weeks (84 days) on production of Form 21 and 23.
- Miscarriage or Medical Termination of Pregnancy (MTP) – payable for 6 weeks (42 days) from the date following miscarriage – on the basis of Forms 8, 10 and 9.
- In the event of the death of the insured woman during confinement leaving behind a child, maternity benefit is payable to her nominee on production of Form 24 (B).
- Maternity benefit rate is double the standard benefit rate, or roughly equal to the average daily wage.

Dependent's Benefit (DB)

The dependents' benefit is payable to the dependents as per section 52 of the act read with provision 6(A) of section 2 in cases where an IP dies as result of EI. The age of dependents, has to be determination either by production of :

- Documentary evidence as specified in regulation 80(2) or
- Age certified by medical officer in charge of government hospital or dispensary.

- The minimum rate of DB w.e.f 1.1.90 is Rs. 14/- per day and these rates of the DB are increased from time to time.

Funeral Expenses

Funeral expenses not exceeding Rs. 1500/- is payable towards expenditure on the funeral of a deceased IP and persons in receipt of periodical payments of PDB.

CHAPTER-14

GENETICS AND HEALTH

Heatlh is a homeostatic condition of the organism in the enviornment. This homeostasis in the form of normal blood pressure, cholesterol level, glucose level, blood molarity, etc. is enclosed by genes.

Genetics is a branch of science dealing with study of heredity and inherited characters.

Causative Factors of Disease
- Social and ecological factors.
- Enviornmental factors.
- Genetic factors.

Predisposition of a person for a disease is determined by phenotype of individual or community.

Gene in Population
- Gene is a unit of heredity.
- It is a specific tiny structure existing in pairs in chromosomes.
- Both useful and deterious genes are present.
- There are about 100,000 structural human genes.
- Alternate forms of a gene are called allele.

Hardy Weinberg Equilibrium :

$$p + q = 1$$

where p = Frequency of A

q = Frequency of a

- Chance that a person will draw anyone of Aa, AA or aa depend on frequency of A unit in gene pool.
- Relative proportion of 3 posible combination will be :

$$p^2 (AA) + 2 pq (Aa) + q^2 (aa)$$

- It is possible to calculate the frequency of heterozygotes in population.

Disturbance of Hardy Weinberg Equilibrium
1. Non random mating
   - Preferential mating (like with like).
2. Selection
   - Mutant allele less likely to pass on to the next generation since its possessor is less likely to have children.
   - selection against recessive alleles is much less effective due to presence of normal genes in carrier.
   - Prenatal counselling has decreased the chance of occurence of mutant genes.
3. Mutation
   - Its ratio is 1 in 1 lakh.
   - It helps in the ability of the species to adopt changing enviornment.
   - Longer is the time elapsed, greater is the likelihood of mutations.

Mutation Rate (MR)
- Dominat disorders : Number of individuals with dominant disorders who don't have family hostory of disease, there,
   MR = (1 − Fitness) × Disease frequency.
- Recessive disorders.
- Survey for mutation rate is difficult due to :
   * Logistic difficulties.
   * Death before assessment.
4. Heterozygous advice − Genes harmful in homozygous state are helpful in carrier state.
5. Geneti drift. − People migrate to new region and may develop new diseases.

INCIDENCE & PREVALENCE
- Only mortality recorded based on I.C.D. or hospital admission.
- Population or hospital based registrations.
- Computerised record linkage in case of siblings and family.
- Monogenic and single gene defect found in early age, causes heavy burden and are relatively difficult to treat.

Genetics and Health

- Multifactorial are more enviornment related and less severe, however burden is more.

Conception to Birth
- 50%-70% pregnant women fail to produce live born babies.
- 50% spontaneous abortion mainly in 1st trimester due to chromosomal abnormalities.

Infancy to Young Age
- 7-9% of population less than 25 years of age have genetic diseases including congenital abnormalities.
- Enviornmental conditions are controlled to some extent.

Middle to Late Age
- Incidence of multifactiorial disorders.
- More than 60% including diabetes mcllitus, hypertension, myocardial infarction, ulcer, thyrotoxicosis, cancer, etc.
- Likely to be enviornmental determinant.

Categories of Genetic Diseases
1. Chromosomal disorders
   - 1 in 200 live birth.
   - Error in chromosomes e.g. deletion, addition, duplication, etc.
   - 6% of still births.
2. Autosomal dominant
   - 1500 autosomal dominant inherited and 1100 are suspected.
   - e.g. Achondroplasia, Huntington's disease, malformation, polycystic kidney, Tuberous sclarosis, etc.
3. Autosomal recessive
   - 600 known and 800 suspected.
   - e.g. Phenylketonuria, Albinism, Taysach's, etc.
4. X-linked dominant
   - Known disorders are less than 100.
   - e.g. Alport's Syndrome, familial hypophosphataemia, etc.
5. X-linked Recessive
   - More than 100 disorders known.
   - e.g. Haemophilia, Hunter Syndrome, etc.
6. Mitochondrial disorder
   - Always inherited from female.

- Mutation in mitochondrial gene can lead to phenotypic defects.
- e.g. Leigh disease, MELAS (mito chondrial encephalopathy, lactose acidosis and stroke like syndrome).

7. Multifactorial disorders
    - It is due to interaction between enviornment and genes.
    - 1 in 20 individuals are affected.
    - e.g. spina bifida, anencephaly, hypertension, diabetes mellitus, schizophrenia, alzheimer's disease, etc.
    - They can have genes which determine whether external influence will result in illness.

8. Non-inherited genetic disorders.
    - e.g. AIDS, ageing, cancer, radiations, etc.

PREVENTIVE MEASURES

1. Health Promotion.
    a) Eugenics : To improve genetic endorsement of human population which can be negative or positive.
        - Negative – e.g. Hitler improved his racetuinking it to be superior.
        - Positive – Mixing people; selection for betterment, e.g. U.S.A. – Getting good breeds & allowing them to settle down.
    b) Euthenics : Improving the envoirnment and genetic interaction by selective manipulation of the enviornment. e.g. mentally retarded can improve their I.Q. by good enviornmental stimulation.

2. Genetic Counselling
    - Face to face communication by which ine can help the person to make decisions and act on them.
        * Prospective : Prediction of problem in family.
        * Retraspective : e.g. after first child abnormality, aims to prevent genetic disorders.

3. Early Diagnosis & Treatment.
    - Prenatal diagnosis.
        * Examination of amniotic fluid.
        * Chrionic villi sampling.
        * Ultrasonography.
        * Culture foetal cells.

- Treatment
    * Termination of pregnancy.
    * Diet improvement.
    * Anti hemolytic globulin.
    * Surgery.
4. Rehabilitation.
5. Disease limitation.
    - Surgical correction.

Genetic Counselling

It is a process of communication which deals with the human problem associated with a genetic disease in the family.
- Helps the person to make decision & act on them.
- Aim is to provide counselling with complete understanding of genetic disease and or problems as posible and all options.
- Psychological support to those already affected.
- For decision making.

Pre-requisite of Physicians for Genetic Counselling :
- Sound knowledge of disease.
- Expertise in genetic counselling.
- Ability to communicate people in simple language with adequate allotment of time, care and sensitivity to the concerned person.
- Must have knowledge of important options.
- Have empathy i.e. warmth, care, sympathy, understanding and insight into the human condition.
- Sensitive to parental guilt.

Guiding Principles :
- Accurate diagnosis.
- Non-directive counselling.
- Concern for individuals.
- Informed counselling.
- Truth in counselling.
- Confidentiality and trust.
- Timing of counselling.
- Duty to convey information about known options.

- Counselling education.
- Duty to re-contact.
- Do not harm.

Indications for Pre-conception Genetic Counselling
- Advanced age.
- Previous fetus or child with genetic disease.
- Infertility history.
- Family history of genetic disease.
- Parental carriers of genetic disease.
    * Ethnic groups where genetic carriers may be present are African (Black), American, European, Japanese, etc.
- Aggravation of genetic disease.
    * E.g. worsening of pulmonary status in cystic fibrosis.
- Consanguinity.
    * Handicapped & Mental retardation in 5-8% of consanguinous couples.
- Enviornmental exposure.
    * Exposure to medication.
    * Illicit drug use.
    * Alcohol, smoking.
    * Mercury, lead, copper exposure.
    * Infection (TORCH).
    * Chemotheraphy.
    * Maternal illness during pregnancy.

LEGAL PROTECTION
1. M.T.P (1971) Act.
2. Prenatal diagnosis technique (Regulation and Prevention of Misuse Act, 1994) – If any abnormality is detected then can go to genetic clinic or medical genetist, gynaecologist (supervised by supreme court).
3. Equal opportunity, protection of rights and full participation Act, 1995 – for person with disabilities. There are more than 6 crore disabled in India.

CHAPTER-15

SOCIAL SCIENCE AND MEDICINE

Social science plays an important role in maintaining health. There is a wide difference in morbidity and mortality between :
- Urban & rural.
- Rich and poor.
- Developed & developing.
- Non-communicable and communicable disease.

Studies under social science are :
- Sociology.
- Social/Cultural anthropology. ⎫ Behavioural science
- Social Psychology. ⎭
- Economics.
- Political science.

Sociology – It deals with knowledge of social institution in state, organised structures, causes and types of varieties of these and social acts and social relationship.

Society – It is not only collection of people but also has commnunication of mental level as aims, aspiration, values and need.

Origin of Society :

- Basic instincts — Hunger and sex are bringing people together.
    * Hunger gives rise to individual survival.
    * Reproduction gives rise to survival as species.
- Living together in same enviornment.
- Having similar activities.
- Biological multiplication.

All of these lead to :
- Establishment of biological network.

- Social institution for physical & mental mutual relations.
- Sense of security.
- Formation of society.

Mile stones in development of society of man are :
1. Attainment of position and law enforcement.
2. Development of thumb with circumserial movement.
3. Development of brain (practice perfection).
4. Nourishment (Breast feeding).
5. Control of fertility (decreased infant birth).
6. Acculturation.
   - Addition of experiences.
   - Development of values.
   - Transfer to coming and next generation.
   - Man becomes a social animal.
   - Man learns from other's experiences.
   - Plans for future.
   - Past experiences.

TYPES OF SOCIAL RELATIONSHIPS

Primary
- People live in defined area.
- Feeling of spontaneity and freedom.
- Husband & wife.
- Parents & child.
- Generally seen in villages.

Secondary
- Duration of contact is short.
- Seen in cities.
- Limited knowledge of each other.
- Feeling of external is always present.
- Formal relations like Doctor patient, customer shopkeeper, author reader, esp. professional groups.
- They are formed due to needs like :
  * Geographical closeness.
  * Solving the problem.
  * Reduce tension.

* Wants to achieve goals.
* Co-operation.
* Some common things in regions.
* Idiology.
* Life-styles.
* Occupations.

TYPES OF RELATIONSHIPS

- Temporary and short – People come for short time or for discussion.
- Small and permanent – Villages, family.
- Big and temporary – People coming for rally/movies.
- Large and permanent – Metropolitan cities.

COMMUNITY

A sociological unit of individual who came together for common interest of satisfying their day to day needs of :

- Geographical demand.
- Sharing common culture.
- Self reliant and specific social structure.

Types

- Rural.
- Urban.
- Urban agglomeration.
- Standard urban area.
- Tribal.

City

It has continuous out growth but within boundaries.

Local factors for outgrowth of cities are :

- Enonomic status.
- Literacy.
- Occupation.
- Knowledge, attitude and practice, belief, culture.
- Values.
- Habits and health status.
- Social stigma.
- Poor accessibility and utilization of services.
- Rural degradation and discrimination.

Impact of balanced Social Development

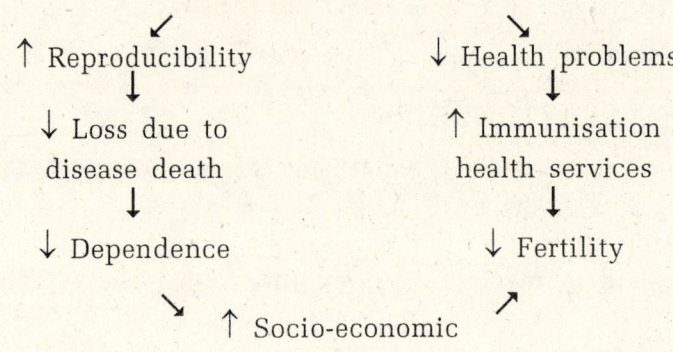

Note : ↑ – Increased
↓ – Decreased

Socio economic classification by Kuppuswami

It takes into consideration 3 factors :
- Education.
- Occupation.
- Income (per capita/per month)

Various levels in education, occupation and income are assigned a particular level and on summing the 3 factors the total score is used in finding the appropriate socio economic class.

Kuppuswami Classification

Education	Occupation	Income (Per capita/month)
Professional degree - 7	Professional - 10	> 800 - 12
B.A./B.S.C./B.Com. - 6	Semi prof. - 6	> 400-799 - 10
Intermediate - 5	Shop owner - 5	> 300-399 - 6
High school - 4	Skilled worker - 4	> 200-299 - 4
Middle school - 3	Semi skilled worker - 3	> 120-199 - 3
Primary/Literate - 2	Unskilled - 2	> 40-199 - 2
Illiterate - 1	Unemployed - 1	< 40 - 1

Total Score

I	Upper class	26 - 29
II	Upper middle class	16 - 25
III	Lower middle class	11 - 15
IV	Upper lower class	5 - 10
V	Lower class	< 5

CHAPTER-16

MENTAL HEALTH

Health is multidimensional and mental aspect is one of the important dimension of the health. Mental health is not mere absence of mental illness. Good mental health is the ability to respond to the many varied experiences of life with flexibility and a sense of purpose. Mental health has been defind as "a state of balance between the individual and the surrounding world, a state of harmony between oneself and others, a coexistence between the realities of the self and that of other people and that of the enviornment."

Psychologists have mentioned the following characteristics as attributes of a mentally healthy person :

a) A mentally healthy person is free from internal conflicts; he is not at "war" with himself.
b) He is well-adjusted, i.e., he is able to get along well with others. He accepts criticism and is not easily upset.
c) He search his identity.
d) He has a strong sense of self esteem.
e) He knows himself, his need, problems and goals (this is known as self-actualization).
f) He has good self-control and balances rationality and emotionality.
g) He faces problems and tries to solve them intelligently i.e., coping with stress and anxiety.

It has been discovered by recent researches that psychological factors can induce all kinds of illness, not simply mental ones, e.g. essential hypertension, peptic ulcer and bronchial asthma. Some major mental illnesses such as depression and schizophrenia have a biological component. It has been infered that there is a behavioural, psychological or biological dysfunction which results in deranged mental equilibrium.

MENTAL ILLNESS

- It affect all age groups.
- 1 : 5 youths of less than 15 years of age suffer from mild to severe disease.
- 17 % of students suffer from anxiety in final year of secondary school.
- In every 40 seconds, one suicide occurs.
- Unipolar depression, bipolar depression, obsessive compulsive disorder and schizophrenia are among 10 leading causes of disability in 1990.
- 10% of school children in Alexandria, Egypt suffer from mental illness.
- The number of mental disorder cases can be reduced on early diagnosis and proper treatment.

Characteristic Features

1. Disturbance in body functions :
   a) Sleep.
   b) Appetite & food intake.
   c) Bowel and bladder movement.
   d) Sexual desire and activity.
2. Changes in mental function :
   a) Behaviour.
      - Irritation, overactive, excitement.
      - Abusive, quarrelsome.
      - Dull, non-active.
      - Funny movements.
   b) Talk and thought.
      - Talkative, mute.
      - Irrelevant, incoherent.
      - Peculiar wrong belief.
      - Delusions (crawling worms, poisoning, etc.).
   c) Emotions
      - Elations.
      - Inappropriate to situation.
      - Laughing, weeping, talking to self.

d) Perception (Disturbance in understanding various stimuli).
- Hallucinations.
  * Sound
  * Light
  * Sight.

e) Memory
- Lose.
- Forgetful.
- Disorientation.
- Difficulty in recognizing.

f) Intelligence and judgement
- Loses reasoning skills.
- Makes mistakes.
- Dull.

g) Level of consciousness.
- Disturbed in brain damage.
- Disorientation to time and place.

3. Changes in individual and social activities :

a) Individual.
- Neglect proper hygiene, clothing, etc.
- Soils clothes, bed, etc.

b) Social
- Lacks participation in social function.
- Embarass others.
- Behaves rudely, abusive, assault, etc.

Types of Mental Illness

1. Severe (Psychoses)
   - Schizophrenia.
   - Maniac depressive psychoses.
   - Organic psychoses.
2. Minor
   - Neurosis.

3. Others
   - Mental retardation.
   - Childhood behavioural problems.
   - Epilepsy.

PSYCHOSIS

Abnormal behaviour.

A) Functional Psychoses

(i) Schizophrenia
   - It is the commonest psychosis.
   - It generally prevails in age group 15-25 years.
   - It is precipitated by stress.
   - It may be hereditery.
   - Person lives in a dream world of his own.

Clinical Features
- Abnormal thinking, perceptions and emotions.
- Delusion – Firmly believed ideas.
- Hallucination – Perceive imaginary voice, image, etc.
- Sad, apathetic, talks to self.
- Sleep disturbance.
- Excitement.

Aetiology
- Multifactorial.
- Hyper sensitive, 'dopamine' system.

Management
- Listen patiently.
- Remove restrains.
- Healthy and proper diet.
- Keep harmful weapons out of reach.
- Family counselling.
- Reassurance.

(i) Episodic happiness and sadness.
- Increased motor ability, talkative, increased irritability under maniac phase.
- Apathy, lack of interest, etc. under depressive phase.
- Insomnia.
- Suicidal ideas.
- Poor appetite.
- Constipation.

B) Organic Psychoses

There is presence of structural damage.
- Disorientation, poor comprehension and poor calculation.
- Memory deficit.
- Emotional liability.
- Self neglect.
- Delirium.
- Dementia.
- Decreased intellectual function, memory and judgement.
- Commonly seen in Alzheimer's disease., T.B., Syphilis, B_{12} deficiency, etc.

NEUROSIS

Person is unable to react normally to life situation.
- Depression.
- Anxiety.
- Sexual neurosis.
- Somatoform disorder.
- Dissociative conversion disorder – Typical sysmptoms of illness without organic pathology are :
    * Paralysis.
    * Fits.
    * Vomitings.
    * Hiccough.
    * Difficult breathing.
    * Does not injure himself.
    * Stressful events.

CAUSES OF MENTAL ILL HEALTH
- Changes or diseases of brain.
- Hereditary factors.
- Stress and strain.
- Social factors.
- Unhappy childhood.
- Unhappy family life.

In India about 6% of population suffer from behavioural problems.

CONTROL

Primary
- Provision of careing and educative atmosphere of development through parents, teachers, etc.
- Youth – Welfare for :
    * Counselling.
    * Information.
    * Employment.
- Social Welfare
    * Literacy compaigns.
    * Poverty alleviation.
- Family life education.
    * Care and support.

Secondary
- Early diagnosis and treatment.
- Child guidance.
- Points to identify are :
    * Excitement, violent behaviour, socially unacceptable manner.
    * Talk excessively or not at all.
    * Express bizarre somatic symptoms.
    * Stopped working without reasons.
    * Talks about one's own life.
    * Complains of plan to be killed by someone.
    * Sleep disturbance for few weeks.
    * Stopped taking into rest in his own hygiene.

NEUROSIS CONTROL

Reduce the duration of mentals illness.

- Day care programme.
  * To improve social skills.
- Half way homes.
  * Short stay homes.
  * For support and guidance.
- Self help tips.
  * For mentally retarded people.
  * Parents share their experiences at training centres.
- Family service programme.
  * Counselling.
  * Home care.
- Industrial therapy centres
  * Work as per capacity.
- Vocational training centres.

Homoeopathic approach

Hahnemann considers mental diseases as one-sided diseases of the chronic type affecting the whole psycho-somatic entity. He discussed mental diseases in Organon's aphorism 210 to 230.

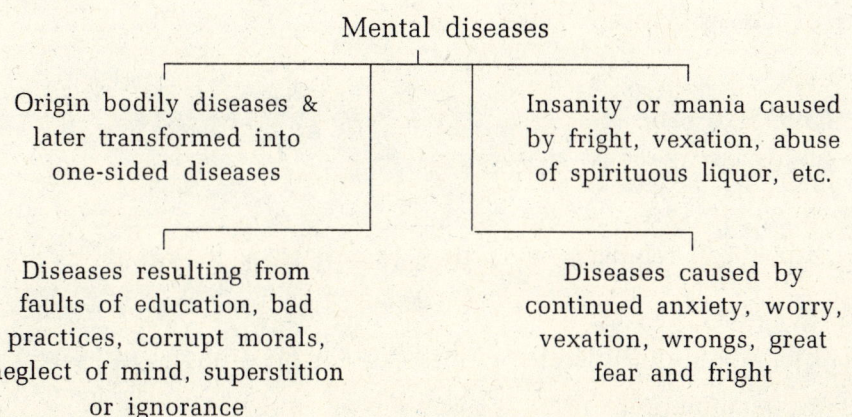

According to symptoms similarity medicines which can be considered are Acon., Arg-n., Hyos., Bell., Ign., Nat-m., Nux-v., Puls. Sil., Staph., Stram., Thuj., Verat., etc.

NATIONAL MENTAL HEALTH PROGRAMME

It was launched in 1995. It operated in 22 districts only.

Objectives
- Ensure availability and accessibility of mental health care.
- Incorporate mental health in general health care.
- Promote community participation.
- Implement training of doctors and paramedical staff.

Services
- Treatment of neurosis and psychosis.
- Rehabilitation.
- Health education.

ALCOHOLISM AND DRUG ABUSE

Drug is defined as "any substance that when taken into the living organism, may modify one or more of its functions" (WHO). Drug abuse is defined as self-administration of a drug for non-medical reasons, in quantities and frequencies which may impair an individual's ability to function effectively and which may result in social, physical, or emotional harm.

Types of Drug Abuse

1. Too much :
   - Excessive use.
   - Increased frequeny of sedatives.
2. Too long :
   - Drug taken regularly more than required e.g. Pethidine.
3. Wrong use :
   - Drug used other than prescribed e.g. Phenobarbitone in epilepsy.
4. Wrong combination :
   - Barbiturates and alcohol may cause death.
5. Wrong drug :
   - Illegal drug usage e.g. heroin, brown sugar, etc.

Reasons for Drug Abuse

1. Curiosity for experimentation.
2. Emotional pressure :
   - Insecurity.
   - Boredom.
   - Relieve tension.
   - Anxiety.
3. Social pressure :
   - Regards for elders, stars, singers etc.
4. Group pressure.
5. Availability.
6. Previous use.
7. Dependence.

Identifications of durg Abuses

1. Academic changes :
   - Poor concentration.
   - Declining performance.
2. Physical changes :
   - Loss of appetite.
   - Insomnia.
   - Weight loss.
   - Temper tantrums.
   - Puffy eyes.
   - Sweaty night.
   - Slurred speech.
   - Red eyes.
   - Injection sites.
3. Withdrawal symptoms.
4. Others :
   - Poor hygiene.
   - Bad stains on clothes.
   - Syringes/needles.
   - Stealing.

CRITERIA FOR SUBSTANCE DEPENDENCE

Maladaptive pattern or distress during twelve months.
1. Tolerance :
   - Need for increased amount.
   - Decreased effect with same amount.
2. Withdrawal :
   - Distress.
3. Substance intake in larger amount for longer period than intended.
4. Persistent desire, unsuccessful attempt to cut down.
5. Extra time spent in activities to obtain substance.
6. Social, occupational and recreational activities decreased.
7. continuous intake despite knowledge of adverse effects.

DIAGNOSTIC CRITERIA FOR ALCOHOLISM

Intoxication :
1. Recent in gestion.
2. Maladaptive behaviour.
3. One or more episodes.

Alcohol Withdrawal :
1. Symptoms after cessation of heavy prolonged use of alcohol.
2. Two or more symptoms/sign within hours or days :
   a. Increased hand tremor.
   b. Insomnia.
   c. Nausea, vomiting.
   d. Transient visual, tactile, auditory hallucinations or illusions.
   e. Psychomotor agitation.
   f. Anxiety.

Aetiology :
1. Genetic factors.
   - Aldehyde dehydrogenase deficiency.
2. Personality disorders.

3. Easy availability, social acceptance of use.
4. Recurrent/chronic anxiety/depression.
5. Recurrent/chronic physical problems.
6. Underlying mental disorders.
7. Family, occupational stress.

Homoeopathic efficacy

Homoeopathic medicines which proved to be efficacious are Agar., Aur., Chin., Crot-h., Lach., Nux-v., Ran-b., Sel., Sut-ac., Sulph., Syph., Tub., Verat., Zinc., etc.

Prevention

A. Primary

1. Legal approach
   - Narcotic drugs and psychotropic substances.
   - Control over production.
   - Restriction/prohibition of advertisements.
   - Anti smoking measures.
   - Dry states.
2. Community approach.
   - Community participation.
   - Youth clubs to compaign against use of drugs.
   - Prohibition of liquor shops.
   - Surveillance.
   - Counselling for youth.
   - Encouragement of recreational activities.

B. Secondary

- Identifications.
- Treatment.
   * Detoxification.
   * Counselling, follow up.
   * Changes in enviornment.
   * Psychotherapy.
   * Mobilise social support, family support.

- Referral.
    - Severe withdrawal symptoms.
    - Severe mental, physical problems.
    - Presence of psychiatric symptoms.
    - severe delirium tremens.
    - Korsakoff's Wernick's encephalopathy.

C. Tertiary
- Rehabilitation
    - Vocational training.
    - Employment programmes.

CHAPTER-17

BIOSTATISTICS

Biostatistics is a statistical method used in planning, collection, compilation, analysis & interpretation of data in the field of medicine, biology & public health.

Uses of Biostatistics

1. To find out normally existing rates of biological processes.
2. To find out the effectiveness of vaccines, drugs etc. by using control studies.
3. To find out the rate of vital events like mortality, morbidity, natality in a population with respect to time.
4. To compare two populations regarding a particular attribute to check if it is real or just a chance occurrence.
5. To evolvise the utilization of various health core facilities.
6. To find out the achievements of various public health programmes.
7. They help in planning implementation and evaluation of public health programmes.

Sources of Data

1. Experimental data from various lab experiments.
2. Health surveys, epidemiological investigations.
3. Records of vital events, hospital records, etc.

Types of Data

It can be various types like quantitative, qualitative, chronological etc.

1. **Quantitative data** – It can be measured numerically. It has a range & certain limits, units, etc.
2. **Discrete data** – when distinct, finite values are taken.
   e.g. – no. of children in family, pulse, B.P.

3. **Continuous data** – Take any value & in a specific interval.
   E.g. – height, weight, temperature, B.P. etc.
4. **Chronological data** – Data pertaining to specific information over a period of time.
   E.g. – variation in rate of growth of population.

There is also another classification which describes two types of data :

1. **Primary Data** – Obtained directly from the individual e.g. Census.
2. **Secondary Data** – Obtained from sources other than the individual e.g. hospital data.

PRESENTATION OF STATISTICAL DATA

After collection the data needs to be sorted out and presented properly for analysis and interpretation. They can be presented using various tables and diagrams like tables, charts, diagrams, graphs, pictures etc.

The diagrams suitable to different types of data are :

I. For quantitative data – histogram, ogive, frequency polygon.

II. For qualitative data :
   (a) Bar diagram.
   (b) Pie diagram.
   (c) Line diagram (shows trend of events).
   (d) Percentage (to study relative importance of components parts of total figure).
   (e) Scatter diagram (to study the relationship black & white 2 quantitative characters).
   (f) Age-sex pyramid (to depict age-sex pattern of community).
   (g) Spot map (to know distribution of events geographically).

Tabulation

One of the simplest means of data presentation. There are 3 types of tables in use.

(1) Simple table

Only one attribute is shown, the frequency of events is small. Easy to understand.

E.g. Table-1 showing health problems during pregnancy.

Table-1 Health problems during pregnancy

Among births during the three years preceding the survey, percentage of mothers experiencing specific health problems during pregnancy by residence, India, 1998-99

Problem during pregnancy	Total
Night blindness	12.1
Blurred vision	21.8
Convulsions not from fever	14.3
Swelling of the legs, body, or face	26.3
Excessive fatigue	43.4
Anaemia	26.5
Vaginal bleeding	3.5
Number of births	32,393

Source : NFHS-2.

(2) Master table

It is a table used to record all the initial readings in a serial wise manner. It becomes very important in the presence of large number of observations with several attributes.

(3) Frequency Distribution Table

Here data is first sorted out into small manageable groups (class intervals) and the small number of events or items (frequency). It is of two types, depending on the data to be presented.

(i) Frequency table for qualitative data here the characteristic is fixed but frequency various e.g.

Table-2 showing assistance during delivery as per NFHS-2.

Table-2 Assistance during delivery

Percent distribution of births during the three years preceding the survey by attendant assisting during delivery, according to selected background characteristics, India, 1998-99

Background characteristic	Attendant assisting during delivery[1]						Total percent	Number of births
	Doctor	ANM/ nurse/ midwife/ LHV	Other health professional	Dai (TBA)	Other	Missing		
Place of delivery								
Public health facility	70.6	28.6	0.1	0.3	0.4	0.0	100.0	5,247
NGO or trust hospital/ clinic	82.7	17.3	0.0	0.0	0.0	0.0	100.0	234
Private health facility	87.2	12.3	0.1	0.2	0.2	0.0	100.0	5,409
Own home	4.7	6.3	0.8	53.4	34.7	0.0	100.0	17,224
Parents' home	9.3	9.4	1.4	50.7	29.3	0.0	100.0	3,945
Other[2]	6.3	10.5	0.0	27.6	25.3	30.3	100.0	333
Total	30.3	11.4	0.6	35.0	22.4	0.3	100.0	32,393

(ii) Frequency distribution table for quantitative data
— Here both characteristic and frequency varies e.g. the following figures are the Hb level in gm% of a class. Construct a frequency distribution table with class interval of 1 gm%.
8, 8.5, 11.6, 11.2, 12.5, 11.4, 8.9, 10.1, 11.2, 8.9, 10.5, 11.6, 12.1, 12.5, 14.8, 9.6, 10.2, 11.6, 11.2, 14.1, 12.4, 8.6, 9.4, 13.2, 14.4, 11.4, 13.9

Hb level in gm%		Frequency (no. of students)
8.0 – 9.0	℟℟	5
9.0 – 10.0	11	2
10.0 – 11.0	111	3
11.0 – 12.0	1111 111	8
12.0 – 13.0	℟℟	4
13.0 – 14.0	11	2
14.0 – 15.0	111	3

Charts and Diagrams

(1) Bar Charts

Bar charts properties :
1. Easy to prepare.
2. Values can be compared visually.
3. Proper class intervals are present.

Types

(i) Simple Bar Chart
— The bars are separated by appropriate space.
e.g. simple bar chart for problems during prenancy (from NFHS-2)

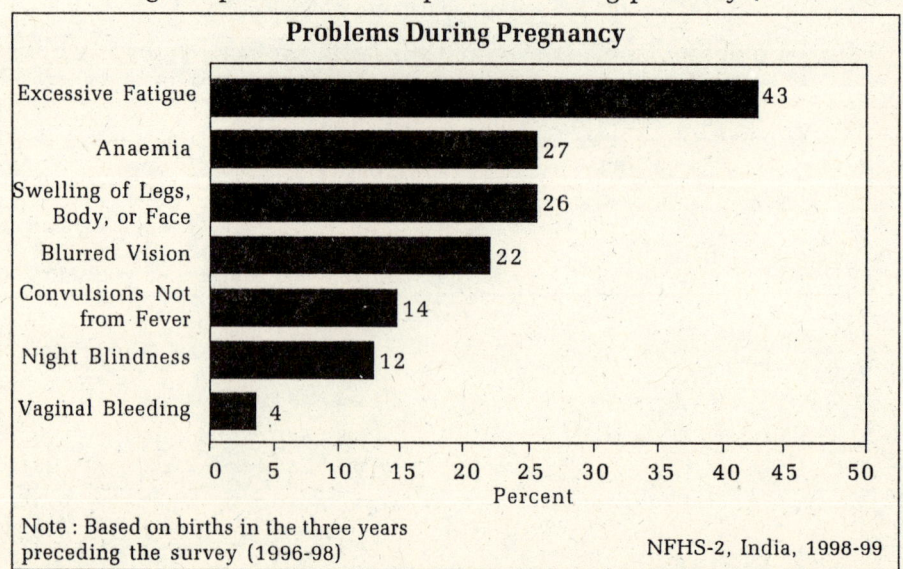

Note : Based on births in the three years preceding the survey (1996-98)
NFHS-2, India, 1998-99

(ii) *Multiple Bar Chart*
– Here two or more bars can be together, helps in easy comparision.

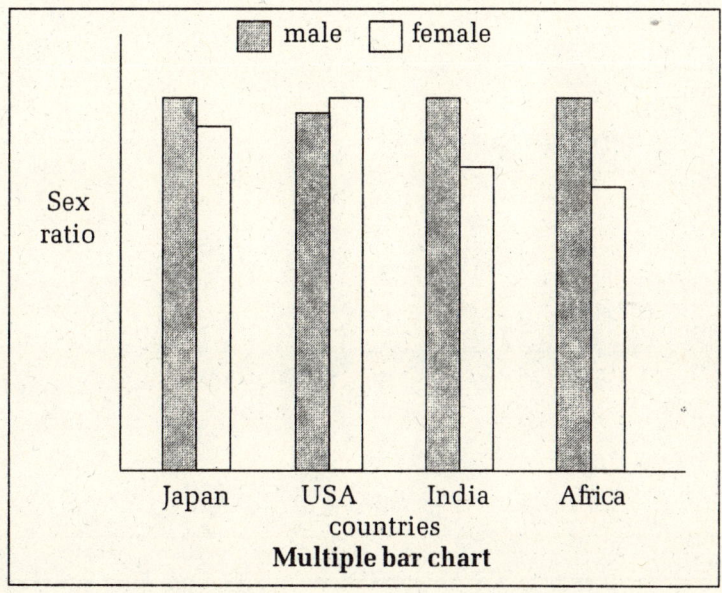

Multiple bar chart

(iii) *Component bar chart*
– bars are divided and each part represents the magnitude or the item.

(2) Histogram

Haemoglobin level in gm%	No. of students
8.0 – 9.0	8
9.0 – 10.0	14
10.0 – 11.0	28
11.0 – 12.0	95
12.0 – 13.0	42
13.0 – 14.0	18
14.0 – 15.0	5

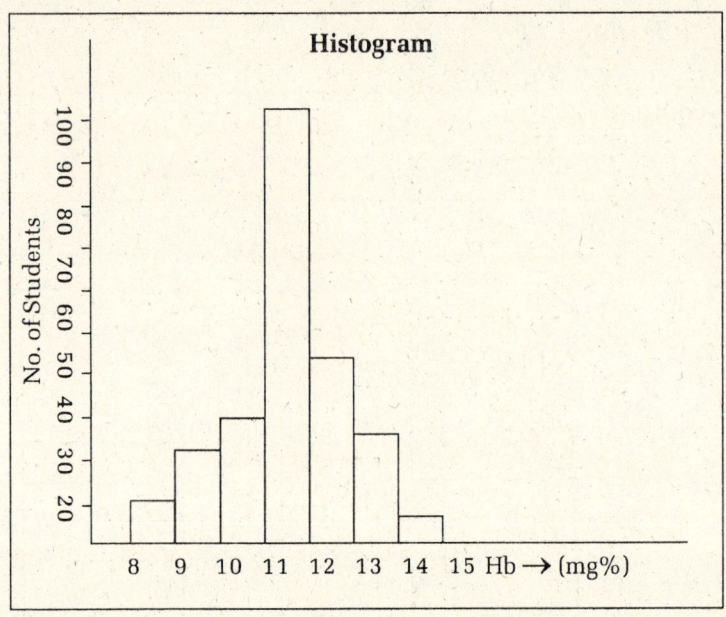

(3) Line Diagram

E.g. Draw a line diagram to show the IMR in rural and urban area.

Year	1971	1976	1981	1985	1991	1992	1993	1994	1995	1996
Total	129	129	110	97	80	79	74	74	74	72
Rural	138	139	119	107	87	85	82	80	80	78
Urban	82	80	62	59	53	53	49	52	48	46

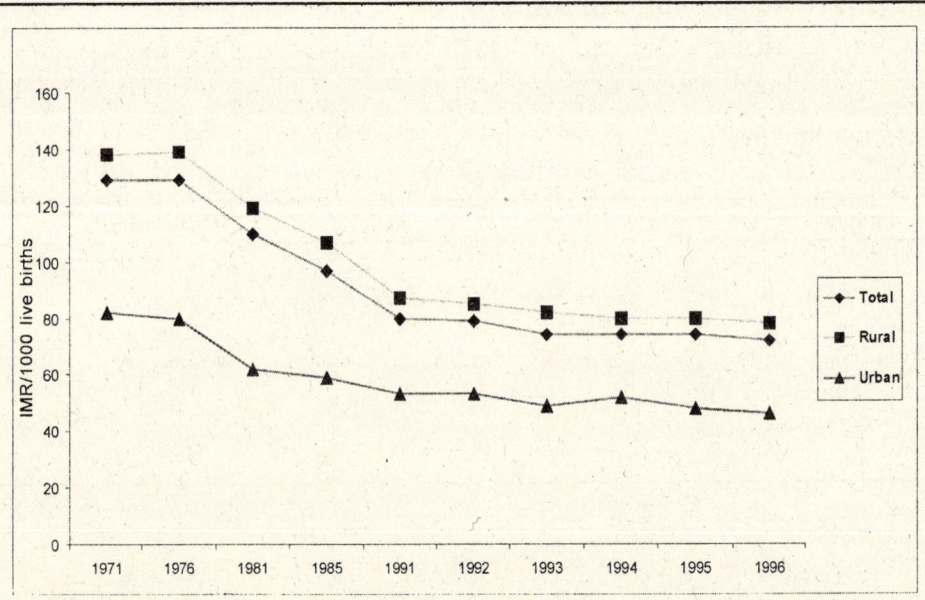

(4) PIE Charts

Different sectors of a circle represent various items, that can then be compared.

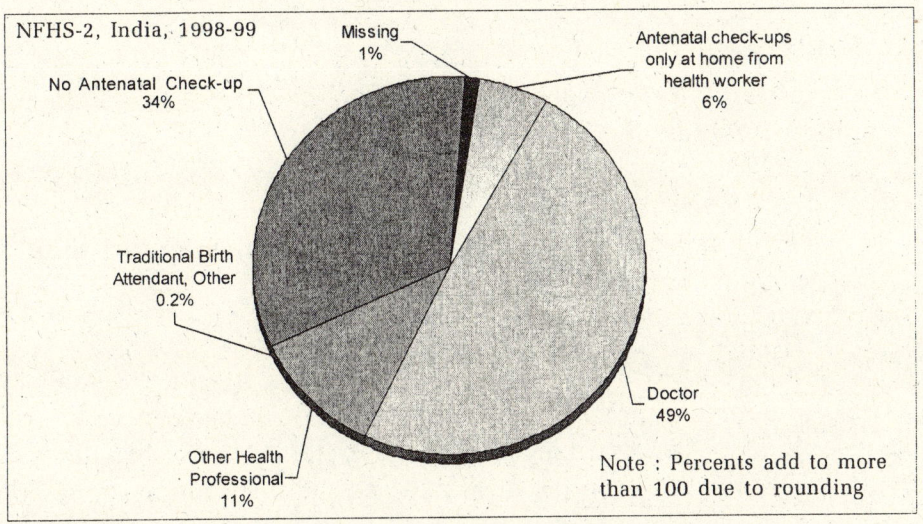

Source of Antenatal Check-Ups During Pregnancy

STATISTICAL AVERAGES

Central tendency indicates a representative or typical value of a whole set of observations around & most values aggregate.

Different methods to measure central tendency are :
(i) Arithmetic Mean
(ii) Median
(iii) Mode

Mean

It is the most useful of all statistical means. But it is influenced by the extremes of values in the data i.e. it is unduly influenced by abnormal values in the distribution. Thus, it is used when the variations in the values are not very large.

It is denoted by a symbol $\bar{x}$.
It is obtained by adding all the values
i.e. $x_1 + x_2 + x_3 \cdots x_4$ also expressed

as σ representing 'summation'. The summation is divided by number of values denoted by

So, Arithmetic mean for $\bar{x} = \frac{\Sigma x}{\eta}$ ungrouped data.

$= \frac{\Sigma fixi}{\Sigma fi}$ for grouped data.

Geometric mean = antilog $\left[\frac{1}{n}\Sigma \log xi\right]$

It is easy to calculate & observe. All observations are considered.

Median

The value of middle observation when data is arranged in the ascending or descending order of magnitude.

Median of grouped data = $\frac{lc + N/2 - Fc}{F\ median} \times lc$

lc = lower boundary of median class (the class interval in & cumulative frequency lies).

Fc = cumulative frequency preceding median class.

Median is sometimes preferable to mean as it is unaffected by abnormally large or small observations. It does not take each value into consideration. It does not depend upon the total & number of items. It is more representative than the mean if a skewed distribution is present.

Mode

It is the commonly occurring value in the distribution of data. It is easy to understand & is not affected by extreme items.

The selection of appropriate measure of central tendency depends on nature of data & purpose of enquiry if no decimals are required (mode), extreme values.

The advantage of mode is that it is easy to understand & is not affected by extreme items. But the exact location is uncertain quite often and not clearly defined. Thus, it is not often used in biological or medical statistics.

E.g. serum albumin levels of 20 pre school children are given below.
2.90, 3.57, 3.73, 3.55, 3.72, 3.88, 2.98, 3.61, 3.75, 3.45
3.71, 3.76, 3.84, 3.30, 3.38, 3.76, 3.61, 3.0, 3.45, 3.76
calculate mean, mode, median

Σx = Sum of all values
 = 70.71 mg%

n = No. of children
 = 20

Mean $\bar{X} = \frac{\Sigma x}{\eta} = \frac{70.71}{20}$

$= 3.54$ g%

Median = 2.9, 2.98, 3.0, 3.30, 3.38, 3.45, 3.45, 3.55, 3.57, 3.61, 3.61, 3.71, 3.71, 3.72, 3.73, 3.75, 3.76, 3.76, 3.76, 3.88.

The value occurring in the middle after placing in ascending order is 3.61 so, median is 3.61 g%.

Mode = Most commonly occurring value i.e. 3.76 (frequency is 3).

MEASURES OF DISPERSION

Definition

Dispersion is the variation with in a group for a particular data.

It is measured by the following :

(i) Range
(ii) Mean deviation
(iii) Standard deviation.

(i) **The Range** – It is the difference between the highest and lowest values in a given sample.

(ii) **The Mean Deviation** – It is the average deviation from the arithmetic mean given by simple formula

$$M.D = \frac{\Sigma (x - \bar{x})}{\eta}$$

(iii) **The Standard Deviation** – It is the root means square deviation. It is represented by sigma 'σ' (S.D). It is given by

$$\sigma = \sqrt{\frac{\Sigma (x - \bar{x})^2}{\eta}}$$

if < 30 then

$$\sigma = \sqrt{\frac{\Sigma (x - \bar{x})^2}{\eta - 1}}$$

e.g. – Diastolic blood pressure measures of three groups having 10 patients in each group are given below.

Groups

A 70, 86, 86, 86, 90, 90, 94, 98, 100

B 70, 84, 85, 86, 87, 93, 95, 99, 100

C 70, 85, 85, 86, 94, 95, 100, 100, 100

Calculated the mean, median, mode, range, average deviation and standard deviation of the above data. Compare them and state in which ground diastatic pressure is more homogeneous.

We have to calculate the deviation from mean as follows :

Group A

x	$\bar{x}$	x - $\bar{x}$	(x - $\bar{x}$)²
70	88.89	18.89	356.8321
86	88.89	2.89	8.3521
86	88.89	2.89	8.3521
86	88.89	2.89	8.3521
90	88.89	1.11	1.2321
90	88.89	1.11	1.2321
94	88.89	5.11	26.1121
98	88.89	9.11	82.9921
100	88.89	11.11	123.4321
800	88.89	55.11	616.8889 ≅ 617

Mean = 800/9 = 88.89
Median = 90
Mode = 86
Range = 100-70 = 30

Mean distribution = $\dfrac{\Sigma(x-\bar{x})}{\eta}$ = 55.219 = 6.12

$$SD = \left(\dfrac{(x-\bar{x})^2}{x-1}\right)^{1/2} = \left(\dfrac{617}{9-1}\right)^{1/2} = 8.78$$

Group B

x	$\bar{x}$	x - $\bar{x}$	(x - $\bar{x}$)²
70	88.7	18.7	349.69
84	88.7	4.7	22.09
85	88.7	3.7	13.69
86	88.7	2.7	7.29
87	88.7	1.7	2.89
93	88.7	4.3	18.49
95	88.7	6.3	39.69
99	88.7	10.3	106.9
100	88.7	11.3	127.69
799	88.7	63.7	687.61

Mean $= \bar{x} = \dfrac{\Sigma x}{\eta} = \dfrac{799}{9} = 88.7$

Median = 87
Mode = not applicable
Range = 100−70=30

Mean distribution $= \dfrac{63.7}{9} = 7.07$

SD $= (687.61/9.1)^{½} = 9.3$

Group C

x	$\bar{x}$	x−$\bar{x}$	(x−$\bar{x}$)²
70	90.7	20.7	428.49
85	90.7	5.7	32.49
85	90.7	5.7	32.49
86	90.7	4.7	22.09
94	90.7	3.3	10.89
95	90.7	4.3	18.49
100	90.7	7.3	86.49
100	90.7	7.3	86.49
100	90.7	7.3	86.49
815	90.7	72.3	804.41

Mean = 815/9 = 90.7
Median = 94
Mode = 100
Range = 100−70=30
Mean deviation = 72.3/9 = 8.033

SD $= (804.41/9 - 1)^{½} = (100.55)^{½} = 10.02$

Comments

Mean deviation & standard deviation increases from group A to C, while arithmetic means are B < A < C.

Homogenous distribution is found in group A (minimum SD).

Coefficient of Variation

Coefficient of variation is relative measure of dispersion

$= \dfrac{SD}{x} \times 100$

It is used when values are measured in different units used → to compare when data shows more variation and to compare 2 different data & different means 2 + SD.

e.g. – Data given below are the measurement of contain organ at autopsy of Indian males, ages 21-30 years. Find the coefficient of variation for all.

	No.	Mean	Range	S.D
Height (cm)	30	164.6	142 – 100	7.64
Weight (kg)	30	43.2	22 – 55	7.48
Brain (g)	14	1317	1100 – 2355	296.0
Heart (G)	30	249.5	110 – 1000	150.0
Liver	30	1200	540 – 2500	376.0

Coefficient of variation = $\dfrac{SD}{X} \times 100$

Height (cm) = coefficient = $\dfrac{7.64}{164.6} \times 100 = 4.64\%$

Weight (kg) = coefficient = $\dfrac{7.48}{43.2} \times 100 = 17.3\%$

Brain (g) = coefficient = $\dfrac{296}{1317} \times 100 = 22.4\%$

Heart (g) = coefficient = $\dfrac{450}{249} \times 100 = 60.2\%$

Liver (g) = coefficient = $\dfrac{376}{1200} \times 100 = 31.3\%$

Normal Distribution

Normal distribution or normal curve is a smooth symmetrical curve of frequency distribution & narrow class intervals. Its shape depends upon number & nature of observations.

In a normal curve % area is represented by

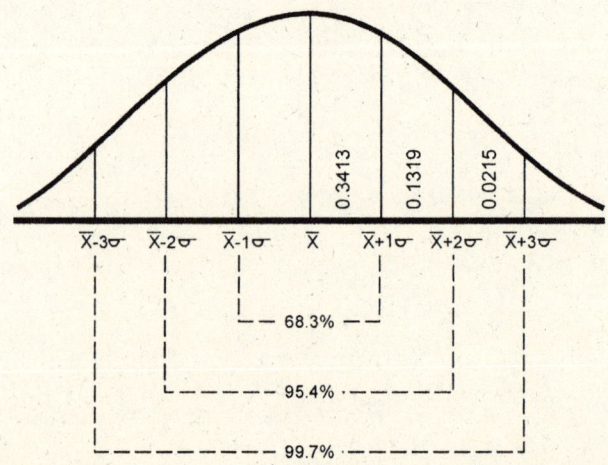

i) $\bar{x} \pm 1SD \to 68.3\%$
ii) $\bar{x} \pm 2SD \to 95.4\%$
iii) $\bar{x} \pm 3SD \to 99.7\%$

Serum calcium of healthy adult persons in a urban area is normally distributed with a mean 10.0 mg. & S.D 0.5 mg.

(i) What proportion of persons are expected to have serum calcium of 9 to 11 mg.

Proportion of people expected to have Ca^{2+} 9-11 mg% $\to \bar{x} \pm 2SD = 10 \pm 2\,(0.4) = $ 9-11 mg%

∴ 95.4% of people are expected to have 9-11 mg% levels.

SAMPLING

Sampling methods – (i) Simple random sampling.
(ii) Systematic random sampling.
(iii) Stratified random sampling.
(iv) Cluster sampling.

Simple Random Sampling

It is done in such a way that each unit has an equal chance of being drawn in a sample. It provides the greatest number of possible samples.

e.g. – To select 26 students out of 75, each is assigned a number. A table of random numbers is used to determine units which are to be included in sample.

Systematic Random Sampling

This is a method of selecting every unit at a particular sampling interval. Each unit in a sampling frame has same chance of being selected but number of possible sample is greatly reduced.

Patients are numbered 1st. A number is selected at random, at a sampling interval.

e.g. Select 8 leprosy patients out of 24 patients from O.P.D register.
First find out the sampling interval 24/8 = 3
∴ Every 3rd patient is selected, starting from say 2.
∴ 2, 5, 8, 11, 14, 17, 20, 23.

Stratified Random Sampling

The sample is deliberately drawn in a systematic way so that each portion of the sample represents a corresponding strata. This is known as stratified sampling. It is useful when one is interested in analysing data by certain characteristics of populations. It is used for heterogenous population. Population is first divided into strata on the basis of characteristics & in the strata population (age, sex, education), then samples are selected randomly from each strata independently account to proportion by any type of sampling method.

i.e. $xi = \dfrac{x}{N} \times Ni$, where

xi = sample size in strata
Ni = population size in strata
x = Total sample size
N = Total population size.

E.g. Select 20 families by stratified sampling method for estimating the incidence rate of TB in and serum area where 60 families are residing.

The total families are divided into 2 groups :
(i) families which have ⩾6 members
(ii) families which have < 6 members.

(i) families which have ⩾6 members :
2B, 3, 4, 5B, 5C, 5B, 6A, 6C, 7A, 7B, 8, 11, 12, 14, 16, 17, 18, 19, 21, 23, 24, 25, 26, 27B, 29, 30A, 30B, 31A, 32, 35, 35A, 37B, 38, 40

(ii) families which have <6 members :
1, 2A, 5A, 6B, 7, 10, 13, 20, 21A, 22B, 27A, 28, 30C, 31A, 35B, 39A, 39C, 39D, 39E

In the given study,

x = 20, N = 60, Ni = 38, N= 22

$\therefore x_1 = \dfrac{20}{60} \times 38 = 12.67 \approx 13$

$x_2 = \dfrac{20}{60} \times 22 = 7.33 \approx 7$

Sampling interval = $\dfrac{60}{20}$ = 3.

Random no. = 1

From 1st strata, =>
2B, 5B, 6A, &B, 12, 16, 19, 24, 27B, 30B, 35, 37A, 40,

$\therefore$ from 2nd strata =>
1, 6B, 13, 22B, 30C, 39A, 39D.

Cluster Sampling

Cluster sampling is used from point of view of administrative convenience. The population is divided into recognizable sub-divisions (clusters) based on geographical contiguity & a sample of each cluster is selected. Interview is taken from each & every unit in the cluster.

It is the method of evaluation commonly used for concurrent evaluation of RCH services. This method is used when units of population are natural groups or clusters such as villages, wards, etc. Accuracy is ± 10% and the confidence interval is 95%.

Advantages are :
(i) Less time consuming.
(ii) Affordable.
(iii) Only a small number of target population is sampled.

Under RCH one district/month is covered in each state to ascertain whether facilities are functioning well & used. Out of 30 clusters – from each cluster 7 mothers who had delineced in last 1 year and 7 children 12-23 months of age are surveyed. First house in each cluster is selected randomly.

$$\text{Coverage} = \frac{210}{\text{elegible children of surveyed houses}} \times 100$$

Use :
(1) Real coverage position when significant part of services is provided by private/voluntary bodies.
(2) Also checks the reported performance reflects date for 1 year prior to date of survey.

e.g. of cluster sampling for immunization coverage survey of the children in a area which is divided into 10 blocks, select 4 blocks from that area by cluster sampling methods. Population of the blocks are given below :

Block	Population	Cumulative frequency
1	250	250
2	600	850
3	425	1275
4	375	1650
5	550	2200
6	400	2600
7	300	2900
8	350	3250
9	450	3700
10	300	4000

Sampling interval (S.I) = $\dfrac{4000}{4 \text{ (no. of blocks reqd.)}}$ = 1000

Now, we take a random number & has → no. of digits ≤ those in S.I.

say x = 800

From cumulative frequency table, we find the block & has this no. – ∴ 2nd Block.

Then, we add x + SI = 1800

This lies in 5th block.

Next no. = 1800 + 1000 = 2800

This lies in 7th block

Next no. = 2800 + 1000 = 3800

This lies in 10th block.

2nd, 5th, 7th, 10th blocks are chosen.

Sampling interval = $\dfrac{\text{Total cumulative population}}{\text{No. of pockets (in cluster)}}$

E.g. immunization coverage.

Pilot Survey
- Small scale survey prior to the main survey to obtain information & will facilitate planning.

Advantage
- Aquantaince to the survey technique.

STANDARD ERROR

Standard error is a parameter used to measure error which results from sampling. It indicates how reliable an estimate of the mean is likely to be.

$$S.E = \dfrac{\sigma}{\sqrt{\eta}}$$

σ = std. deviation

η = sample size

It enables us to judge whether the mean of a given sample is within the set confidence limits or not.

Confidence interval

It is constituted by the limits between a multiple of S.D on either side of mean i.e. between 2 confidence limits. It means that area of normal

curve includes the values defined by confidence limits = $\bar{x} \pm 2\sigma$ = 95% of values of distribution are included between the limits $x \pm 2\sigma$
∴ probability of a reading falling outside 95% confidence limits is 5% (1 in 20) → [P = 0.05].

In 1999, a random sample of 1000 men between 40-60 years was selected from a particular community for assessment of CHD. 100 of these men were Aged & CHD. Calculate SE & 95% CI of prevalence of CHD among all men residing here.

SE of population = $\sqrt{\dfrac{pq}{n}}$ where

p = Men with CHD
q = Men with CHD.
n = Sample size.

$$SE = \left(\dfrac{100 \times 900}{1000}\right)^{1/2} = 9.48$$

∵ 95% CI is taken → ∴ 2 S.D are considered.
∴ 95% CI prevalence of CHD = x ± 2S.E
= 100 ± 2(9.48)
= 81 to 119

TESTS OF SIGNIFICANCE

Following are the tests of significance :
(a) Standard error of the mean or simply standard error.
(b) Standard error of proportion.
(c) Standard error of difference.
(d) Standard error of difference between two proportions.
(e) chi - square test.
(f) t - test.

(i) Standard error of proportion = $\sqrt{\dfrac{pq}{n}}$

p, q are proportions

(ii) Standard error of difference between two mean = $\sqrt{\dfrac{\sigma_1^2}{n_1} + \dfrac{\sigma_2^2}{n_2}}$

(iii) Standard error of difference between two proportions

= $\sqrt{\dfrac{p_1 q_1}{n_1} + \dfrac{p_2 q_2}{n_2}}$

CHI – SQUARE TEST (χ^2 test)

It provides a method of testing the significance of difference between two proportions. We can understand it by following a example :

In a clinical trial to assess the value of new method of treatment (A) in comparison with old method (B). Patients were divided at random into two groups of 257 patients treated by method A, 41 died and 244 patients treated by method B 64 died.

Can you draw the conclusion that both methods are equally effective.

Basically for qualitative data we use chi-square test.

Method	No. treated	No. died	No. survived
A	257 (r_1)	41 (c)	216 (a)
B	244 (r_2)	+ 64 (d)	180 (b)
	501 (x)	a50 (c_2)	396 (c_1)

Step 1 : Null hypothesis for chi – square test → No diff. between effect of the 2 methods.

$$x^2 = \frac{(ad-bc)^2}{r_1 r_1 \, c_1 c_2} \times \eta$$

$$= \frac{(216 \times 64 - 180 \times 41)^2}{257 \times 244 \times 396 \times 105} \times 501 = 7.98$$

Step 2 : Degree of freedom = (c-1) (R-1)
C = no. of columns = (2-1) (2-1)
= 1
R = no. of rows

Step 3 : On referring to x^2 table & 1° of freedom the value of x^2 for a probability of 0.05 is 3.84

∴ observed value (7.98) is much higher, the null hypothesis is not valid.

=> method A is superior to method B.

Coefficient of Correlation

$$r = \frac{\Sigma \, (x-\bar{x}) \, (y-\bar{y})}{\sqrt{\Sigma \, (x-\bar{x})^2 \, \Sigma \, (y-\bar{y})^2}}$$

Biostatistics

1. The temperature and pulse rate of 5 patients is as under :

S.no.		1	2	3	4	5
Temperature (F)	x	98	99	100	103	105
Pulse rate	y	72	80	88	96	104

Does any relationship exist between temperature & pulse rate, If yes state what type of relationship is there? Also find the pulse rate if temperature is 100° F.

x = temp., y = pulse

coeff. of corr., $r = \dfrac{\sum(x-\bar{x})(y-\bar{y})}{\left(\sum(x-\bar{x})^2 \sum(y-\bar{y})^2\right)^{1/2}}$

= (-3.2) (-18) + (-2.2) (-10) + (-0.2)(8) + (1.8)(6) + (3.8)(14)

$\div \left[\left((-3.2)^2 + (-2.2)^2 + (-10) + (-0.2)^2 + (-1.8)^2 + (-3.8)^2\right) \right.$
$\left. \left[(-18)^2 + (-10)^2 + 8^2 + 6^2 + 14^2\right]\right]^{1/2}$

$= \dfrac{142}{\sqrt{23616}} = \dfrac{42}{153.5} = 0.93$

since r is near 1, it indicates a strong +ve association between temp. & pulse rate.

Temp. 100°F → pulse rate

$y = \bar{y} + b(x - \bar{x})$ where $b = \dfrac{\sum(x=\bar{x})(y=\bar{y})}{\sum(x-\bar{x})^2}$

$= 90 + \dfrac{142}{32.8} \times (100 - 101.2)$

= 90 − 5.196 = 84.804

∴ If temp. = 100°F, then pulse rate = 85 beats/min.

2. To study the possible association between oral contraceptive use and the occurrence of rheumatoid arthritis (RA) an investigator selected 100 women with a confirmed diagnosis of RA and 200 women undergoing treatment at the same medical facility for other musculoskeletal conditions as subjects. The medical records of all subjects (prior to the date of first diagnosis) were reviewed for evidence of oral contraceptive use. The results are summarized in the table below :

	Rheumatoid Arthritis		
Oral contraceptive use	Present	Absent	Totals
User	40 (a)	120 (b)	160
Non-user	60 (c)	80 (d)	140
Totals	100	200	300

a) What type of study design was employed?
b) Calculate and interpret the OR. Can RR be directly calculated from the results of this study? Why?
c) Is there a statistically significant association between oral contraceptive use and occurrence or rheumatoid arthritis?

a) Case control study (retrospective study).
b) Odds ratio (OR) is measure of strength of association between risk factor & outcome.

$$OR = ad/bc = \frac{40 \times 80}{120 \times 60} = 0.44$$

∴ OC use showed a risk of having RA 0.44 times that of not using it.

Relative risk (RR) cannot be calculated directly from a case control study because it does not provide incidence rates as there is no appropriate denominator or population at risk to calculate these rates. RR can be exactly determined from a cohort (prospective) study.

c) Is there a statistically significant association between OC use & occurrence of RA?

Null hypothesis – No association between OC use and RA occurrence.

$$x^2 = \frac{(ad-bc)^2}{r_1 r_2 c_1 c_2} \times n = \frac{(40 \times 80 - 120 \times 60)^2}{100 \times 200 \times 160 \times 140} \times 300$$

$$= 10.71$$

Degree of freedom = (2-1) (2-1) = 1

Referring to χ^2 table & degree of freedom = 1, value of χ^2 for probability of 0.05 = 3.84

∴ Observed when (10.71) is much higher, null hypothesis is not true.
∴ There is significant association between OC use & RA

Vital & Health Statistics Exercise

Q.1 The maternal mortality rate, infant mortality rate and the Perinatal mortality rate a community having a population of 60,000 were found to be 8, 120 & 65 per thousand live births respectively, considering this mortality to be high, more MCH services were provided in that community. Next year the following data was observed.

(1) Mother's death due to complication of Pregnancy = 9
(2) Death in less than one year age = 180
(3) Death in the first 7 days of life = 58
(4) Birth rate = 30/1000
(5) Still births weighing more than 1000 gms. at birth = 50. Calculate the rates & comment on the effectiveness of MCH services.

A.1 No. of live births = Birth rate × population

$$= \frac{30}{1000} \times 60,000 = 1800$$

1) MMR = No. of maternal deaths/Total no. of live births × 1000

$$= \frac{9}{1800} \times 1000 = 5/100 \text{ live births}$$

2) IMR = Deaths < 1 yr. of age/Total no. of live births × 1000

$$= \frac{180}{1800} \times 1000 = 100/1000$$

3) PMR = Late fetal deaths + early neonatal deaths/×1000
Total live births > 1000 g at birth
= Still births + deaths with in 7 days age/ ×1000
live births + still births

$$= \frac{58+50}{1800+50} \times 1000 = 58.38/1000 \text{ live births.}$$

∴ MMR, IMR, PMR → all decreased from 8→5, 120→100, 65→58.38 per 1000 live births respectively, thereby proving that MCH services in that area are effective.

Q.2 The population of a village according to the census 1981 and 1991 was 15,000 & 21,000 respectively. Estimate mid year population for 1997.

A.2 Census → 1st March

To calculate mid-yr. population :

i) Natural increase method : Difference between number of births & immigration & number of deaths & emigration. This is not possible in developing countries because accurate records are not present.

ii) Arithmetic progression method → Based on the assumption that each year population increases equally.

$P_t = P_o + Rt$ where

P_t = Population at req. time (t years after last census)

P_o = Population at last census.

R_t = Annual growth rate (for 4 months if mid-year population – on 1st July is to be taken).

iii) Geometric progression method → Based on assumption that there is constant growth.

Use of log tables is required.

$Pt = Po (1+R)^t$

In this case → Census – on 1st March
mid-year population – 1st July.
(∴ 4 months)

Mid-year population of 1997 = Population of 1997 till March 14 July (4 months = 1/3rd of annual population)

Growth rate (R) = 21,000 – 15,000/10 years = 600/year.

Mid-year population of 1997(Pt)

= 21000 (Po) + (600×6 + 1/3 × 600)

= 21000 + 3800

= 24,800

Mid-year population of 1997 is 24,800.

b) Population of Delhi as per 1st March 1981 was 62,20,000. As per 1st March 1991 it was 94,21,000.

i) In 1996, : R = 94,21,000 – 62,20,000/10 = 3,20,100

Mid-year population

= 94,21,00 + (3,20,100 × 5 + 1/3 × 3,20,100)

= 11,128,200.

ii) In 2001

Mid-year population = 94,21,000 + (3,20,100 × 10 + 1,06,700)

= 12,728,700

Q.3 In a small town of 40,000 population 500 primary and 2000 secondary cases of a disease were recorded.

i) What is the ratio of Primary to Secondary cases?
ii) What is the proportion of secondary cases?
iii) What is the Primary attack rate in the town?
iv) What is the secondary attack rate?

Biostatistics

A.3 i) Ratio of 1° to 2° cases = $\dfrac{500}{2000}$ = 1:4

(ii) 1° attack rate = No. of 1° cases/Total pop. × 100

$$= \dfrac{500}{4,000} \times 100 = 1.25\%$$

(iv) Secondary attack rate = $\dfrac{\text{Number of 2° cases}}{\text{Total no. of susceptible}} \times 100$

$$= \dfrac{20,000}{40,000 - 500} \times 100 = 5.06\%$$

Q.4 Calculate the gross reproduction rate of the data given below where the sex-ratio of female births to male births 1:1.

Age Group	S.R.	No. of women in the age Gp.	No. of live Births in a year	Age-specific fertility rates
15–19	0.97	250	50	50/150 = 2.20
20–24	0.97	450	135	135/450 = 0.30
25–29	0.96	425	136	136/425 = 0.32
30–34	0.96	400	100	100/400 = 0.25
35–39	0.95	240	36	36/240 = 0.15
40–44	0.94	200	14	14/200 = 0.07

A.4

Age Group (years)	No. of women in each age group	No. of live Births	Age-specific fertility rates
15–19	250	25	25/250 = 0.1
20–24	450	67.5	67.5/450 = 0.15
25–29	425	68	0.16
30–34	400	50	0.125
35–39	240	18	0.075
40–44	200	7	0.035

Sex ratio = 1:1

$$\text{GRR} = \sum (\text{female live births in age group/No. of} \times \text{CI women in age group})$$

$$= \dfrac{\text{TFR}}{2} \quad (\because \text{sex ratio} = 1:1)$$

$$= \left(\dfrac{25}{250} + \dfrac{67.5}{450} + \dfrac{68}{425} + \dfrac{50}{400} + \dfrac{18}{240} + \dfrac{7}{200}\right) \times \dfrac{5}{2}$$

$$= 1.6125$$

Q.5 Data – Total population of the Town – 50,000

Age Group	No. of women in the age Gp.	No. of live births in each age Gp.	ASFR	No. of female live births in each age Gp.	Survival of age
15–19	2000	80	$\frac{80}{2000} \times 1000$	40	0.97
20–24	1500	300	$\frac{300}{1500} \times 1000$	150	0.97
25–29	1500	250	$\frac{250}{1500} \times 1000$	125	0.96
30–34	1500	200	$\frac{200}{1500} \times 1000$	100	0.96
35–39	1500	50	$\frac{50}{1500} \times 1000$	25	0.95
40–44	2000	20	$\frac{20}{2000} \times 1000$	10	0.94
Total	10,000	900	Sum = 1.29	450	–

From the given data :

(1) Calculate net reproduction rate.
(2) Enumerate other fertility indicators which can be calculated.
(3) Compare the calculated NRR with national NRR for any year (specify the year of comparison) and target for health for all by 2000 AD.

A.5 (a) $NRR = \sum \left(\frac{\text{Female live births}}{\text{No. of females}} \times \text{survival of age group} \right) \times CI$

$= \left[\left(\frac{40}{200} \times 0.97 + \frac{150}{1500} \times 0.97 + \frac{125}{1500} \times 0.96 \right. \right.$

$\left. \left. + \frac{100}{1500} \times 0.96 + \frac{10}{2000} \times 0.94 + \frac{25}{1500} \times 0.95 \right) \right] \times 5$

$= 1.404$

(b) Other fertility indicators :
- Birth rate
- GFR
- GMFR
- Age-specific fertility rate
- Age-specific marital fertility rate
- Pregnancy rate
- Abortion rate & ratio

- TFR
- GRR
- NRR
- Child-woman ratio
- Abortion rate & ratio.

(c) NRR in 1990 = 1.5

Here, given NRR = 1.404

Target for HFA by 2000 is of NRR = 1 & is equivalent to attaining replacement levels. This can be achieved only if CPR is at least 60%.

Q.6.

Age Group	Population of age group village A	B	Deaths in age group A	B	Standard population
0-1	60	260	04	25	300
1-9	600	1250	03	08	2300
10-19	840	750	08	08	2200
20-59	1200	2500	06	12	4500
60 & above	300	250	30	15	700
	3000	5000	51	68	10,000

Calculate :

(i) Death rate of both villages & Compare.

(ii) Age specific death rates for both the villages compare and Comment.

(iii) Age adjusted death rate of both villages calculate and compare.

A.6. (i) Death rate of village A = $\dfrac{57}{3000} \times 1000 = 17/1000$

Death rate of village B = $\dfrac{68}{5000} \times 1000 = 13.6/1000$

Village A => Total population = 3000
            No. of deaths   = 51

Village B => Total population = 5000
            No. of deaths   = 68

Age Group	Expected deaths A	B	Total
0-1	66.67	< 100	A = 144.94
1-9	5	< 6.4	B = 137.8
10-19	9.52	< 10.67	
20-59	5	> 4.8	
60 & above	100	> 60	

DR of village A > DR of village B.

ii) Age-specific death rate = $\dfrac{\text{No. of deaths in age gp.}}{\text{population in age group}} \times 1000$

(comparison in table)

iii) Age-adjusted death rate = $\dfrac{\text{Total expected deaths}}{\text{Total std. population}} \times 1000$

Village A = Std. DR = $\dfrac{144.94}{10,000} \times 1000 = 14.49/1000$

Village B = $\dfrac{137.8}{10,000} \times 1000 = 13.78/1000$

∴ Std. DR of village A > Std. DR of village B.

Q.7. In a group of 5000 industrial workers there were 75 deaths during A particular year.
  a) Calculate standard mortality ratio for industrial workers, by using following data.
  b) Compare the health status of the industrial worker with the General population in data.

DATA

Age Group	Industrial worker population	Expected deaths	Deaths	General population death rates (per 1000)
15–24	500	$\dfrac{2 \times 500}{1000} = 1$		2.0
25–34	1000	$\dfrac{3 \times 1000}{1000} = 3$		3.0
35–44	2000	$\dfrac{4.5 \times 2000}{1000} = 9$		4.5
45–54	1000	$\dfrac{5 \times 1000}{1000} = 5$		5.0
55–64	500	$\dfrac{30 \times 500}{1000} = 15$		30.0
Total	5,000	33	75	

A.7.a) Expected deaths = $\dfrac{\text{Death rate of gen. popu.}}{1000} \times \text{Popu. of workers}$

SMR = $\dfrac{\text{Observed deaths}}{\text{Expected deaths}} \times 100 = \dfrac{75}{33} \times 100 = 227$

b) Since the value is greater than 100, occupation causes greater mortality rate.

CHAPTER-18

HEALTH PLANNING, MANAGEMENT AND ECONOMICS

Planning and management are also important in the field of health sciences. These two not only help in improving the quality and efficiency of health care services but also help to tackle several health problems with the help of limited resources.

HEALTH PLANNING

In general, planning has 3 main components :
(a) Plan formulation,
(b) Execution and
(c) Evaluation.

Health Planning as per WHO is defined as :

"The orderly process of defining community health problems, identifying unmet needs and surveying the resources to meet them, establishing priority goals that are realistic and feasible and projecting administrative action to accomplish the purpose of the proposed programme."

Resources

The term resources is used to describe the manpower, money, materials, skills knowledge, techniques and time needed for plan execution in order to reach the specified objectives.

Planning Cycle

Planning cycle is the sequence involving all the necessary steps involved in plan formulation, execution and evaluation.

Basic Steps of Planning Cycle are :
1. Analysis of health situation.
2. Defining programme objectives.

3. Assessing the resources available.
4. Assigning priorities among objectives.
5. Formulation of alternate programmes.
6. Selection of best programme.
7. Programme implementation.
8. Monitoring.
9. Evaluation.

Determinants of health planning
1. Epidemiology/Demographic profile.
2. Resources – economic aspect i.e. financial, money, material, manpower and time.
3. Policies – a political determinants.
4. Scientific and technological availability.

Necessity of Planning
- To optimise the resources available, the best effective manner.
- Effective functioning of organising sectors.

Planning process or cycle
3 Phases :
1. Diagnostic Phase.
2. Implementive Phase.
3. Evaluative Phase.

1. Identification of problem, magnitude and amount. Identification of various solution for part problem. Identification of most appropriate solution problem.
2. Implement of services.
3. Evaluation and modification of services.

MANAGEMENT
Definition
- An effort to attain the future objective by a rational determination in the present of requisite resources, personal, procedure needed to achieve those objective.
- Process of determining future action through credible strategies for achieving the stated objective.

Requisite
1. Political stability – policies due to changes in & the parties, there

are no fruitful implementation of objectives. It also affect economical stability.
2. Political Will – towards the dislike leprosy, T.B.
3. Presence of appropriate health infrastructure.

Obstacles
1. Political unstability.
2. Lack of resources and economics.
3. Lack of participation by health experts and trained personal.
4. Lack of group dynamics (co-operation between the people of a organisation).

Objectives
Laissez Faire. Opposite to Planning. i.e. without any planning health status improves itself or
1. For improvement of organisation pattern in relation to health centre.
2. Spread
   - The development of needed new health services.
   - Strengthen the services.
   - Improving the utilisation of services.
3. To discourage the programmes not needed.
4. To improve the quality of health care through better coordination.
5. To eliminate the duplication of health services among the govt. and non-govt. services especially implemented for Delhi.
   - C.G.H.S.
   - Delhi administrative hospital.
   - M.C.D.
   - Doctor population ratio 1.6/1000 population is important to assess the requirement, but > in urban areas.
   - 75% rural population = 20.25% physician supply, i.e. to have better geographical distribution of services.
6. Survey – for evaluating the utilization of services.

Management : Tools and Techniques
1. P.P.B.S. – Programme Planning and Budget System.
2. System analysis/System approach.
3. Operation research.

4. P.E.R.T. – Programme evaluation and review technique.
5. Gantt chart.

P.P.B.S.
1. **Resorces** – Procedure made for better utilization of resources. Appropriate allocation of resources is the main object.
   e.g. for disease control and eradication : N.M.E.P.
   - Planning.
   - Appropriate allocation of resources.
2. **System approach** – It is more of management tool rather than planning tool. It is related to shading of various elements in particular system and evaluate the ratio or actual and expected output.
   e.g. A.P.I. < .2%.
3. **Operation research** – These are made into various aspect of operative system and finding the optimal solution to tackle the problem.
   e.g. – Pulse polio programme.
   Vaccine procurement – till consumer cold chain.
4. **P.E.R.T.** – It is required for people of High level in a organization – It is a graphical detailed representation of a programme.
   - A method of making future activities so if any modification if required can be achieved & the help of experts.
5. **Gantt Chart**
   - Time activity analysis in the implementation of planned programme. So that the desired objects are met in set of already decided time-limit e.g. programme month (find the limit).

Management methods based on behavioural sciences

1. Organisational Design

It should meet the health needs and demands of the people. It should be reviewed every few years and updated with the existing problems and latest technology.

2. Personnel Management

All the fundamental techniques like proper methods of selection, training & motivation; division of responsibility; incentives for better work; opportunities for promotion and professional advancement, etc., contribute to the efficiency of health service delivery.

3. Communication

Better communication at different levels like between the doctor and the patient; doctor and nurse; health ministry and the government, etc. contribute to effective functioning of an organisation.

4. Information Systems

The functions of information system consist of collection, classification, transmission, storage, retrieval, transformation and display of information for the management of the health system.

5. Management by Objectives (MBO)

Objectives are set forth for different units and subunits to prepare their own plan of action – usually on a short term basis.

HEALTH ECONOMICS

Introduction

Economics revolve around the study of markets or exchange between producers and consumers and that production and consumption are among the most fundamental activities of human being. Economists are trained to examine problems of allocation of scarce resources. Economist focuses on how to do the most with the available resources and who is benefited and who looses from the activity.

Economics applied to the health field is known as *Health Economics*. Health economics seeks inter alia to quantify over time, the resources used in health service delivery, its organization and financing : the efficiency with which the resource are allocated and used for health purposes and the effects of preventive, curative and rehabilitative services on individual and national productivity.

The field of health economics emerged due to very high growth in national health expenditure. Health sector poses formidable challenge to economists due to extreme situation of scarcity and unique complexities. Central concern of medicine is to go into the causes and treat the ill health. Health economics can contribute to the understanding of and solution to the myriad of problems facing health sector.

There are important gains in the health status during last few decades. However much remains to be done to achieve the health targets. Tight budget, inadequate access to primary health care facilities, inefficient production, inefficient consumer pattern, poor quality of health care, changing disease profile and persistent high fertility rate are among the causes and manifestations of malfunctioning system. Health economics helps in understanding the problems and improving efficiency of health services.

Efficiency/Effectiveness	Model
(i) Input.	Output.
(ii) Means.	Results.
(iii) Money/Resources.	Health benefit.
(iv) Amount of money generated, allocated, distributed and utilized.	No. of cases prevented, cured, rehabilitated and saved.

Provision and Utilization of Health Services (Govt. and Private)

- Health care is provided to the people mainly by public and private health sectors.
- By and large government sector is providing free health services and private sector is charging fees for service.
- About 80% of the O.P.D. patients are seeking medical care from private practitioners whereas 80% of the indoor patients are admitted to the government hospitals.

Health Financing

The resources are scarce. It is estimated that Rs. 22,000 crores are required to achieve some of the set targets. In the annual budget of the year 1996-1997. Rs. 1515.00 crores was allocated for health sector. Out of the total budget approximately 3% is allocated to health sector. In terms of G.D.P. it is around 1.3% and along with household expenditure it is around 6% of G.D.P. in our country as compared to 12% spent by U.S.A. and U.K. Out of total government expenditure 25% is spent by the central government and the state governments spend 75%.

The expenditure by the state government varies from state to state. More than 60% is incurred on providing curative services and only 26% for preventive services and remaining on administrative expenses. About 67% of the resources spent have gone to urban areas. There is 93% to 97% expenditure on revenue and only 3% to 7% on capital. Of the revenue expenditure, about 60% goes to salaries and 15% to 30% for supplies and rest on other aspects of health care delivery system.

Additional money is required to meet rising cost of health care due to escalation of prices, increase in salaries, increase in cost of material and supplies, advancement of technology, need and demand for better quality care. Hence resources have to be generated. government alone is not a position to meet the needs.

The resources can be generated by launching the schemes like (a) health insurance (b) user charges, and (c) other innovative approaches. Regulated privatization would attract more patients releasing pressure and money from public sector. There are advantages and disadvantages of each of the scheme and controversies regarding all these approaches.

Efficient utilization of resources

Efficient utilization can be achieved through allocation efficiency and internal efficiency.

Allocation efficiency is concerned with the allocation of resources to the production of output, which yield the highest value from their use. Thus existing mal-distribution of resources between primary and tertiary health care sectors or preventive and curative health care services needs to be corrected to improve efficiency and results. Allocating more funds for preventive and promotive services can save more lives. It is wiser approach to prevent diseases than allowing diseases to occur and treat them.

It is recommended by the experts that the Primary Health Care budget should be at least 1.0% of G.D.P. instead of 0.65% (Currently).

It may be emphasized that to save as health service cost is not a valid objective. The objective must be realizing the same benefits from the lower cost so as to increase benefits without adding to the cost.

Neighbouring developing countries have better health indicators with less percent of G.D.P. expenditure on health care e.g. Sri Lanka, Maldives, etc.

Internal efficiency is concerned with the avoidance of waste. Such wastage may be caused by deficient administration, a lack of managerial capabilities. Due to under funding of specific complementary output such as drug, fuel and working vehicle would lead to non-functioning of the manpower or ineffective treatment leading to inefficiency wastages. Another example is bulk purchase of drugs of limited use or early expiry and under utilization of equipments purchased at heavy price according to reports, equipments worth hundred of crores are lying idle in many hospitals.

To improve the efficiency the health professional there is a need to orient himself and become *cost conscious*. However, it must be properly understood that becoming cost conscious does not mean saving of the money for the sake of saving.

Cost Accounting

Cost accounting is the application of costing and cost accounting principles, methods and technique. It is essential for efficient operations of the hospital or programme. It carried out periodically and methodically to help the hospital/health administration in :

i) Determining actual cost of operating each department service.
ii) Cost of hospitalization per day.
iii) Detecting wasteful of expenditure.

Following cost analysis can be undertaken :

Cost Object

A unit of service for which we wish to know the cost. As this becomes more specific, the cost accounting methodology become more complex.

Direct and indirect cost

Direct cost applies to only one cost that is directly linked with the service e.g. cost of X-rays film is direct cost and cost spent on machine, manpower, electricity, and other services required to produce X-rays is indirect cost.

Household cost

Cost incurred by the beneficiaries to seek health care, e.g. expenditure incurred on transport, etc. by the patient.

Full cost analysis

Total amount of money spent on particular health service/programme.

Unit cost analysis

Amount of expenditure incurred on each unit of service, e.g. cost of vaccination of one child.

Opportunity cost

The money otherwise could have been earned during the lost time or opportunity, or due to restriction of budget, allocation from the programme is withdrawn leading to loss of the programme.

Fixed cost

The cost incurred irrespective of volume of service provided, e.g. cost incurred on building, equipment, salary, etc.

Variable cost

Cost which is dependent on volume of service. Cost incurred on drugs, reagents, etc., would increase, as the number of patients treated increases.

Marginal cost

Extra cost incurred to produce one more positive result.

Setting a price (Pricing)

By using fixed and variable cost calculation, the price of the service can be set. Profit can be estimated or subsidies can be worked out.

By taking into consideration all the costs, input can be calculated. The input-output ratios can be obtained to find out the efficiency and take corrective measures to improve the efficiency. Efficiency is obtained when more results are produced with same inputs (time, person, money) or same results are obtained with less input.

The outcome can be studied in term of cost effectiveness i.e. number of case prevented, treated a lives saved by spending particular amount of money.

To take a decision regarding introduction of new programme, e.g. vaccination programme.

Cost of input and amount of money saved which otherwise spent on treatment and other aspects of the patients care to be taken into consideration.

Estimations and projections can be made which will help health policy makers and managers in decision-making.

Cost containment

Cost of the health services can be reduced without affecting results by taking containment measures such as :

- Buy prudently, stock minimally, issue accurately and spent frugally.
- Prevent pilferage and wastage by internal auditing and effective supervision.

- Reduction of 20% of cost on medicine can be achieved without impairing the quality of care and maintaining patient satisfaction.

Physician can play important role in cost containment by :
- Reducing number of investigation.
- Reducing number of drug prescription.
- Equally effective cheaper alternatives.
- Reducing average length of stay in the hospital.
- Strengthening scheduling of patient and staff.
- Developing cheaper and innovative technology.

Thus by generating additional resources, reallocating the resources, taking cost containment measures and avoiding wastages by applying cost evaluating techniques; resources can be efficiently utilized to provide cost effective health services and health services benefits can be obtained at lower cost.

Key message
- The objective of health care is to save lives, prevent and cure disease, promote and maintain health, by providing quality care to all.
- No cost is too great, when it comes to saving a human life but saving money out of extra expenditure may save another life.
- Health care is oriented to the health needs, service expectation and people's aspiration and not profit oriented.

Message
- Become cost conscious.
- Avoid wastages.
- Adopt better management skills, technology and approaches to improve health services.

NATIONAL HEALTH POLICY (1983)

National Health Policy, Government of India, Ministry of Health & Family Welfare, New Delhi, 1983.

Introduction
1. The Constitution of India envisages the establishment of a new social order based on equality, freedom, justice and the dignity of the individual. It aims at the elimination of poverty, ignorance and ill-health and directs

the state to raise the level of nutrition, standard of living of its people and improvement of public health as among its primary duties, securing the health and strength of workers, men and women, specially ensuring that children are given opportunities and facilities to develop in a healthy manner.

1.2. Since the inception of the planning process in the country, the successive five year plans have been providing the framework within which the states may develop their health services infrastructure, facilities for medical education, research, etc. Similar guidance has sought to be provided through the discussions and conclusions arrived at in the joint conferences of the central Councils of Health and Family Welfare and the National Development Council. Besides, central legislation has been enacted to regulate standards of medical education, prevention of food adulteration, maintenance of standards in the manufacture and sale of certified drugs, etc.

1.3. While the broad approaches contained in the successive plan documents and discussion in the forums referred to in para 1.2 may have generally served the needs of the situation in the past, it is felt that an integrated, comprehensive approach towards the future development of medical education, research and health services requires to be established to serve the actual health needs and priorities of the country. It is in this context that the need has been felt to evolve a National Health Policy.

Our heritage

2. India has a rich, centuries-old heritage of medical and health sciences. The philosophy of ayurveda and the surgical skills enunciated by Charaka and Shusharuta bear testimony to our ancient tradition in the scientific health care of our people. The approach of our ancient medical systems was of a holistic nature, which took into account all aspects of human health and disease. Over the centuries, with the intrusion of foreign influences and mingling of cultures, various systems of medicine evolved and have continued to be practised widely. However, the allopathic system of medicine has, in a relatively short period of time, made a major impact on the entire approach to health care and pattern of development of the health services infrastructure in the country.

Progress achieved

3. During the last three decades and more, since the attainment of independence, considerable progress has been achieved in the promotion of the health status of our people. Smallpox has been eliminated; plague

is no longer a problem; mortality from cholera and related diseases has decreased and malaria brought under control to a considerable extent. The mortality rate per thousand of population has been reduced from 27.4 to 14.8 and the life expectancy at birth has increased from 32.7 to over 52. A fairly extensive network of dispensaries, hospitals and institutions providing specialised curative care has developed and a large stock of medical and health personnel, of various levels, has become available. Significant indigenous capacity has been established for the production of drugs and pharmaceuticals, vaccines, sera, hospital equipments, etc.

The existing picture

4. In spite of such impressive progress, the demographic and health picture of the country still constitutes a cause for serious and urgent concern. The high rate of population growth continues to have an adverse effect on the health of our people and the quality of their lives. The mortality rates for women and children are still distressingly high; almost one third of the total deaths occur among children below the age of 5 years; infant mortality is around 129 per thousand live births. Efforts at raising the nutritional levels of our people have still to bear fruit and the extent and severity of malnutrition continues to be exceptionally high. Communicable and non-communicable diseases have still to be brought under effective control and eradicated. Blindness, leprosy and T.B. continue to have a high incidence. Only 31% of the rural population has access to potable water supply and 0.5% enjoys basic sanitation.

4.1. High incidence of diarrhoeal diseases and other preventive and infectious diseases, specially amongst infants and children, lack of safe drinking water and poor environmental sanitation, poverty and ignorance are among the major contributory causes of the high incidence of disease and mortality.

4.2. The existing situation has been largely engendered by the almost wholesale adoption of health manpower development policies and the establishment of curative centres based on the Western models, which are inappropriate and irrelevant to the real needs of our people and the socio-economic conditions obtaining in the country. The hospital-based disease, and cure-oriented approach towards the establishment of medical services has provided benefits to the upper crusts, of society, specially those residing in the urban areas. The proliferation of this approach has been at the cost of providing comprehensive primary health care services to the entire population, whether residing in the urban or the rural areas.

Furthermore, the continued high emphasis on the curative approach has led to the neglect of the preventive, promotive, public health and rehabilitative aspects of health care. The existing approach, instead of improving awareness and building up self-reliance, has tended to enhance dependency and weaken the community's capacity to cope with its problems. The prevailing policies regarding the education and training of medical and health personnel, at various levels, has resulted in the development of a cultural gap between the people and the personnel providing care. The various health programmes have, by and large, failed to involve individuals and families in establishing a self-reliant community. Also, over the years, the planning process has become largely oblivious of the fact that the ultimate goal of achieving a satisfactory health status for all of our people cannot be secured without involving the community in the identification of their health needs and priorities as well as in the implementation and management of the various health and related programmes.

Need for evolving a health policy – the revised 20-Point Programme

5. India is committed to attain the goal of "Health for All by the Year 2000 A.D." through the universal provision of comprehensive primary health care services. The attainment of this goal requires a thorough overhaul of the existing approaches to the education and training of medical and health personnel and the reorganisation of the health services infrastructure. Furthermore, considering the large variety of inputs into health, it is necessary to secure the complete integration of all plans for health and human development with the overall national socio-economic development process, specially in the more closely health related sectors, e.g. drugs and pharmaceuticals, agriculture and food production, rural development, education and social welfare, housing, water supply and sanitation, prevention of food adulteration, maintenance of prescribed standards in the manufacture and sale of drugs and the conservation of the environment. In sum, the contours of the National Health Policy have to be evolved within a fully integrated planning framework which seeks to provide universal, comprehensive primary health care services, relevant to the actual needs and priorities of the community at a cost which the people can afford, ensuring that the planning and implementation of the various health programmes is through the organised involvement and participation of the community, adequately utilising the services being rendered by private voluntary organisations active in the health sector.

5.1. It is also necessary to ensure that the pattern of development of the health services infrastructure in the future fully takes into account the revised 20-Point Programme. The said programme attributes very high priority to the promotion of family planning as a people's programme, on a voluntary basis; substantial augmentation and provision of primary health care facilities on a universal basis; control of leprosy, T.B. and blindness; acceleration of welfare programmes for women and children; nutrition programmes for pregnant women, nursing mothers and children, especially in the tribal, hill and backward areas. The programme also places high emphasis on the supply of drinking water to all problem villages, improvements in the housing and environments of the weaker sections of society; increased production of essential food items; integrated rural developments; spread of universal elementary education; expansion of the public distribution system, etc.

Population stabilisation

6. Irrespective of the changes, no matter how fundamental, that may be brought about in the over-all approach to health care and the restructuring of the health services, not much headway is likely to be achieved in improving the health status of the people unless success is achieved in securing the small family norm, through voluntary efforts, and moving towards the goal of population stabilisation. In view of the vital importance of securing the balanced growth of the population, it is necessary to enunciate, separately, a national population policy.

Medical and Health Education

7. It is also necessary to appreciate that the effective delivery of health care services would depend very largely on the nature of education, training and appropriate orientation towards community health of all categories of medical and health personnel and their capacity to function as an integrated team, each of its members performing given tasks within a coordinated action programme. It is, therefore, of crucial importance that the entire basis and approach towards medical and health education, at all levels, is reviewed in terms of national needs and priorities as well as the curricular and training programmes restructured to produce personnel of various grades of skill and competence, who are professionally equipped and socially motivated to deal effectively with day-to-day problems, within the existing constraints.

Towards this end, it is necessary to formulate, separately, a national medical and health education policy which (i) sets out the changes required to be brought about in the curricular contents and training programme of medical and health personnel, at various levels of functioning; (ii) takes into account the need for establishing the extremely essential inter-relations between functionaries of various grades; (iii) provides guidelines for the production of health personnel on the basis of realistically assessed manpower requirements; (iv) seeks to resolve the existing sharp regional imbalances in their availability; and (v) ensures that personnel at all levels are socially motivated towards the rendering of community health services.

Need for providing primary health care with special emphasis on the preventive, promotive and rehabilitative aspects

8. Presently, despite the constraint of resources, there is disproportionate emphasis on the establishment of curative centres – dispensaries, hospitals, institutions for specialist treatment – the majority of which are located in the urban areas of the country. The vast majority of those seeking medical relief have to travel long distance to the nearest curative centre, seeking relief for ailments which could have been readily and effectively handled at the community level. Also, for want of a well established referral system, those seeking curative care have the tendency to visit various specialist centres, thus further contributing to congestions, duplication of efforts and consequential waste of resources. To put an end to the existing all-round unsatisfactory situation, it is urgently necessary to restructure the health services within the following broad approach :

(i) To provide, within a phased, time-bound programme a well dispersed network of comprehensive primary health care services, integrally linked with the extension and health education approach which takes into account the fact that a large majority of health functions can be effectively handled and resolved by the people themselves, with the organised support of volunteers, auxiliaries, para-medics and adequately trained multi-purpose workers of various grades of skill and competence, of both sexes. There are a large number of private, voluntary organisations active in the health field, all over the country. Their services and support would require to be utilised and intermeshed with the governmental efforts, in an integrated manner.

(ii) To be effective, the establishment of the primary health care approach would involve large scale transfer of knowledge, simple skill ana technologies to health volunteers, selected by the communities and enjoying their confidence. The functioning of the front line workers, selected by the community would require to be related to definitive action plans for the translation of medical and health knowledge into practical action, involving the use of simple and inexpensive interventions which can be readily implemented by persons who have undergone short periods of training. The quality of training of these health guides/workers would be of crucial importance to the success of this approach.

(iii) The success of the decentralised primary health care system would depend vitally on the organised building up of individual self-reliance and effective community participation; on the provision of organised, back-up support of the secondary and territory levels of the health care services, providing adequate, logistical and technical assistance.

(iv) The decentralisation of services would require the establishment of a well worked out referral system to provide adequate expertise at the various levels of the organisational set-up nearest to the community, depending upon the actual needs and problems of the area, and thus ensure against the continuation of the existing rush towards the curative centres in the urban areas. The effective establishment of the referral system would also ensure the optimal utilisation of expertise at the higher levels of the hierarchical structure. This approach would not only lead to the progressive improvement of comprehensive health care services at the primary level but also provide timely attention to those who are in need of urgent specialist care, whether they live in the rural or the urban areas.

(v) To ensure that the approach to health care does not merely constitute a collection of disparate health interventions but consists of an integrated package of services seeking to tackle the entire range of poor health conditions, on a broad front, it is necessary to establish a nation-wide chain of sanitary-cum-epidemiological stations. The location and functioning of these stations may be between the primary and secondary levels of the hierarchical structure, depending upon the local situations and other relevant considerations. Each such station would require suitably trained staff equipped to identify, plan and provide preventive, promotive and mental health care services. It would be beneficial, depending upon the local situations, to establish such stations at the Primary Health Centres. The district health organisation should have, as an integral part of its set-up, a well organised epidemiological unit to coordinate and superintend the functioning of the field stations. These stations would participate in the integrated action plans to eradicate and control diseases, besides tackling specific local environmental health problems.

In the urban agglomerations, the municipal and local authorities should be equipped to perform similar functions, being supported with adequate resources and expertise, to deal effectively with the local preventable public health problems. The aforesaid approach should be implemented and extended through community participation and contributions, in whatever form possible, to achieve meaningful results within a time-bound programme.

(vi) The location of curative centres should be related to the populations they serve, keeping in view the densities of population, distances, topography and transport connections. These centres should function within the recommended referral system, the gamut of the general specialities required to deal with the local disease patterns being provided as near to the community as possible and at the secondary level of the hierarchical organisation. The concept of domiciliary care and the field-camps approach should be utilised to the fullest extent, to reduce the pressures on these centres, specially in efforts relating to the control and eradication of blindness, tuberculosis, leprosy, etc.

(vii) Special, well-coordinated programmes should be launched to provide mental health care as well as medical care and the physical and social rehabilitation of those who are mentally retarded, deaf, dumb, blind, physically disabled, infirm and aged. Also, suitably organised of various disabilities.

(viii) In the establishment of the re-organised services, the first priority should be accorded to provide services to those residing in the tribal, hill and backward areas as well as to endemic disease affected populations and the vulnerable sections of the society.

(ix) In the re-organised health services scheme, efforts should be made to ensure adequate mobility of personnel, at all level of functioning.

(x) In the various approaches, set out in (i) to (ix) above, organised efforts would be required to fully utilise and assist in the enlargement of the services being provided by private voluntary organisations active in the health field. In this context, planning encouragement and support would also require to be afforded to fresh voluntary efforts, specially those which seek to serve the needs of the rural areas and the urban slums.

Re-orientation of the existing health personnel

9. A dynamic process of changes and innovation is required to be brought about in the entire approach to health manpower development, ensuring the emergence of fully integrated bands of workers functioning within the "Health Team" approach.

Private practice by governmental functionaries

National Health Policy

10. It is desirable for the states to take steps to phase out of system of private practice by medical personnel in government service, providing at the same time payment of appropriate compensatory no-practising allowance. The states would require to carefully review the existing situation, with special reference to the availability and dispersal of private practitioners, and take timely decisions in regard to this vital issue.

Practitioners of indigenous and other systems of medicine and their role in health care

11. The country has a large stock of health manpower comprising of private practitioners in various systems, for example, ayurveda, unani, siddha, homoeopathy, yoga, naturopathy, etc. This resource has not so far been adequately utilized. The practitioners of these various systems enjoy high local acceptance and respect and consequently exert considerable influence on health beliefs and practise. It is, therefore, necessary to initiate organised measures to enable each of these various systems of medicine and health care to develop in accordance with its genius. Simultaneously, planned efforts should be made to detail the functioning of the practitioners of these various systems and integrate their service at the appropriate levels, within specified areas of responsibility and functioning, in the over-all health care delivery system, specially in regard to the preventive, promotive and public health objectives. Well considered

NATIONAL HEALTH POLICY (2002)

steps would also be required to move towards a meaningful phased integration of the indigenous and the modem systems.

1. Introductory

1.1. A National Health Policy was last formulated in 1983, and since then there have been marked changes in the determinant factors relating to the health sector. Some of the policy initiatives outlined in the N.H.P.-1983 have yielded results, while, in several other areas, the outcome has not been as expected.

1.2. The N.H.P.-1983 gave a general exposition of the policies which required recommendation in the circumstances then prevailing in the health sector. The noteworthy initiatives under that policy were :-

(i) A phased, time-bound programme for setting up a well-dispersed network of comprehensive primary health care services, linked with extension and health education, designed in the context of the ground reality that elementary health problems can be resolved by the people themselves;

(ii) Intermediation through 'Health volunteers' having appropriate knowledge, simple skills and requisite technologies;

(iii) Establishment of a well-worked out referral system to ensure that patient load at the higher levels of the hierarchy is not needlessly burdened by those who can be treated at the decentralized level;

(iv) An integrated net-work of evenly spread speciality and super-speciality services; encouragement of such facilities through private investments for patients who can pay, so that the draw on the governments facilities is limited to those entitled to free use.

1.3. Government initiatives in the pubic health sector have recorded some noteworthy successes over time. Smallpox and guinea worm disease have been eradicated from the country; polio is on the verge of being eradicated; leprosy, kala azar, and filariasis can be expected to be eliminated in the foreseeable future. There has been a substantial drop in the total fertility Rate and Infant Mortality Rate. The success of the initiatives taken in the public health field are reflected in the progressive improvement of many demographic/epidemiological/infrastructural indicators over time - (Table-1).

Table-1
Achievements Through The Years -1951-2000

Indicator	1951	1981	2000
Demographic Changes			
Life Expectancy	36.7	54	64.6(R.G.I.)
Crude Birth Rate	40.8	33.9(S.R.S.)	26.1(99 S.R.S.)
Crude Death Rate	25	12.5(S.R.S.)	8.7(99 S.R.S.)
I.M.R.	146	110	70(99 S.R.S.)
Epidemiological Shifts			
Malaria (cases in million)	75	2.7	2.2
Leprosy cases per 10,000 population	38.1	57.3	3.74
Small pox (no. of cases)	>44,887	Eradicated	
Guineaworm (no. of cases)		>39,792	Eradicated
Polio		29709	265
Infrastructure			
S.C./P.H.C./C.H.C.	725	57,363	1,63,181 (99-R.H.S.)
Dispensaries & Hospitals(all)	9209	23,555	43,322 (95-96-C.B.H.I.)
Beds (Pvt. & Public)	117,198	5,69,495	8,70,161 (95-96-C.B.H.I.)
Doctors (Allopathy)	61,800	2,68,700	5,03,900 (98-99-M.C.I.)
Nursing Personnel	18,054	1,43,887	7,37,000 (99-I.N.C.)

1.4. While noting that the public health initiatives over the years have contributed significantly to the improvement of these health indicators, it is to be acknowledged that public health indicators/disease-burden statistics are the outcome of several complementary initiatives under the wider umbrella of the developmental sector, covering rural development, agriculture, food production, sanitation, drinking water supply, education, etc. Despite the impressive public health gains as revealed in the statistics in Table-1, there is no gainsaying the fact that the morbidity and mortality levels in the country are still unacceptably high. These unsatisfactory health indices are, in turn, an indication of the limited success of the public health system in meeting the preventive and curative requirements of the general population.

1.5. Out of the communicable diseases which have persisted over time, the incidence of malaria staged a resurgence in the 1980s before stabilising at a fairly high prevalence level during the 1990s. Over the years, an increasing level of insecticide-resistance has developed in the malarial vectors in many parts of the country, while the incidence of the more deadly P. falciparum malaria has risen to about 50 percent in the country as a whole. In respect of T.B., the public health scenario has not shown any significant decline in the pool of infection amongst the community, and there has been a distressing trend in the increase of drug resistance to the type of infection prevailing in the country. A new and extremely virulent communicable disease – H.I.V./A.I.D.S. – has emerged on the health scene since the declaration of the N.H.P.-1983. As there is no existing therapeutic cure or vaccine for this infection, the disease constitutes a serious threat, not merely to public health but to economic development in the country. The common water-borne infections – gastroenteritis, cholera, and some forms of hepatitis – continue to contribute to a high level of morbidity in the population, even though the mortality rate may have been somewhat moderated.

1.6. The period after the announcement of N.H.P.- 83 has also seen an increase in mortality through life-style' diseases – diabetes, cancer and cardiovascular diseases. The increase in life expectancy has increased the requirement for geriatric care. Similarly, the increasing burden of trauma cases is also a significant public health problem.

1.7. Another area of grave concern in the public health domain is the persistent incidence of macro and micro nutrient deficiencies, especially among women and children. In the vulnerable sub-category of women and the girl child, this has the multiplier effect through the birth of low birth weight babies and serious ramifications of the consequential mental and physical retarded growth.

1.8. N.H.P.-1983, in a spirit of optimistic empathy for the health needs of the people, particularly the poor and under-privileged, had hoped to provide 'Health for All by the year 2000 AD', through the universal provision of comprehensive primary health care services. In retrospect, it is observed that the financial resources and public health administrative capacity which was possible to marshal, was far short of the necessities to achieve such an ambitious and holistic goal. Against this backdrop, it is felt that it would be appropriate to pitch N.H.P.-2002 at a level consistent with our realistic expectations about financial resources, and about the likely increase in public health administrative capacity. The recommendations of N.H.P.-2002 will, therefore, attempt to maximize the broad-based availability of health services to the citizenry of the country on the basis of realistic considerations of capacity. The changed circumstances relating to the health sector of the country since 1983 have generated a situation in which it is now necessary to review the field, and to formulate a new policy framework as the National Health Policy-2002. N.H.P.-2002 will attempt to set out a new policy framework for the accelerated achievement of public health goals in the socio-economic circumstances currently prevailing in the country.

2. Current Scenario

2.1 Financial Resources

2.1.1 The public health investment in the country over the years has been comparatively low, as the percentage of G.D.P. has declined from 1.3 percent in 1990 to 0.9 percent in 1999. The aggregate expenditure in the Health sector is 5.2 percent of the G.D.P. Out of this, about 17 percent of the aggregate expenditure is public health spending, the balance being out-of-pocket expenditure. The central budgetary allocation for health over this period, as a percentage of the total central budget, has been stagnant at 1.3 percent, while that in the states has declined from 7.0 percent to 5.5 percent. The current annual per capita public health expenditure in the country is no more than Rs. 200. Given these statistics, it is no surprise that the reach and quality of public health services has been below the desirable standard. Under the constitutional structure, public health is the responsibility of the states. In this framework, it has been the expectation that the principal contribution for the funding of public health services will be from the resources of the states, with some supplementary input from central resources. In this backdrop, the contribution of central resources to the overall public health funding has been limited to about 15 percent. The fiscal resources of the state governments are known to be very inelastic. This is reflected in the declining percentage of state resources allocated to the health sector out of the state budget. If the decentralized pubic health services in the country are to improve significantly, there is a need for the injection of substantial resources into the health sector from the central government budget. This approach is a necessity – despite the formal constitutional provision in regard to public health, – if the state public health services, which are a major component of the initiatives in the social sector, are not to become entirely moribund. The N.H.P.-2002 has been formulated taking into consideration these ground realities in regard to the availability of resources.

2.2 Equity

2.2.1 In the period when centralized planning was accepted as a key instrument of development in the country, the attainment of an equitable regional distribution was considered one of its major objectives. Despite this conscious focus in the development process, the statistics given in Table-2 clearly indicate that the attainment of health indices has been very uneven across the rural – urban divide.

Table-2
Differentials in Health Status Among states

Sector	Population B.P.L. (%)	I.M.R./ per 1000 Live Births (1999-S.R.S.)	<5Mortality per (N.F.H.S. II)	Weight for Age-% of Children Under-3 years (<-2S.D.)	M.M.R./ Lakh (Annual Report 2000)	Leprosy cases per 10000 population	Malaria +ve Cases in year 2000 (in thousands
INDIA	26.1	70	94.9	47	408	3.7	2200
Rural	27.09	75	103.7	49.6	–	–	–
Urban	23.62	44	63.1	38.4	–	–	–
Better Performing States							
Kerala	12.72	14	18.8	27	87	0.9	5.1
Maharashtra	25.02	48	58.1	50	1.5	3.1	138
T.N.	21.12	52	63.3	37	79	4.1	56
Low Performing States							
Orissa	47.15	97	104.4	54	498	7.05	483
Bihar	42.60	63	105.1	54	707	11.83	132
Rajasthan	15.28	81	114.9	51	607	0.8	53
U.P.	31.15	84	122.5	52	707	4.3	99
M.P.	37.43	90	137.6	55	498	3.83	528

Also, the statistics bring out the wide differences between the attainments of health goals in the better-performing states as compared to the low-performing states. It is clear that national averages of health indices hide wide disparities in public health facilities and health standards in different parts of the country. Given a situation in which national averages in respect of most indices are themselves at unacceptably low levels, the wide inter-state disparity implies that, for vulnerable sections of society in several states, access to public health services is nominal and health standards are grossly inadequate. Despite a thrust in the N.H.P.-1983 for making good the unmet needs of public health services by establishing more public health institutions at a decentralized level, a large gap in facilities still persists. Applying current norms to the population projected for the year 2000, it is estimated that the shortfall in the number of S.Cs/P.H.Cs/C.H.Cs is of the order of 16 percent. However, this shortage is as high as 58 percent when disaggregated for C.H.Cs only. The N.H.P-2002 will need to address itself to making good these deficiencies so as to narrow the gap between the various states, as also the gap across the rural-urban divide.

2.2.2. Access to, and benefits from, the public health system have been very uneven between the better-endowed and the more vulnerable sections of society. This is particularly true for women, children and the socially disadvantaged sections of society. The statistics given in Table-3 highlight the handicap suffered in the health sector on account of socio-economic inequity.

Table-3
Differentials in Health status Among Socio-Economic Groups

Indicator	Infant Mortality/1000	Under 5 Mortality/1000	% Children Underweight
India	70	94.9	47
Social Inequity			
Scheduled Castes	83	119.3	53.5
Scheduled Tribes	84.2	126.6	55.9
Other Disadvantaged	76	103.1	47.3
Others	61.8	82.6	41.1

2.2.3 It is a principal objective of N.H.P.-2002 to evolve a policy structure which reduces these inequities and allows the disadvantaged sections of society a fairer access to public health services.

2.3 Delivery of National Public Health Programmes

2.3.1 It is self-evident that in a country as large as India, which has a wide variety of socio-economic settings, national health programmes have to be designed with enough flexibility to permit the state public health administrations to craft their own programme package according to their needs. Also, the implementation of the national health programme can only be carried out through the state governments' decentralized public health machinery. Since, for various reasons, the responsibility of the central government in funding additional public health services will continue over a period of time, the role of the central government in designing broad-based public health initiatives will inevitably continue. Moreover, it has been observed that the technical and managerial expertise for designing large-span public health programmes exists with the central government in a considerable degree; this expertise can be gainfully utilized in designing national health programmes for implementation in varying socio-economic settings in the states. With this background, the N.H.P.-2002 attempts to define the role of the central government and the state governments in the public health sector of the country.

2.3.2.1. Over the last decade or so, the government has relied upon a 'vertical' implementational structure for the major disease control programmes. Through this, the system has been able to make a substantial dent in reducing the burden of specific diseases. However, such an organizational structure, which requires independent manpower for each disease programme, is extremely expensive and difficult to sustain. Over a long time-range, 'vertical' structures may only be affordable for those diseases which offer a reasonable possibility of elimination or eradication in a foreseeable time-span.

2.3.2.2. It is a widespread perception that, over the last decade and a half, the rural health staff has become a vertical structure exclusively for the implementation of family welfare activities. As a result, for those public health programmes where there is no separate vertical structure, there is no identifiable service delivery system at all. The policy will address this distortion in the public health system.

2.4. The State of Public Health Infrastructure

2.4.1. The delineation of N.H.P.-2002 would be required to be based on an objective assessment of the quality and efficiency of the existing public health machinery in the field. It would detract from the quality of the exercise if, while framing a new policy, it was not acknowledged that the existing public health infrastructure is far from satisfactory. For the outdoor medical facilities inexistence, funding is generally insufficient; the presence of medical and para-medical personnel is often much less than that required by prescribed norms; the availability of consumables is frequently negligible; the equipment in many public hospitals is often obsolescent and unusable; and, the buildings are in a dilapidated state. In the indoor treatment facilities, again, the equipment is often obsolescent; the availability of essential drugs is minimal; the capacity of the facilities is grossly inadequate, which leads to over-crowding, and consequentially to a steep deterioration in the quality of the services. As a result of such inadequate public health facilities, it has been estimated that less than 20 percent at the population, which seek O.P.D. services, and less than 45 percent of that which seek indoor treatment, avail of such services in public hospitals. This is despite the fact that most of these patients do not have the means to make out-of-pocket payments for private health services except at the cost of other essential expenditure for items such as basic nutrition.

2.5. Extending Public Health Services

2.5.1. While there is a general shortage of medical personnel in the country, this shortfall is disproportionately impacted on the less-developed and rural areas. No incentive system attempted so far, has induced private medical personnel to go to such areas; and, even in the public health sector, the effort to deploy medical personnel in such under-served areas, has usually been a losing battle. In such a situation, the possibility needs to be examined of entrusting some limited public health functions to nurses, paramedics and other personnel from the extended health sector after imparting adequate training to them.

2.5.2. India has a vast reservoir of practitioners in the Indian Systems of Medicine and Homoeopathy, who have undergone formal training in their own disciplines. The possibility of using such practitioners in the implementation of state/central government public health programmes, in order to increase the reach of basic health care in the country, is addressed in the N.H.P.-2002.

2.6. Role of Local Self-Government Institutions

2.6.1. Some states have adopted a policy of devolving programmes and funds in the health sector through different levels of the Panchayati Raj Institutions. Generally, the experience has been an encouraging one. The adoption of such an organisational structure has enabled need-based allocation of resources and closer supervision through the elected representatives. The policy examines the need for a wider adoption of this mode of delivery of health services, in rural as well as urban areas, in other parts of the country.

2.7. Norms for Health Care Personnel

2.7.1. It is observed that the deployment of doctors and nurses, in both public and private institutions, is ad-hoc and significantly short of the requirement for minimal standards of patient care. This policy will make a specific recommendation in regard to this deficiency.

2.8. Education of Health Care Professionals

2.8.1. Medical and dental colleges are not evenly spread across various parts of the country. Apart from the uneven geographical distribution of medical institutions, the quality of education is highly uneven and in several instances even sub-standard. It is a common perception that the syllabus is excessively theoretical, making it difficult for the fresh graduate to effectively meet even the primary health care needs of the population. There is a general reluctance on the part of graduate doctors to serve in areas distant from their native place. N.H.P.-2002 will suggest policy initiatives to rectify the resultant disparities.

2.8.2.1. Certain medical disciplines, such as molecular biology and gene-manipulation, have become relevant in the period after the formulation of the previous National Health Policy. The components of medical research in recent years have changed radically. In the foreseeable future such research will rely increasingly on the new disciplines. It is observed that the current under-graduate medical syllabus does not cover such emerging subjects. The policy will make appropriate recommendations in respect of such deficiencies.

2.8.2.2. Also, certain speciality disciplines – anesthesiology, radiology and forensic medicine – are currently very scarce, resulting in critical deficiencies in the package of available public health services. This policy will recommend some measures to alleviate such critical shortages.

2.9. Need for specialists in 'public health' and 'family medicine'

2.9.1. In any developing country with inadequate availability at health services, the requirement at expertise in the areas at 'public health' and 'family medicine' is markedly more than the expertise required for other clinical specialities. In India, the situation is that public health expertise is non-existent in the private health sector, and far short of requirement in the public health sector. Also, the current curriculum in the graduate/post-graduate courses is outdated and unrelated to contemporary community needs. In respect of 'family medicine', it needs to be noted that the more talented medical graduates generally seek specialization in clinical disciplines, while the remaining go into general practice. While the availability of postgraduate educational facilities is 50 percent of the total number of qualifying graduates each year, and can be considered adequate, the distribution of the disciplines in the postgraduate training facilities is overwhelmingly in favour of clinical specializations. N.H.P.-2002 examines the possible means for ensuring adequate availability of personnel with specialization in the 'public health' and 'family medicine' disciplines, to discharge the public health responsibilities in the country.

2.10. Nursing Personnel

2.10.1. The ratio of nursing personnel in the country vis-a-vis doctors/beds is very low according to professionally accepted norms. There is also an acute shortage of nurses trained in super-speciality disciplines for deployment in tertiary care facilities. N.H.P.-2002 addresses these problems.

2.11. Use of Generic Drugs and Vaccines

2.11.1. India enjoys a relatively low-cost health care system because of the widespread availability at indigenously manufactured generic drugs and vaccines. There is an apprehension that globalization will lead to an increase in the costs of drugs, thereby leading to rising trends in overall health costs. This policy recommends measures to ensure the future health security of the country.

2.12. Urban Health

2.12.1. In most urban areas, public health services are very meagre to an extent that there is no uniform organizational structure. The urban population in the country is presently as high as 30 percent and is likely to go up to around 33 percent by 2010. The bulk of the increase is likely to take place through migration, resulting in slums without any infrastructure support. Even the meagre public health services which are available do not percolate to such unplanned habitations, forcing people to avail of private health care through out-of-pocket expenditure.

2.12.2. The rising vehicle density in large urban agglomerations has also led to an increased number of serious accidents requiring treatment in well-equipped trauma centres. N.H.P.-2002 will address itself to the need for providing this unserved urban population a minimum standard of broad-based health care facilities.

2.13. Mental Health

2.13.1. Mental health disorders are actually much more prevalent than is apparent on the surface. While such disorders do not contribute significantly to mortality, they have a serious bearing on the quality of life of the affected persons and their families. Sometimes, based on religious faith, mental disorders are treated as spiritual affliction. This has led to the establishment of unlicensed mental institutions as an adjunct to religious institutions where reliance is placed on faith cure. Serious conditions of mental disorder require hospitalization and treatment under trained supervision. Mental health institutions are woefully deficient in physical infrastructure and trained manpower. N.H.P.-2002 will address itself to these deficiencies in the public health sector.

2.14. Information, Education and Communication

2.14.1. A substantial component of primary health care consists of initiatives for disseminating to the citizenry, public health-related information. I.E.C. initiatives are adopted not only for disseminating curative guidelines (for the T.B., malaria, leprosy, cataract, blindness programmes), but also as part of the effort to bring about a behavioural change to prevent H.I.V./A.I.D.S. and other life-style diseases. Public health programmes, particularly, need high visibility at the decentralized level in order to have an impact. This task is difficult as 35 percent of our country's population is illiterate. The present IEC strategy is too fragmented, relies too heavily on the mass media and does not address the needs of this segment of the population. It is often felt that the effectiveness of I.E.C. programmes is difficult to judge; and consequently it is often asserted that accountability, in regard to the productive use of such funds, is doubtful. The policy, while projecting an I.E.C. strategy, will fully address the inherent problems encountered in any I.E.C. programme designed for improving awareness and bringing about a behavioural change in the general population.

2.14.2 It is widely accepted that school and college students are the most impressionable targets for imparting information relating to the basic principles of preventive health care. The policy will attempt to target this group to improve the general level of awareness in regard to 'health-promoting' behaviour.

2.15 Health Research

2.15.1 Over the years, health research activity in the country has been very limited. In the government sector, such research has been confined to the research institutions under the Indian Council of Medical Research, and other institutions funded by the states/central government. Research in the private sector has assumed some significance only in the last decade. In our country, where the aggregate annual health expenditure is of the order of Rs. 80,000 crores, the expenditure in 1998-99 on research, both public and private sectors, was only of the order of Rs. 1,150 crores. It would be reasonable to inter that with such low research expenditure, it is virtually impossible to make any dramatic break-through within the country, by new molecules and vaccines; also, without a minimal back-up of applied and operational research, it would be difficult to assess whether the health expenditure in the country is being incurred through optimal applications and appropriate public health strategies. Medical research in the country needs to be focused on therapeutic drugs/vaccines for tropical diseases, which are normally neglected by international pharmaceutical companies on account of their limited profitability potential. The thrust will need to be in the newly-emerging frontier areas of research based on genetics, genome-based drug and vaccine development, molecular biology, etc. N.H.P.-2002 will address these inadequacies and spell out a minimal quantum of expenditure for the coming decade, looking to the national needs and the capacity of the research institutions to absorb the funds.

2.16 Role of the Private Sector

2.16.1 Considering the economic restructuring underway in the country, and over the globe, in the last decade, the changing role of the private sector in providing health care will also have to be addressed in this policy. Currently, the contribution of private health care is principally through independent practitioners. Also, the private sector contributes significantly to secondary-level care and some tertiary care. It is a widespread perception that private health services are very uneven in quality, sometimes even sub-standard. Private health services are also perceived to be financially exploitative, and the observance of professional ethics is noted only as an exception. With the increasing role of private health care, the implementation of statutory regulation, and the monitoring of minimum standards of diagnostic centres/medical institutions becomes imperative. The policy will address the issues regarding the establishment at a comprehensive information system, and based on that the establishment of a regulatory mechanism to ensure the maintaining of adequate standards by diagnostic centres/medical institutions, as well as the proper conduct of clinical practice and delivery of medical services.

2.16.2 Currently, non-governmental service providers are treating a large number of patients at the primary level for major disease. However, the treatment regimens followed are diverse and not scientifically optimal, leading to an increase in the incidence of drug resistance. This policy will address itself to recommending arrangements which will eliminate the risks arising from inappropriate treatment.

2.16.3 The increasing spread of information technology raises the possibility of its adoption in the health sector. N.H.P.-2002 will examine this possibility.

2.17 The Role of Civil Society

2.17.1 Historically, it has been the practice to implement major national disease control programmes through the public health machinery of the state/central governments. It has become increasingly apparent that certain components of such programmes cannot be efficiently implemented merely through government functionaries. A considerable change in the mode of implementation has come about in the last two decades, with the increasing involvement of N.G.Os. and other institutions of civil society. It is to be recognized that widespread debate on various public health issues has, in fact, been initiated and sustained by N.G.Os. and other members of the civil society. Also, an increasing contribution is being made by such institutions in the delivery of different components of public health services. Certain disease control programmes require close interaction with the beneficiaries for regular administration of drugs; periodic carrying out of pathological tests; dissemination of information regarding disease control and other general health information. N.H.P.-2002 will address such issues and suggest policy instruments for the implementation of public health programmes through individuals and institutions of civil society.

2.18 National Disease Surveillance Network

2.18.1 The technical network available in the country for disease surveillance is extremely rudimentary and to the extent that the system exists, it extends only up to the district level. Disease statistics are not flowing through an integrated network from the decentralized public health facilities to the state/central government health administration. Such an arrangement only provides belated information, which, at best, serves a limited statistical purpose. The absence of an efficient disease surveillance network is a major handicap in providing a prompt and cost-effective health care system. The efficient disease surveillance network set up for Polio and H.I.V./A.I.D.S. has demonstrated the enormous value of such a public health instrument. Real-time information on focal outbreaks of common communicable diseases – malaria, G.E., cholera and J.E. – and the seasonal trends of diseases, would enable timely intervention, resulting in the containment of the thrust of epidemics. In order to be able to use an integrated disease surveillance network for operational purposes, real-time information is necessary at all levels of the health administration. The policy would address itself to this major systemic shortcoming in the administration.

2.19 Health Statistics

2.19.1 The absence of a systematic and scientific health statistics database is a major deficiency in the current scenario. The health statistics collected are not the product of a rigorous methodology. Statistics available from different parts of the country, in respect of major diseases, are often not obtained in a manner which make aggregation possible or meaningful.

2.19.2.1 Further, the absence of proper and systematic documentation of the various financial resources used in the health sector is another lacuna in the existing health information scenario. This makes it difficult to understand trends and levels of health spending by private and public providers at health care in the country, and, consequently, to address related policy issues and to formulate future investment policies.

2.19.2.2 N.H.P.-2002 will address itself to the programme for putting in place a modern and scientific health statistics database as well as a system of national health accounts.

2.20 Women's Health

2.20.1 Social, cultural and economic factors continue to inhibit women from gaining adequate access even to the existing public health facilities. This handicap does not merely affect women as individuals; it also has an adverse impact on the health, general well-being and development of the entire family, particularly children. This policy recognises the catalytic role of empowered women in improving the overall health standards of the community.

2.21 Medical Ethics

2.21.1 Professional medical ethics in the health sector is an area which has not received much attention. Professional practices are perceived to be grossly commercial and the medical profession has lost its elevated position as a provider of basic services to fellow human beings. In the past, medical research has been conducted within the ethical guidelines notified by the Indian Council of Medical Research. The first document containing these guidelines was released in 1960, and was comprehensively revised in 2001. With the rapid developments in the approach to medical research, a periodic revision will no doubt be more frequently required in future. Also, the new frontier areas of research – involving gene manipulation, organ/human cloning and stem cell research – impinge on visceral issues relating to the sanctity of human life and the moral dilemma of human intervention in the designing of life forms. Besides this, in the emerging areas of research, there is the uncharted risk of creating new life forms, which may irreversibly damage the environment as it exists today. N.H.P.-2002 recognises that this moral and religious dilemma, which was not relevant even two years ago, now pervades mainstream health sector issues.

2.22 Enforcement of Quality Standard for Food and Drugs

2.22.1 There is an increasing expectation and need of the citizenry for efficient enforcement of reasonable quality standards for food and drugs. Recognizing this, the policy will make an appropriate policy recommendation on this issue.

2.23 Regulation of Standards in Para Medical

2.23.1 It has been observed that a large number of training institutions have mushroomed, particularly in the private sector, for para medical personnel with various skills – Lab. technicians, Radio diagnosis technicians, Physiotherapists, etc. Currently, there is no regulation/monitoring, either of the curriculae of these institutions, or of the performance of the practitioners in these disciplines. This policy will make recommendations to ensure the standardization of such training and the monitoring of actual performance.

2.24 Environmental and Occupational Health

2.24.1 The ambient environmental conditions are a significant determinant of the health risks to which a community is exposed. Unsafe drinking water, unhygienic sanitation and air pollution significantly contribute to the burden of disease, particularly in urban settings. The initiatives in respect of these environmental factors are conventionally undertaken by the participants, whether private or public, in the other development sectors. In this backdrop, the policy initiatives and the efficient implementation of the linked programmes in the health sector, would succeed only to the extent that they are complemented by appropriate policies and programmes in the other environment-related sectors.

2.24.2 Work conditions in several sectors of employment in the country are sub-standard. As a result, workers engaged in such employment become particularly vulnerable to occupation-linked ailments. The long-term risk of chronic morbidity is particularly marked in the case of child labour. N.H.P.-2002 will address the risk faced by this particularly vulnerable section of society.

2.25 Providing Medical Facilities to Users from Overseas

2.25.1 The secondary and tertiary facilities available in the country are of good quality and cost-effective compared to international medical facilities. This is true not only of facilities in the allopathic disciplines, but also of those belonging to the alternative systems of medicine, particularly ayurveda. The policy will assess the possibilities of encouraging the development of paid treatment-packages for patients from overseas.

2.26 The Impact of Globalization on the Health Sector

2.26.1 There are some' apprehensions about the possible adverse impact of economic-globalisation on the health sector. Pharmaceutical drugs and other health services have always been available in the country at extremely inexpensive prices. India has, established a reputation around the globe for the innovative development of original process patents for the manufacture of a wide-range of drugs and vaccines within the ambit of the existing patent laws. With the adoption of Trade Related Intellectual Property Rights (T.R.I.P.S.), and the subsequent alignment of domestic patent laws consistent with the commitments under T.R.I.P.S., there will be a significant shift in the scope of the parameters regulating the manufacture of new drugs/vaccines. Global experience has shown that the introduction of a T.R.I.P.S.-consistent patent regime for drugs in a developing country results in an across-the-board increase in the cost of drugs and medical services. N.H.P.-2002 will address itself to the future imperatives of health security in the country, in the post-T.R.I.P.S. era.

2.27 Inter-Sectoral Contribution to Health

2.27.1 It is well recognized that the overall well-being of the citizenry depends on the synergistic functioning of the various sectors in the socio-economy. The health status of the citizenry would, inter alia, be dependent on adequate nutrition, safe drinking water, basic sanitation, a clean environment and primary education, especially for the girl child. The policies and the mode of functioning in these independent areas would necessarily overlap each other to contribute to the health status of the community. From the policy perspective, it is therefore imperative that the independent policies of each of these inter-connected sectors, be in tandem, and that the interface between the policies of the two connected sectors, be smooth.

2.27.2 Sectoral policy documents are meant to serve as a guide to action for institutions and individual participants operating in that sector. Consistent with this role, N.H.P.-2002 limits itself to making recommendations for the participants operating within the health sector. The policy aspects relating to inter-connected sectors, which, while crucial, fall outside the domain of the health sector, will not be covered by specific recommendations in this policy document. Needless to say, the future attainment of the various goals set out in this policy assumes a reasonable complementary performance in these inter-connected sectors.

2.28 Population Growth and Health Standards

2.28.1 Efforts made over the years for improving health standards have been partially neutralized by the rapid growth of the population. It is well recognized that population stabilization measures and general health initiatives, when effectively synchronized, synergistically maximize the socio-economic well-being of the people. Government has separately announced the 'National Population Policy-2000'. The principal common features covered under the National Population Policy-2000 and N.H.P.-2002, relate to the prevention and control of communicable diseases; giving priority to the containment of H.I.V./A.I.D.S. infection; the universal immunization of children against all major preventable diseases; addressing the unmet needs for basic and reproductive health services, and supplementation of infrastructure. The synchronized implementation of these two policies – National Population Policy – 2000 and National Health Policy-2002 – will be the very cornerstone of any national structural plan to improve the health standards in the country.

2.29 Alternative Systems of Medicine

2.29.1 Under the overarching umbrella of the national health frame work, the alternative systems of medicine – Ayurveda, Unani, Siddha and Homoeopathy-have a substantial role. Because of inherent advantages, such as diversity, modest cost, low level of technological input and the growing popularity of natural plant-based products, these systems are attractive, particularly in the underserved, remote and tribal areas. The alternative systems will draw upon the substantial untapped potential of India as one of the eight important global centers for plant diversity in medicinal and aromatic plants. The policy focuses on building up credibility for the alternative systems, by encouraging evidence-based research to determine their efficacy, safety and dosage, and also encourages certification and quality-marking of products to enable a wider popular acceptance of these systems of medicine. The policy also envisages the consolidation of documentary knowledge contained in these systems to protect it against attack from foreign commercial entities by way of malafide action under patent laws in other countries. The main components of N.H.P.-2002 apply equally to the alternative systems of medicines. However, the policy features specific to the alternative systems of medicine will be presented as a separate document.

3. Objectives

3.1 The main objective of this policy is to achieve an acceptable standard of good health amongst the general population of the country. The approach would be to increase access to the decentralized public health system by establishing new infrastructure in deficient areas, and by upgrading the infrastructure in the existing institutions. Overriding importance would be given to ensure a more equitable access to health services across the social and geographical expanse of the country. Emphasis will be given to increase the aggregate public health investment through a substantially increased contribution by the central government. It is expected that this initiative will strengthen the capacity of the public health administration at the state level to render effective service delivery. The contribution of the private sector in providing health services would be much enhanced, particularly for the population group which can afford to pay for services. Primacy will be given to preventive and first-line curative initiatives at the primary health level through increased sectoral share of allocation. Emphasis will be laid on rational use of drugs within the allopathic system. Increased access to tried and tested systems of traditional medicine will be ensured. Within these broad objectives, N.H.P.-2002 will endeavour to achieve the time-bound goals mentioned in Table-4.

Table-4
Goals to be achieved by 2000-2015

Eradicate Polio and Yaws	2005
Eliminate Leprosy	2005
Eliminate Kala Azar	2010
Eliminate Lymphatic Filariasis	2015
Achieve Zero level growth of H.I.V./A.I.D.S.	2007
Reduce Mortality by 50% on account of T.B., Malaria and Other Vector and Water Borne diseases	2010
Reduce Prevalence of Blindness to 0.5%	2010
Reduce I.M.R. to 30/1000 and M.M.R. to 100/Lakh	2010
Increase utilization of public health facilities from current level of <20 to >75%	2010
Establish an integrated system of surveillance, National Health Accounts and Health Statistics.	2005
Increase health expenditure by government as a % of G.D.P. from the existing 0.9% to 2.0%	2010
Increase share of central grants to Constitute at least 25% of total health spending	2010
Increase state Sector Health spending from 5.5% to 7% of the budget	2005
Further increase to 8%	2010

4. N.H.P.-2002 – Policy Prescriptions

4.1 Financial Resources

4.1.1 The paucity of public health investment is a stark reality. Given the extremely difficult fiscal position of the state governments, the central government will have to play a key role in augmenting public health investments. Taking into account the gap in health care facilities, it is planned, under the policy to increase health sector expenditure to 6 percent of G.D.P., with 2 percent of G.D.P. being contributed as public health investment, by the year 2010. The state governments would also need to increase the commitment to the health sector. In the first phase, by 2005, they would be expected to increase the commitment of their resources to 7 percent of the budget; and, in the second phase, by 2010, to increase it to 8 percent of the budget. With the stepping up of the public health investment, the central government's contribution would rise to 25 percent from the existing 15 percent by 2010. The provisioning of higher public health investments will also be contingent upon the increase in the absorptive capacity of the public health administration so as to utilize the funds gainfully.

4.2 Equity

4.2.1 To meet the objective of reducing various types of inequities and imbalances – inter-regional; across the rural – urban divide; and between economic classes – the most cost-effective method would be to increase the sectoral outlay in the primary health sector. Such outlets afford access to a vast number of individuals, and also facilitate preventive and early stage curative initiative, which are cost effective. In recognition of this public health principle, N.H.P.-2002 sets out an increased allocation of 55 percent of the total public health investment for the primary health sector; the secondary and tertiary health sectors being targeted for 35 percent and 10 percent respectively. The Policy projects that the increased aggregate outlays for the primary health sector will be utilized for strengthening existing facilities and opening additional public health service outlets, consistent with the norms for such facilities.

4.3 Delivery of National Public Health Programmes

4.3.1.1 This policy envisages a key role for the central government in designing national programmes with the active participation of the state governments. Also, the policy ensures the provisioning of financial resources, in addition to technical support, monitoring and evaluation at the national level by the centre. However, to optimize the utilization of the public health infrastructure at the primary level, N.H.P.-2002 envisages the gradual convergence of all health programmes under a single field administration. Vertical programmes for control of major diseases like T.B., malaria, H.I.V./A.I.D.S., as also the R.C.H. and Universal Immunization Programmes, would need to be continued till moderate levels of prevalence are reached. The integration of the programmes will bring about a desirable optimisation of outcomes through a convergence of all public health inputs. The policy also envisages that programme implementation be effected through autonomous bodies at state and district levels. The interventions of state health departments may be limited to the overall monitoring of the achievement of programme targets and other technical aspects. The relative distancing of the programme implementation from the state Health Departments will give the project team greater operational flexibility. Also, the presence of state government officials, social activists, private health professionals and M.L.As./M.Ps. on the management boards of the autonomous bodies will facilitate well-informed decision-making.

4.3.1.2   The Policy also highlights the need for developing the capacity within the state public health administration for scientific designing of public health projects, suited to the local situation.

4.3.2   The policy envisages that apart from the exclusive staff in a vertical structure for the disease control programmes, all rural health staff should be available for the entire gamut of public health activities at the decentralized level, irrespective of whether these activities relate to national programmes or other public health initiatives. It would be for the head of the district health administration to allocate the time of the rural health staff between the various programmes, depending on the local need. N.H.P.-2002 recognizes that to implement such a change, not only would the public health administrators be required to change their mindset, but the rural health staff would need to be trained and reoriented.

4.4 The state of Public Health Infrastructure

4.4.1.1   As has been highlighted in the earlier part of the policy, the decentralized public health service outlets have become practically dysfunctional over large parts of the country. On account of resource constraints, the supply of drugs by the state governments is grossly inadequate. The patients at the decentralized level have little use for diagnostic services, which in any case would still require them to purchase therapeutic drugs privately. In a situation in which the patient is not getting any therapeutic drugs, there is little incentive for the potential beneficiaries to seek the advice of the medical professionals in the public health system. This results in there being no demand for medical services, so medical professionals and paramedics often absent themselves from their place of duty. It is also observed that the functioning of the public health service outlets in the four Southern states - Kerala, Andhra Pradesh, Tamil Nadu and Karnataka – is relatively better, because some quantum of drugs is distributed through the primary health system network, and the patients have a stake in approaching the public health facilities. In this backdrop, the policy envisages kick-starting the revival of the primary health system by providing some essential drugs under central government funding through the decentralized health system. It is expected that the provision of essential drugs at the public health service centres will create a demand for other professional services from the local population, which, in turn, will boost the general revival of activities in these service centres. In sum, this initiative under N.H.P.-2002 is launched in the belief that the creation of a beneficiary interest in the public health system, will ensure a more effective supervision of the public health personnel through community monitoring, than has been achieved through the regular administrative line of control.

4.4.1.2 This policy recognizes the need for more frequent in-service training of public health medical personnel, at the level of medical officers as well as paramedics. Such training would help to update the personnel on recent advancements in science, and would also equip them for their new assignments, when they are moved from one discipline of public health administration to another.

4.4.1.3 Global experience has shown that the quality of public health services, as reflected in the attainment of improved public health indices, is closely linked to the quantum and quality of investment through public funding in the primary health sector. Table-5 gives statistics which clearly show that standards of health are more a function of the accurate targeting of expenditure on the decentralised primary sector (as observed in China and Sri Lanka), than a function of the aggregate health expenditure.

Table-5
Public Health Spending in select Countries

Indicator	%Population with income of<$1 day	Infant Mortality Rate/1000	% Health Expenditure to G.D.P.	% Public Expenditure on Health to Total Health Expenditure
India	44.2	70	5.2	17.3
China	18.5	31	2.7	24.9
Sri Lanka	6.6	16	3	45.4
U.K.	–	6	5.8	96.9
U.S.A.	–	7	13.7	44.1

Therefore the policy, while committing additional aggregate financial resources, places great reliance on the strengthening of the primary health structure for attaining improved public health outcomes on an equitable basis. Further, it also recognizes the practical need for levying reasonable user-charges for certain secondary and tertiary public health care services, for those who can afford to pay.

4.5 Extending Public Health Services

4.5.1.1 This policy envisages that, in the context of the availability and spread of allopathic graduates in their jurisdiction. state governments would consider the need for expanding the pool of medical practitioners to include a cadre of licentiates of medical practice, as also practitioners of Indian Systems of Medicine and Homoeopathy. Simple services/procedures can be provided by such practitioners even outside their disciplines, as part of the basic primary health services in under-served areas. Also, N.H.P.-2002 envisages that the scope of the use of paramedical manpower of allopathic disciplines, in a prescribed functional area adjunct to their current functions, would also be examined for meeting simple public health requirements. This would be on the lines of the services rendered by nurse practitioners in several developed countries. These extended areas of functioning of different categories of medical manpower can be permitted, after adequate training, and subject to the monitoring of their performance through professional councils.

4.5.1.2 N.H.P.-2002 also recognizes the need for states to simplify the recruitment procedures and rules for contract employment in order to provide trained medical manpower in under-served areas. State governments could also rigorously enforce a mandatory two-year rural posting before the awarding of the graduate degree. This would not only make trained medical manpower available in the underserved areas, but would offer valuable clinical experience to the graduating doctors.

4.6 Role of Local Self-government Institutions

4.6.1 N.H.P.-2002 lays great emphasis upon the implementation of public health programmes through local self-government institutions. The structure of the national disease control programmes will have specific components for implementation through such entities. The policy urges all state governments to consider decentralizing the implementation of the programmes to such institutions by 2005. In order to achieve this, financial incentives, over and above the resources normatively allocated for disease control programmes, will be provided by the central government.

4.7 Norms for Health Care Personnel

4.7.1 Minimal statutory norms for the deployment of doctors and nurses in medical institutions need to be introduced urgently under the provisions of the Indian Medical Council Act and Indian Nursing Council Act, respectively. These norms can be progressively reviewed and made more stringent as the medical institutions improve their capacity for meeting better normative standards.

4.8 Education of Health Care Professionals

4.8.1.1 In order to ameliorate the problems being faced on account of the uneven spread of medical and dental colleges in various parts of the country, this policy envisages the setting up of a Medical Grants Commission for funding new government Medical and Dental Colleges in different parts of the country. Also, it is envisaged that the Medical Grants Commission will fund the upgradation of the infrastructure of the existing government Medical and Dental Colleges of the country, so as to ensure an improved standard of medical education.

4.8.1.2 To enable fresh graduates to contribute effectively the provision of primary health services as the physician of first contact, this policy identifies a significant need to modify the existing curriculum. A need-based, skill-oriented syllabus, with a more significant component of practical training, would make fresh doctors useful immediately after graduation. The policy also recommends a periodic skill-updating of working health professionals through a system of continuing medical education.

4.8.2 The policy emphasises the need to expose medical students through the undergraduate syllabus, to the emerging concerns for geriatric disorders, as also to the cutting edge disciplines of contemporary medical research. The policy also envisages that the creation of additional seats for post-graduate courses should reflect the need for more manpower in the deficient specialities.

4.9 Need for Specialists in 'Public Health' and 'Family Medicine'

4.9.1 In order to alleviate the acute shortage at medical personnel with specialization in the disciplines of 'public health' and 'family medicine', the policy envisages the progressive implementation of mandatory norms to raise the proportion of postgraduate seats in these discipline in medical training institutions, to reach a stage wherein ¼th of the seats are earmarked for these disciplines. It is envisaged that in the sanctioning of post-graduate seats in future, it shall be insisted upon that a certain reasonable number of seats be allocated to 'public health' and 'family medicine'. Since the 'public health' discipline has an interface with many other developmental sectors, specialization in public health may be encouraged not only for medical doctors, but also for non-medical graduates from the allied fields of public health engineering, microbiology and other natural sciences.

4.10 Nursing Personnel

4.10.1.1 In the interest of patient care, the policy emphasizes the need for an improvement in the ratio of nurses vis-a-vis doctors/beds. In order to discharge their responsibility as model providers of health services, the public health delivery centres need to make a beginning by increasing the number of nursing personnel. The policy anticipates that with the increasing aspiration for improved health care amongst the citizens, private health facilities will also improve their ratio of nursing personnel vis a-vis doctors/beds.

4.10.1.2 The policy lays emphasis on improving the skill-level of nurses, and on increasing the ratio of degree-holding nurses vis-a-vis diploma-holding nurses. N.H.P.-2002 recognizes a need for the central government to subsidize the setting up, and the running of, training facilities for nurses on a decentralized basis. Also, the policy recognizes the need for establishing training courses for super-speciality nurses required for tertiary care institutions.

4.11 Use of Generic Drugs and Vaccines

4.11.1.1 This policy emphasizes the need for basing treatment regimens, in both the public and private domain, on a limited number of essential drugs of a generic nature. This is a prerequisite for cost-effective public health care. In the public health system, this would be enforced by prohibiting the use of proprietary drugs, except in special circumstances. The list of essential drugs would no doubt have to be reviewed periodically to encourage the use of only essential drugs in the private sector the imposition of fiscal disincentives would be resorted to. The production and sale of irrational combinations of drugs would be prohibited through the drug standards statute.

4.11.1.2 The National Programme for Universal Immunization against preventable diseases requires to be assured of an uninterrupted supply of vaccines at an affordable price. To minimize the danger arising from the volatility of the global market, and thereby to ensure long-term national health security, N.H.P.-2002 envisages that not less than 50% of the requirement of vaccines/sera be sourced from public sector institutions.

4.12 Urban Health

4.12.1.1 N.H.P.-2002 envisages the setting up of an organised urban primary health care structure. Since the physical features of urban settings are different from those in rural areas, the policy envisages the adoption of appropriate population norms for the urban public health infrastructure. The structure conceived under N.H.P.-2002 is a two-tiered one: the primary centre is seen as the first-tier, covering a population of one lakh, with a dispensary providing an O.P.D. facility and essential drugs, to enable access to all the national health programmes; and a second-tier of the urban health organisation at the level of the government general hospital, where reference is made from the primary centre. The policy envisages that the funding for the urban primary health system will be jointly borne by the local self-government institutions and state and central governments.

4.12.1.2   The policy also envisages the establishment of fully-equipped 'hub-spoke' trauma care networks in large urban agglomerations to reduce accident mortality.

4.13 Mental Health

4.13.1.1   N.H.P.-2002 envisages a network of decentralised mental health services for ameliorating the more common categories of disorders. The programme outline for such a disease would involve the diagnosis of common disorders, and the prescription of common therapeutic drugs, by general duty medical staff.

4.13.1.2   In regard to mental health institutions for indoor treatment of patients, the policy envisages the upgrading of the physical infrastructure of such institutions at central government expense so as to secure the human rights of this vulnerable segment of society.

4.14 Information, Education and Communication

4.14.1   N.H.P.-2002 envisages an I.E.C. policy, which maximizes the dissemination of information to those population groups which cannot be effectively approached by using only the mass media. The focus would therefore be on the inter-personal communication of information and on folk and other traditional media to bring about behavioural change. The I.E.C. programme would set specific targets for the association of P.R.Is./N.G.Os./Trusts in such activities. In several public health programmes, where behavioural change is an essential component, the success of the initiatives is crucially dependent on dispelling myths and misconceptions pertaining to religious and ethical issues. The community leaders, particularly religious leaders, are effective in imparting knowledge which facilitates such behavioural change. The programme will also have the component of an annual evaluation of the performance of the non-governmental agencies to monitor the impact of the programmes on the targeted groups. The central/state government initiative will also focus on the development of modules for information dissemination in such population groups, who do not normally benefit from the more common media forms.

4.14.2   N.H.P.-2002 envisages giving priority to school health programmes which aim at preventive-health education, providing regular health check-ups, and promotion of health-seeking behaviour among children. The school health programmes can gainfully adopt specially designed modules in order to disseminate information relating to 'health' and 'family life'. This is expected to be the most cost-effective intervention as it improves the level of awareness, not only of the extended family, but the future generation as well.

4.15 Health Research

4.15.1   This policy envisages an increase in government-funded health research to a level of 1 percent of the total health spending by 2005; and thereafter, up to 2 percent by 2010. Domestic medical research would be focused on new therapeutic drugs and vaccines for tropical diseases, such as T.B. and malaria, as also on the sub-types of H.I.V./A.I.D.S. prevalent in the country. Research programmes taken up by the government in these priority areas would be conducted in a mission mode. Emphasis would also be laid on time-bound applied research for developing operational applications. This would ensure the cost-effective dissemination of existing/future therapeutic drugs/vaccines in the general population. Private entrepreneurship will be encouraged in the field of medical research for new molecules/vaccines, infer alia, through fiscal incentives.

4.16 Role of the Private Sector

4.16.1.1   In principle, this policy welcomes the participation of the private sector in all the areas of health activities – primary, secondary or tertiary. However, looking at the past experience of the private sector, it can reasonably be expected that its contribution would be substantial in the urban primary sector and the tertiary sector, and moderate in the secondary sector. This policy envisages the enactment of suitable legislation for regulating minimum infrastructure and quality standards in clinical establishments/medical institutions by 2003. Also, statutory guidelines for the conduct of clinical practice and delivery of medical services are targeted to be developed over the same period. With the acquiring of experience in the setting and enforcing of minimum quality standards, the policy envisages graduation to a scheme of quality accreditation of clinical establishments/medical institutions, for the information of the citizenry. The regulatory/accreditation mechanisms will no doubt also cover public health institutions. The policy also encourages the setting up of private insurance instruments for increasing the scope of the coverage of the secondary and tertiary sector under private health insurance packages.

4.16.1.2 In the context of the very large number of poor in the country, it would be difficult to conceive an exclusive government mechanism to provide health services to this category. It has sometimes been felt that a social health insurance scheme, funded by the government, and with service delivery through the private sector, would be the appropriate solution. The administrative and financial implications of such an initiative are still unknown. As a first step, this policy envisages the introduction of a pilot scheme in a limited number of representative districts, to determine the administrative features of such an arrangement, as also the requirement of resources for it. The results obtained from these pilot projects would provide material on which future public health policy can be based.

4.16.2 N.H.P.-2002 envisages the co-operation of the non-governmental practitioners in the national disease control programmes so as to ensure that standard treatment protocols are followed in their day-to-day practice.

4.16.3 This policy recognizes the immense potential of information technology applications in the area of tele-medicine in the tertiary health care sector. The use of this technical aid will greatly enhance the capacity for the professionals to pool their clinical experience.

4.17 The Role of Civil Society

4.17.1 N.H.P.-2002 recognizes the significant contribution made by N.G.Os. and other institutions of the civil society in making available health services to the community. In order to utilize their high motivational skills on an increasing scale, this policy envisages that the disease control programmes should earmark not less than 10% of the budget in respect of identified programme components, to be exclusively implemented through these institutions. The policy also emphasizes the need to simplify procedures for government – civil society interfacing in order to enhance the involvement of civil society in public health programmes. In principle, the state would encourage the handing over of public health service outlets at any level for management by N.G.Os. and other institutions of civil society, on an 'as-is-where-is' basis, along with the normative funds earmarked for such institutions.

4.18 National Disease Surveillance Network

4.18.1 This policy envisages the full operationalization of an integrated disease control network from the lowest rung of public health administration to the central government, by 2005. The programme for setting up this network will include components relating to the installation of data-base handling hardware; I.T. inter-connectivity between different tiers of the network; and in house training for data collection and interpretation for undertaking timely and effective response. This public health surveillance network will also encompass information from private health care institutions and practitioners. It is expected that real-time information from outside the government system will greatly strengthen the capacity of the public health system to counter focal outbreaks of seasonal diseases.

4.19 Health Statistics

4.19.1.1 The policy envisages the completion of baseline estimates for the incidence of the common diseases – T.B., malaria, blindness – by 2005. The policy proposes that statistical methods be put in place to enable the periodic updating of these baseline estimates through representative sampling, under an appropriate statistical methodology. The policy also recognizes the need to establish, in a longer time-frame, baseline estimates for non-communicable diseases, like C.V.D., cancer, diabetes; and accidental injuries, and communicable diseases, like hepatitis and J.E. N.H.P.-2002 envisages that, with access to such reliable data on the incidence of various diseases, the public health system would move closer to the objective of evidence-based policy-making.

4.19.1.2 Planning for the health sector requires a robust information system, inter-alia, covering data on service facilities available in the private sector. N.H.P.-2002 emphasises the need for the early completion of an accurate data-base of this kind.

4.19.2 In an attempt at consolidating the data base and graduating from a mere estimation of the annual health expenditure, N.H.P.-2002 emphasises the need to establish national health accounts, conforming to the 'source-to-users' matrix structure. Also, the policy envisages the estimation of health costs on a continuing basis. Improved and comprehensive information through national health accounts and accounting systems would pave the way for decision-makers to focus on relative priorities, keeping in view the limited financial resources in the health sector.

4.20 Women's Health

4.20.1 N.H.P.-2002 envisages the identification of specific programmes targeted at women's health. The Policy notes that women, along with other under-privileged groups, are significantly handicapped due to a disproportionately low access to health care. The various policy recommendations of N.H.P.-2002, in regard to the expansion of primary health sector infrastructure, will facilitate the increased access of women to basic health care. The policy commits the highest priority of the central government to the funding of the identified programmes relating to woman's health. Also, the policy recognizes the need to review the staffing norms of the public health administration to meet the specific requirements of women in a more comprehensive manner.

4.21 Medical Ethics

4.21.1.1 N.H.P.-2002 envisages that, in order to ensure that the common patient is not subjected to irrational or profit-driven medical regimens, a contemporary code of ethics be notified and rigorously implemented by the Medical Council of India.

4.21.1.2 By and large, medical research within the country in the frontier disciplines, such as gene-manipulation and stem cell research, is limited. However, the policy recognises that a vigilant watch will have to be kept so that the existing guidelines and statutory provisions are constantly reviewed and updated.

4.22 Enforcement of Quality Standards for Food and Drugs

4.22.1 N.H.P.-2002 envisages that the food and drug administration will be progressively strengthened, in terms of both laboratory facilities and technical expertise. Also, the policy envisages that the standards of food items will be progressively tightened up at a pace which will permit domestic food handling/manufacturing facilities to undertake the necessary upgradation of technology so that they are not shut out of this production sector. The policy envisages that ultimately food standards will be close, if not equivalent, to Codex specifications; and that drug standards will be at par with the most rigorous ones adopted elsewhere.

4.23 Regulation of Standards in Paramedical Disciplines

4.23.1 N.H.P.-2002 recognises the need for the establishment of statutory professional councils for paramedical disciplines to register practitioners, maintain standards of training, and monitor performance.

4.24 Environmental and Occupational Health

4.24.1 This policy envisages that the independently-stated policies and programmes of the environment-related sectors be smoothly interfaced with the policies and the programmes of the health sector, in order to reduce the health risk to the citizens and the consequential disease burden.

4.24.2 N.H.P.-2002 envisages the periodic screening of the health conditions of the workers, particularly for high-risk health disorders associated with their occupation.

4.25 Providing Medical Facilities to Users from Overseas

4.25.1 To capitalize on the comparative cost advantage enjoyed by domestic health facilities in the secondary and tertiary sectors, N.H.P.-2002 strongly encourages the providing of such health services on a payment basis to service seekers from overseas. The providers of such services to patients from overseas will be encouraged by extending to their earnings in foreign exchange, all fiscal incentives, including the status at "deemed exports", which are available to other exporters of goods and services.

4.26 Impact of Globalisation on the Health Sector

4.26.1 The policy takes into account the serious apprehension, expressed by several health experts, of the possible threat to health security in the post-T.R.I.P.S. era, as a result of a sharp increase in the prices of drugs and vaccines. To protect the citizens of the country from such a threat, this policy envisages a national patent regime for the future, which, while being consistent with T.R.I.P.S., avails of all opportunities to secure for the country, under its patent laws, affordable access to the latest medical and other therapeutic discoveries. The policy also sets out that the government will bring to bear its full influence in all international forums – U.N., W.H.O., W.T.O., etc. – to secure commitments on the part of the nations of the globe, to lighten the restrictive features of T.R.I.P.S. in its application to the health care sector.

5. Summation

5.1 The grafting of a National Health Policy is a rare occasion in public affairs when it would be legitimate, indeed valuable, to allow our dreams to mingle with our understanding of ground realities. Based purely on the clinical facts defining the current status of the health sector, we would have arrived at a certain policy formulation; but, buoyed by our dreams, we have ventured slightly beyond that in the shape of N.H.P.-2002, which, in fact, defines a vision for the future.

5.2 The health needs of the country are enormous and the financial resources and managerial capacity available to meet them, even on the most optimistic projections, fall somewhat short. In this situation, N.H.P.-2002 has had to make hard choices between various priorities and operational options. N.H.P.-2002 does not claim to be a road-map for meeting all the health needs of the populace of the country. Further, it has to be recognized that such health needs are also dynamic, as threats in the area of public health keep changing over time. The policy, while being holistic, undertakes the necessary risk of recommending differing emphasis on different policy components. Broadly speaking, N.H.P.-2002 focuses on the need for enhanced funding and an organizational restructuring of the national public health initiatives in order to facilitate more equitable access to the health facilities. Also, the policy is focused on those diseases which are principally contributing to the disease burden – T.B., malaria and blindness from the category of historical diseases; and H.I.V./A.I.D.S. from the category of 'newly emerging diseases'. This is not to say that other items contributing to the disease burden of the country will be ignored; but only that the resources, as also the principal focus of the public health administration, will recognize certain relative priorities. It is unnecessary to labour the point that under the umbrella of the macro-policy prescriptions in this document, governments and private sector programme planners will have to design separate schemes, tailor-made to the health needs of women, children, geriatrics, tribals and other socio-economically under-served sections. An adequately robust disaster management plan has to be in place to effectively cope with situations arising from natural and man-made calamities.

5.3 One nagging imperative, which has influenced every aspect of this policy, is the need to ensure that 'equity' in the health sector stands as an independent goal. In any future evaluation of its success or failure, N.H.P.-2002 would wish to be measured against this equity norm, rather than any other aggregated financial norm for the health sector. Consistent with the primacy given to 'equity', a marked emphasis has been provided in the policy for expanding and improving the primary health facilities, including the new concept of the provision of essential drugs through central funding. The policy also commits the central government to an increased under-writing of the resources for meeting the minimum health needs of the people. Thus, the policy attempts to provide guidance for prioritizing expenditure, thereby facilitating rational resource allocation.

5.4 This policy broadly envisages a greater contribution from the central budget for the delivery of public health services at the state level. Adequate appropriations, steadily rising over the years, would need to be ensured. The possibility of ensuring this by imposing an earmarked health cess has been carefully examined. While it is recognized that the annual budget must accommodate the increasing resource needs of the social sectors, particularly in the health sector, this policy does not specifically recommend an earmarked health cess, as that would have a tendency of reducing the space available to Parliament in making appropriations looking to the circumstances prevailing from time to time.

5.5 The policy highlights the expected roles of different participating groups in the health sector. Further, it recognizes the fact that, despite all that may be guaranteed by the central government for assisting public health programmes, public health services would actually need to be delivered by the state administration, N.G.Os. and other institutions of civil society. The attainment of improved health levels would be significantly dependent on population stabilisation, as also on complementary efforts from other areas of the social sectors – like improved drinking water supply, basic sanitation, minimum nutrition, etc. – to ensure that the exposure of the populace to health risks is minimized.

5.6 Any expectation of a significant improvement in the quality of health services, and the consequential improved health status of the citizenry, would depend not only on increased financial and material inputs, but also on a more empathetic and committed attitude in the service providers, whether in the private or public sectors. In some measure, this optimistic policy document is based on the understanding that the citizenry is increasingly demanding more by way of quality in health services, and the health delivery system, particularly in the public sector, is being pressed to respond. In this backdrop, it needs to be recognized that any policy in the social sector is critically dependent on the service providers treating their responsibility not as a commercial activity, but as a service, albeit a paid one. In the area of public health, an improved standard of governance is a prerequisite for the success of any health policy.

TENTH FIVE YEAR PLAN (2002-2007)

To improve the health status of the population, and the monitorable targets for the Tenth Five Year Plan and beyond are as follows :

1. Reduction of poverty ratio by 5 per cent points by 2007, and by 15 per cent points by 2012.
2. All children in school by 2003; all children to complete 5 years of schooling by 2007.
3. Reduction in gender gaps in literacy and wage rates by at least 50 per cent by 2007.
4. Reduction in the decadal rate of population growth between 2001 and 2011 to 16.2 per cent.
5. Increase in literacy rate to 75 per cent within the plan period.
6. Reduction of infant mortality rate to 45 per cent 1000 live births by 2007 and to 28 by 2012.
7. Reduction of maternal mortality ratio to 2 per 1000 live births by 2007 and to 1 by 2012; and
8. All villages to have sustained access to potable drinking water within the Plan period.

CHAPTER-19

HEALTH EDUCATION

HEALTH EDUCATION

Education is the process by which behavioural changes take place in individual as a result of experiences which he has under gone.

Health education is a process of bringing about a change from undesirable health fraction to desirable health by bringing about the change in the knowledge and behaviour of the people by their own efforts.

The definition given by W.H.O. states that Health education as a process & effects change in health practices of people & in the knowledge & attitude related to such change.

a) It is a process involving the results of many processes.

Step :
- Identify needs.
- Collecting necessary information.
- Selecting program objectives.
- Planning the program & the people.
- Suitable methods and media.
- Implementation.
- Evaluation.

b) Involves efforts by people.

c) Concerned with establishing or inducing change in knowledge, attitude and behaviour that promote healthier living.

Objectives of Health Education

1. Informing people – To improve the scientific knowledge of people about prevention of disease and promotion of health.

2. Motivating people – People must be motivated to change their habits and way of living as people make their own choices about health matters.
3. Guiding into action – To give scientific knowledge to people so that hey can use such knowledge got the betterment of community then their own participation and others and promotion concerned & healthy life style prevention. Supportive aim at raising the competence of individuals.

Supportive activations :
1. Identified for successful implementation of primary health care.
2. Successful commonly participation.

Goals :

1. To encourage people to adopt and sustain healthy life style and practices.
2. Promotion of proper use and utilization of health services available to the people.
3. Promote individual and community participation to achieve health development.
4. To provide effective and balanced :
   - Education;
   - Public health;
   - Health care and allied.
5. Extend benefit to high rest.
6. Adoption of new idea :

   Awareness
   ↓
   Interest
   ↓
   Evaluation
   ↓
   Trial
   ↓
   Satisfaction
   ↓
   Adoption
   ↓
   Feedback

Methods of Health Education
- Soil – people.
- Seeds – health factor (based on scientific knowledge and healthfulness).
- Sower – transmitted means (must be attractive and acceptable.

Contents of Health Education
Following are the essential contents of health education :
1. Human Biology.
2. Nutrition.
3. Hygiene and Sanitation.
4. Knowledge about disease, their control and prevention.
5. Mental Health.
6. Social Health.

Principles of Health Education
1. Leaders. We involve leaders because :
   - We learn best from leaders.
   - Give useful contribution in Health Education work.
   - Know existing culture and change habits and practices.
2. Interest.
3. Community Participation.
4. Motivation.
5. Comprehension.
6. Reinforcement.
7. Good Presentation.
8. Easy to understand, learn.
9. Learning by doing.
10. Feed back.

Practice of Health Education
1. Audio visual aids :
   - Auditory Aids – e.g. Radio, tape recorder, etc.
   - Visual Aids – e.g. Charts, models, slides, film strips, etc.
   - Combined A-V aids – e.g. Television, cinema, etc.

2. Methods in health communication
   I. Individual approach
      - Personal contact.
      - Home visits.
      - Personal letters.
   II. Group approach
      - Lectures.
      - Demonstrations.
      - Discussion methods.
         * Group discussion.
         * Panel discussion.
         * Symposium.
         * Workshop.
         * Conferences.
         * Seminars.
         * Role play.
   III. Mass approach
      - Television.
      - Radio.
      - Newspaper.
      - Printed material.
      - Direct mailing.
      - Posters.
      - Health museums & exhibitions.
      - Folk methods.
      - Internet.

HEALTH COMMUNICATION

Communication referes to the countless ways that humans have of keeping in touch with one another. The term Health communication is often used synonymously with Health education.

Communication may be :
- One way communication.
- Two way communication.
- Verbal communication.
- Non-verbal communication.

- Formal and informal communication.
- Visual communication.
- Tele communication and internet.

Functions of Health Communication

1. Information
Provide scientific knowledge to people about health problems and how to maintain and promote health.

2. Education
Increases the knowledge and awareness about diseases.

3. Motivation
It is the power that drives a person from within to act. The individual is motivated to translate health information into personal behaviour and life style for their own health.

4. Persuasion
Persuasion is the art of winning friends and influencing people so that people may change life style and modify the risk factors of disease.

5. Counselling
Counselling is the process that can help people understand better and deal with their problems and comunicate better with those with whom they are emotionally involved.

Common skill :
1. Non-verbal communication.
2. Active listening.
3. Asking question.
4. Paraphrasing.
   - Identifying and reflecting feelings.
   - Appropriate use of silence.

Advanced common skill :
1. Focussing.
2. Interpretation.
3. Problem solving.
4. Repeat & reserving.
5. Confronting – a difficult skill, done & good rapport.

6. Supporting and modelling behaviour.
7. Summarising.

6. Raising Morale

Communication make an attempt to raise the morale i.e. capacity of a group of people (or team) to pull together persistently or consistently.

7. Health Development

Communicatin diffuses knowledge in respect of the goals of development and prepare the people for the roles expected of them.

8. Health organisation

Vertical or horizontal communications within an organization depicts the degree of freedom in the internal communication network.

CHAPTER-20

HEALTH CARE OF COMMUNITY

HEALTH CARE OF COMMUNITY

Health care is an extensive phenomenon which not just include medical care but a number of other services for health promotion and maintenance.

It has been defined as a multitude of services rendered to individuals, families or communities by the agents of the health services or professions, for the purpose of promoting, maintaining, monitoring or restoring health.

Health has been declared as an universal human right thereby it becomes a duty of the governments to provide essential health care to all the people.

Levels of Health Care

There are 3 levels of health care, primary, secondary and tertiary care.

(1) Primary Health Care

It represents the first level of contact between individual, (community) and health care system.

Primary health care has been defined as "essential health care based on practical, scientifically sound and socially acceptable methods and technology universally accessible to individuals and families in the community through their full participation and at a cost that the community and the country can afford to maintain at every stage of their development in the spirit of self determination.

The entire success of health care delivery system depends on how effective is the level of primary care. It is close to the people and most of their problems can be dealt at this level only.

In India primary health care is provided by Primary Health Centres (P.H.C.), sub-centers working through health workers male and female, village health guide, trained dais, etc.

(2) Secondary Care Level

It comes when the primary care level is unable to provide the solution to the health problems of the individuals. It works as 1st referral level and is provided by the district hospitals and Community Health Centres (C.H.C.).

(3) Tertiary Care Level

It is the highest level of health care. And is used only for complex and difficult cases. Here specialized faculties like advanced diagnostic and treatment procedures, good technical knowledge etc. are available. It is provide by national level institutes as A.I.I.M.S., medical colleges hospitals and other specialized institutes

A new revolution began in the field of health care after Alma-Ata International conference 1978. The primary health care was defined as :

"**Primary Health Care** is a practical approach to making essential **health care** universally accessible to individuals and families in the community in an acceptable and affordable way and with their full participation...

"It means much more than the mere extension of basic **health** services...

"having the aim of using only those technologies that have really proved their worth and can be afforded...

"delivered by community **health** workers who understand the real **health** needs of the communities they serve and have the confidence of the people".

Elements of Primary Health Care

Eight essential components of primary health care are :
1. Education about prevailing health problems and the methods of their prevention and control.
2. Promotion of food supply and proper nutrition.
3. An adequate supply of safe water and basic sanitation.
4. Maternal and child health care, including family planning.
5. Provision for essential drugs.

6. Appropriate treatment of common diseases and injuries.
7. Prevention and control of locally endemic diseases.
8. Immunization against major infectious diseases.

Key Principles of Primary Health Care

(1) Care should be aimed at the most needy groups.

The principle put forward the need for equity resources should be distributed, according to need, with more going to the more needy e.g.

- Some population groups are below the poverty line, such as the landless and jobless, refugees and squatters. They the rural dwellers and the squatters in the urban shanty towns. They are not only poor but live with few or no services including health services.
- Some groups are more vulnerable to disease, especially children under five, pregnant and nursing women.
- Some are invisible to the planners e.g. nomadic minorities in the settled countries.

(2) P.H.C. should include a range of essential, appropriate activities.

A number of vertical programmes have tried to combat diarrhoea, malaria, measles or malnutrition usually in children under five. The sad fact is that tackling one problem may stop children dying of that problem but they then die of something else and in the same numbers. A range of services is necessary.

Integration of these services is also important or the village health worker can end up trying to carry out the plans of twelve different programmes each with its own land rover, twice-yearly supervision, records, etc. Here founders need to co-ordinate.

(3) Care should be accessible and acceptable to everybody.

Health services must be shared equally by all people irrespective of their ability to pay, and all (rich or poor, urban or rural) must access to health services.

(4) There should be full community participation and P.H.C. should be contributing to the self reliance and self determination of communities.

Most programmes intend that the communities will participate and most create some kind of structure to make it possible, usually village P.H.C. committees. However, there are some problems.

First, a programme of community education and mobilisation, to give people the information and skills they need to make good choices, can take up to three months per village and few programmes will budget for this time and investment.

Second, most programmes are not prepared to delegate any serious power or decision making. For example, most P.H.C. programmes invite the community to join in the identification of priority problems, but since the programmes are funded from health budgets, they usually can do little if the community sees the need for a road as a priority. Honesty from the beginning is essential. The priorities of women can be buried at several stages of the consultation process or they can be brought forward through conscious effort.

Where the community involvement is poor the P.H.C. activities which are most successful are the ones such as immunisation. Here the community does not need to have active, organised involvement it only has to turn up and stand still for a few minutes. The activities which do much less well are those in which active, co-ordinated participation over time is essential. Think of what the community would need to do in order to tackle malnutrition in the small children or raise the age of arranged marriages for their daughters.

(5) **P.H.C. should be integrated both with other parts of the health programme and with other development sectors.**

P.H.C. should involve all sectors related to health and aspects of national and community development, in particular agriculture, animal husbandary, food, industry, education, housing, public works, communication and other sectors.

Functions of Primary Health Care

1. Curative Care

(a) Treatment of common diseases and injuries.
(b) Provision of essential drugs.
(c) Reproductive health and mother and child health (M.C.H.).

2. Static P.H.C. Programmes

(a) Expanded programme of immunisation (E.P.I.).

This is sometimes now called Universal Child Immunisation (U.C.I.) because U.N.I.C.E.F. provides a lot of finding and tends to see mothers only in relation to children.

The six targeted diseases are :
1. Diptheria – It is the D of D.P.T.
2. Whooping cough – It is the P of D.P.T.
3. Tetanus – It is the T of D.P.T. The main danger is neonatal tetanus, which has to be prevented by immunising mothers before the birth with at least 2 tetanus toxoid injections (T.T.).
4. Polio – Immunised by Oral Polio Vaccine (O.P.V.).
5. Tuberculosis – B.C.G. vaccine.
6. Measles.

Children
- B.C.G. : At birth or soon after.
- D.P.T. and O.P.V. : At 2,3 and 4 months.
- Measles : At 9 months.
- Boosters : D.P.T. and O.P.V. at 18 months or 1 year after the 3rd D.P.T. and O.P.V..

Women aged 15-45
First T.T. : At first contact or early during pregnancy.
Second T.T. : Four weeks after the first T.T.
Third T.T. : At least 6 months after the second T.T. or during the next pregnancy.
Fourth T.T. : At least 1 year after the third T.T. or during the next pregnancy.
Fifth T.T. : At least 1 year after the fourth T.T. or during the next pregnancy.

The schedule demands five contacts between the health services and a baby in its first year.

National and Regional Level Responsibilities
(a) Importation of vaccines in good condition and their distribution so that they are used before expiry date.

Maintenance of the cold chain. Vaccines have to be kept between 0 and 8 degrees centigrade during storage and transport. The cold chain might be following :
- Refrigerated storage facilities in the Capital, then
- Transport in refrigerated lorries to hospitals, then
- Storage in fridges run on electricity, then

- Transport by land rover in insulated boxes to health centres, then
- Transport to mobile clinic on motor bike in insulated box, then

(b) Antenatal, Perinatal and Postnatal Care Part of Mother and Child Health (M.C.H.)

Village Level

Workers needed : Trained Traditional Birth Attendants.

Activities

Antenatal
- Advice on T.T. injections.
- Advice on nutrition, rest, etc.
- Screening of high risk pregnancies to professionals.

Perinatal
- Clean deliveries.
- No internal examination.
- Sterile cord – cutting.
- Organisation of transport for complications.

Postnatal
- Establishing breast-feeding quickly.
- Advice on rest, food, warmth.
- Checks problems.
- Advice on family planning.

(c) Family Planning, including abortions and help for couples who cannot conceive.

Hospital Level

Surgical facilities can be used for Voluntary Surgical Contraception (V.S.C.) male and female.
- I.U.Ds. and Norplants.
- Unblocking blocked tubes in infertile women.
- Abortions (if legal) menstrual extractions D and C's.

Hospital can also :
- Screen women for oral contraceptives.
- Provides oral contraceptives, condoms and Sepo-Provera.
- Examine, diagnose and treat infertile couples.
- Advise about induced abortions if legal.
- Advise about traditional FP methods (not usually done).

Village Level

Activities :

- Distribute condoms through Village Health Worker.
- Encourage breast feeding.
- Distribute oral contraceptives to screened women through the T.Bs.
- Give advise on traditional methods.
- Advise infertile couples on rhythm method etc. and refer if unsuccessful.
- Inform about induced abortions, if legal.
- Encourage debate on age of marriage for girls.

3. Interventions to Improve Nutritional Status

(a) *Protein – Calorie Malnutrition* :

Primary Health Care programmes are still looking for ways of reducing this problem. The most common intervention is the serial weighing of children using individual Road to Health Cards but to be effective this needs to be linked to good education and behaviour change.

Hospital Level

- Nutrition Rehabilitation Centres.
- Rehabilitation of extremely malnourished children.
- Education of mothers for proper feeding.
- Small weaning – food factories.

Health Centre Level

- Nutrition Rehabilitation Centres.
- Rehabilitation of extremely malnourished children.
- Education of mothers in poor feeding.
- Serial weighing and identification of moderately malnourished children.
- Health education sessions.
- Cooking demonstrations : little evidence of over all effectiveness.
- Distribution of food supplements.

Village Level

- Encouraging good nutrition for pregnant women.

- Upper arm circumference measuring and identification of malnourished children.
- Health Education results depend on quality.
- "Food aid" – communal meals or food supplement distribu-tion.
- Identification of strategies for each family with a malnourished child.
- Increasing family food production.
- Encouraging the making and selling of high – protein energy snacks.
- Identification and referral of serious cases of malnutrition.

(b) *Micro – Nutrients* :

This section covers the three nutrients most commonly lacking in whole communities :

- Vitamin A : Its deficiency is a major cause of blindness.
- Vitamin D : Its deficiency causes rickets.
- Iodine : Its deficiency causes goiters, and mental deficiency.

Iron and Folic acid is also important for pregnant women.

National Level

Activities :

- Reinforcement of all commercial salt with Iodine.
- Reinforcement of all commercial oils with vitamins A and D.

P.H.C. Level

Activities :

- Distribution of vitamin A regularly to pregnant and lactating mothers and children under 5, by injection capsules or drops. This can be a part of E.P.I. programme.
- Distribution of Iodine regularly through injections.
- Educate community on vitamin A sources, especially for the pregnant women and children.
- Distribution on exposure to sunlight in vitamin-D deficient areas.
- Encouraging gorging on seasonal fruits such as mangoes, etc. since vitamin A is stored by the body.
- Encourage growth of vitamin A rich crops.
- Encourage exposure of children to sunlight.

Village Level

Activities :

- Encourage use of supplementation programme, if there is one.
- Education on exposure to sunlight in vitamin D deficient areas.
- Educate community on sources of vitamin A especially for pregnant women and children.
- Encourage gorging on seasonal fruits such as mangoes since Vitamin A is stored in the body.
- Encourage growth of Vitamin A rich crops.

4. Health Promotion

Health promotion is the process of helping people to adopt healthier patterns of behaviour.

Terminology : The term Health Education, is still used, but some people feel it implies only a part of the process of giving information and motivation. The term Health Promotion which has come from A.I.D.S. field, is commonly fashionable. Information, Education and Communication (I.E.C.) is used in the Family Planning field. The newest name is Behavioral change and communication.

Classic Health Education describes the kind of short talks to groups of mothers which are given so often in P.H.C., about nutrition or preventing diarrhoea or whatever, often these talks are, top-down and one way examples of the "empty bottles" approach that sees people as empty bottles, which only need to be filled up with scientific knowledge for them to change behaviour.

So the approach is to provide some new information and motivation for change, it might start by considering sessions on F.P. or malaria, in an M.C.H. clinic and conclude that :

- This information is directed at mother, but cannot help if husbands or mothers-in-law make decisions. These people must be offered an information session as well, and at a good time.

Health Education may be used where community mobilisation is a better way to go if malaria is the problem, a community can reduce infection with weed cleaning and smoke. Means and materials are also important for malaria control, they need medicines, mosquito nets and the money to buy them.

National and Regional Level
Activities :
- Mass campaigns with specific messages carried in one direction by mass media on E.P.I. or F.P.
- Social marketing; treating a health product as a sellable article, mainly used for condoms, the product is given an attractive name and image geared at a specific target group and advertised; many outlets.

(District) Health Centre Level with Outpatient Clinics
Acquiring skills and materials
- Adaptation of educational materials.
- Ensuring that all H.C. staff are informed educations and good examples of health behaviour.

Routine Health Promotion
- Group talks to mothers on normal P.H.C. topics.
- Food demonstrations.
- One to one talks.
- Routine actions such as cleaning the grounds.

Activities involving special actors and beneficiaries
- School education.
- Organisation and support of groups with specific functions; e.g. peer group education. On AIDS, education of communities to accept ex-leprosy patients, street the theatre groups educating about alcohol misuse.

Village Level
Activities :
- Group talks to mothers on normal P.H.C. topics.
- Food demonstrations.
- One to one support of individuals e.g. mothers with malnourished children non-compliant.
- Patients being treated for T.B.

5. Prevention and Control of common Local Diseases
(a) *Malaria*

Hospital Level
Activities :
- Monitoring region for foci of infection and any development of resistance to medicines.

- Monitoring developments in new medicine regions and treatments.
- Laboratory check on symptomatic diagnosis.
- Monitoring for malaria after blood-transfusions.

Health Centre Level with Outpatient Clinics

Activities :
- Good supervision of village health workers, ensuring medicine supply, good symptomatic diagnosis and appropriate referral.
- Laboratory checks on symptomatic diagnosis.
- Distributing malaria prophylaxis to pregnant women and small children.
- Monitoring state of pregnancy.

Mobile Clinics

- Distributing malaria prophylaxis to pregnant women and small children.
- Monitoring state of pregnant women.

Village Level

1) Reducing Breeding places
- Clearance village of weeds.
- Clearance village of prddling keeping well, surrounding tidy, filling in holes in the ground, removing broken pieces of pots, old tim etc.
- Building household soak pits.
- Tidying fringes of lakes and where still water is lying.
- For small ponds not used for drinking, putting tiny amounts of oil to form thin surface layer.

2) Killing mosquitoes

Spraying is much less popular now as over all it proved to be ineffective, mosquitoes become resistant to D.D.T. and it hurts the food chain. There are safer alternatives which can be sprayed on interior walls of houses disruptive for the village as everyone has to move out for the day.

3) Reducing Biting
(a) Strategies for the whole household.
- Putting smoky herbs on the fire.

- Metal meshes on windows and doors.
- Planting mosquito – repellent mats.
- One double mosquito net for the pregnant women and small children, works longer if impregnated with pyrethrum even when full of holes expensive but cost effective.

4) **Identifying and Treating infection Quickly**
- Trained and supervised Village Health Worker with medicines.
- Trained Traditional Birth Addendant and Village Health Worker distributing malaria prophylaxis to pregnant women and small children if Govt. policy.
- The community educated to act if any child or pregnant woman has a fever.

(b) Sexually Transmitted Diseases including A.I.D.S.

National and Regional Level (may be working with hospitals)
- Development of mass health promotion programmes.
- Important distribution of condoms and other material.
- Support of innovative approaches to prevention, support of P.W.A's, etc.
- Organisation of safe blood supplies.
- Making of difficult policy decisions e.g. – resources spent on dying children with A.I.D.S.
- Integrating A.I.D.S. programme with others especially family planning programes.
- Monitoring other S.T.D's. especially with migrant labour.

(District) Health Centre Level with outpatient and Outreach Services

Providing the following services either directly or through supporting special projects.

Health Education in B.C.C.
- In school, churches, among street kids, directed at husbands.
- Promoting and distributing condoms and correct teaching of proper condom use.
- Developing new media traditional, theatre and comics.
- Supplying sex workers with condoms advice and work alternatives.
- Make help the other STD's easy to get especially for returning migrant labourers and sex workers.

- Testing and counselling.
- Education to encourage women and "worried well" to seek advice by removing stigma and have A.I.D.S. counselling in integrated clinics, not S.T.D. clinics using fast and precise tests.
- Providing high quality counselling and follow up for H.I.V. + people.
- Support for H.I.V. + people, P.W.A.'s and families.
- Support for PWA's and families at home, provision of materials.
- Support of orphans and careers.

Village Level

Activities :

- Education on prevention.
- V.H.M. distribution of condoms and proper teaching of their correct use.
- Reducing prejudice about P.W.A.'s.
- Support of P.W.A.'s and families at home.
- Education of husbands, especially migrant labourers, which includes the importance of other S.T.D.'s.
- Advice on family planning/condom use to couples, where one is HIV positive.
- Supplying condoms to any, sex worker in the community.

Activities for T.B.A.

- Using gloves to prevent self infection.
- Advice on Family Planning for HIV positive women.

(c) ***Diarrhoea***

National and Regional Level, with Hospital

- Ensuring supply of drugs and equipment.
- Treating the severe cases.
- Investigating indigenous teas used for diarrhoea and incorporating them if effective in treatment patterns.
- Investigating in the water and sanitation sector.

Health Centre Level with Outpatient Clinics

Activities :

- Motivate the specialists to provide quality water and latrines to villages.

- Carrying out some educational tasks as Village Health Guide.
- Following WHO AIB/C/DI treatment plan treatment.
- With IV if necessary, symptomatic treatment of dysentery, referral if fever high.

Activities for Village Health Worker :
- Prevention of diarrhoea.
- Getting drinking and household water sources protected and safe.
- Checking that water is scooped out cleanly and pot kept covered.
- Motivating mothers to use soap for hand washing after defecation, and after cleaning children who have defecated and before cooking or serving food.
- Motivating mothers to keep small children on clean mat.
- Motivating mothers to construct dish-rack above ground etc.
- Motivating mothers to clean up after children, dogs etc. have defecated etc.
- Motivating mothers to construct a dish-rack above ground etc.

Prevention of dehydration, malnutrition or death.
- Educating every mother to take action if child has diarrhoea, to check with the VHM, to continue breast feeding and giving normal foods and liquids; to know how to prepare and use sugar-salt mixture.
- Prepare and use basic salt-sugar mix.
- Knowing local medicines for diarrhoea.
- Knowing signs of moderate dehydration and that O.R.S. packets should be used.
- Knowing signs of severe dehydration and other symptoms that require referral.

(d) *Tuberculosis*

National and Regional Level

Activities :
- Committing country to sustained T.B. control activities.
- Ensuring regular, uninterrupted supply of all essential anti T.B. drug.

Hospital and Health Centre Level

Activities :
- Laboratory confirmation of diagnosis by examining sputum.

Health Care of Community   443

- Treatment : DOTS – (Directly Observed Treatment Short Course) now takes only six to eight months for the first two months patients can stay in the community but take daily medicines in front of a health worker.
- Recording and reporting.

Village Level

Activities by Village Health Worker

- Symptomatically identifying possible cases.
- Monitoring members of the same household.
- Motivating patients to continue treatment and visiting non-compliers.
- Motivating community to get children vaccinated.

(e) **Leprosy**

National and Regional Level

Activities :

- Laboratory confirmation of diagnosis.
- Treatment : Multi-drug treatment now takes 6 months or one year depending or the national regime. Although medication is oral, sled-effects are possible so the patients has to come to a hospital once a month.
- Rehabilitation of advanced cases with missing limbs, etc.
- Finding alternatives to long stay institutions for burnt-out cases.

Village Level

Activities by village health worker with village committee.

- Routine mass checks for symptom.
- Individual symptomatic identification of possible cases.
- Monitoring of members of the same household.
- Education to remove the fear of leprosy and of sufferers.
- Rehabilitation of institutionalised but curved community members.

6. Safe Water and Sanitation

"Water and sanitation is one of the primary drivers of public health. I often refer to it as 'Health 101', which once we can secure access to clean water and to adequate sanitation facilities for all people, irrespective of their living conditions, a huge battle against all kinds of diseases will be won." *Dr. LEE Jong-wook, Director-General, World Health Organization.*

Diarrhoea

- 1.8 million people die every year from diarrhoeal diseases (including cholera); 90% are children under 5, most countries.
- 88% of diarrhoeal disease is attributed to unsafe water supply, inadequate sanitation and hygiene.
- Improved water supply reduces diarrhoea morbidity by between 6% to 25%, if severe outcomes are included.
- Improved sanitation reduces diarrhoea morbidity by 32%.
- Hygiene interventions including hygiene education and promotion of hand washing can lead to a reduction of diarrhoea up to 45%.
- Improvements in drinking-water quality through household water treatment, such as chlorination at point of used reduction of diarrhoea episodes by between 35% and 39%.

Malaria

- 1.3 million people die of malaria each year, 90% of whom are children under 5.
- There are 396 million episodes of malaria every year, most of the disease burden is in Africa south of the Saha.

Hepatitis A

- There are 1.5 million cases of clinical hepatitis A every year.

Arsenic

- In Bangladesh, between 28 and 35 million people consume drinking-water with elevated levels of their drinking water.
- The number of cases of skin lesions related to drinking water in Bangladesh is estimated at 1.5 million.
- Arsenic contamination of ground water has been found in many countries, including Argentina, Bangladesh, China, Mexico, Thailand and the United States.
- The key to prevention is reducing consumption of drinking water with elevated levels of arsenic, by identifying arsenic water sources or by using arsenic removal systems.

Fluorosis

- Over 26 million people in China suffer from dental fluorosis due to elevated fluoride in their drinking water.

Health Care of Community

- In China, over 1 million cases of skeletral fluorosis are thought to be attributable to drinking-water.
- The principal mitigation strategies include exploitation of deep-seated water, use of river water, reservoir const. defluoridation.

Driving Forces

Access to water supply as of 2002

- In 2002, 1.1 billion people lacked access to improved water sources, which represented 17% of the global population.
- Over half of the world's population has access to improved water through household connections or yard tap.
- Of the 1.1 billion without improved water sources, nearly two thirds live in Asia.
- In sub-Saharan Africa, 42% of the population is still without improved water.
- In order to meet the water supply MDG target, an additional 260,000 people per day up to 2015 should gain and water sources.
- Between 2002 and 2015, the world's population is expected to increase every year by 74.8 million people.

Access to sanitation as of 2002

- In 2002, 2.6 billion people lacked access to improved sanitation, which represented 42% of the world's population.
- Over half of those without improved sanitation – nearly 1.5 billion people – live in China and India.
- In sub-Saharan Africa sanitation coverage is a mere 36%.
- Only 31% of the rural inhabitants in developing countries have access to improved sanitation, as opposed 73%.
- In order to meet the sanitation MDG target, and additional 370,000 people per day upto 2015 should gain access sanitation.

Emergencies and disasters

- Almost two billion people were affected by natural disasters in the decade of the 20th century, 86% of them by droughts.
- Flooding increases the ever-present health threat from contamination of drinking-water systems from inadequate industrial waste and by refuse dumps.

- Droughts cause the most ill-health and death because they often trigger and exacerbate malnutrition and famine to adequate water supplies.
- Disaster management requires a continuous chain of activities that includes prevention, preparedness, emergency and recovery.

Water resources developments

- The development of water resources continues in an accelerated pace to meet the food, fibre and energy needs population of 8 billion by 2025.
- Lack of capacity for health impact assessment transfers hidden costs to the health sector and increases the dis local communities.
- Environment management approaches for health need to be incorporated into strategies for integrated water management.

The Global Response

Millennium Development Goals (MDGs)

By including water supply, sanitation and hygiene in the MDGs, the world community has acknowledged the importance as development interventions and has set a series of goals and targets.

Goal – 7. Ensure environmental sustainability

- Target 9 : Integrate the principles of sustainable development into country policies and program and reverse the environmental resources.
- Target 10 :
  (i) Halve by 2015, the proportion of people without sustainable access to safe drinking water and basic sanitation.
  (ii) Integrate sanitation into water resources management strategies.
- Target 11 : Have achieved by 2020, a significant improvement in the lives of at least 100 million slum dwellers.

Goal – 4. Reduce child mortality

- Target 5 : Reduce by two-thirds, between 1990 and 2015, the under-five mortality rate.

Goal – 6. Combat HIV/AIDS, malaria, and other diseases
- Target 8 : Have halted by 2015 and begun to reverse the incidence of malaria and other major diseases.

Water for Life Decade : 2005-2015
- UN declares 2005-2015 "water for life" as the International Decade for Action and set's the world agenda on a water-related issues.

Sailient quotes

"We shall not finally defeat AIDS, tuberculosis, malaria, or any of the other infectious diseases that plague the developing have also won the battle for safe drinking water, sanitation and basic health care."

"The human right to water entitles everyone to sufficient, safe, acceptable, physically accessible and affordable water for domestic uses."

General Comment No. 15 (2002) : The Right to Water.

Encouraged its success in rapidly improving access to safe water through the introduction of one standard, quality-control design (the India Mark II), the Indian government applied the same approach to sanitation. In 1986 a Technology Advisory comprising representatives from the Indian Government, UNDP, UNICEF and the World Bank, recommended one standard urban on-site sanitation, the double vault pour flush latrine.

The Centrally-Sponsored Rural Sanitation Programme provided 100% subsidy for this latrine for Scheduled Castes, Schedule landless labourers. Subsidies for other user groups were decided by the respective states.

Achievements in coverage and use were low. The cost of the double vault permanent model was relatively high and the for construction, with little attention given to demand creation, loan repayment where applicable, or to user participation in such siting, superstructure design or future maintenance needs. Coverage in the rural areas through government support hardly in 1980 to 2.7% in 1992. The greater part of progress - to 11% in 1989 - was achieved by households who preferred and private sector.

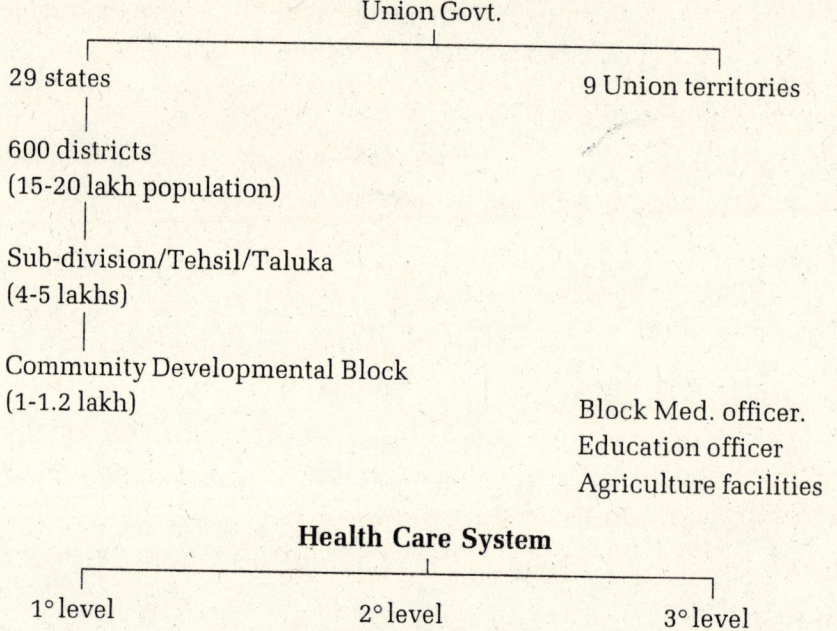

- Health problems.
- Population problems.
- Common disease problems.
- Enviornmental sanitation problems.

In 1992, following a National Seminar on Rural Sanitation, the Goverment launched a new strategy. Subsidies for houshold line were reduced to 80% and the policy stressed participation of householders in the choice of four latrine options with difficult also directed implementing agencies, both government and non-governmental organisations, to use 10% of the government and hygiene education. Implementation remained driven by the implementing agencies.

This changed in the policy guidelines of 2001 when the programme moved to a 'Total Sanitation Campaign' with an emphsized educating rural households without sanitation about the importance of having and using sanitary latrines. Interested household flat subsidy of Rs. 500-600, depending on the type of latrine. The implementing agencies can set up outlets where household required materials.

State Governments decide which agencies can implement the programme under a separate bank account – various government, NGOs and CBOs, district water and sanitation missions, etc. Community Governments (Panchayats) can also carry out the communities, together with local committees. The latter approach is the state policy in Kerala developed in cooperation with sanitation in West Bengal has been promoted to rural households directly through NGOs and CBOs.

The Total Sanitation Campaign is part of the Sector Reforms Project introduced in April 1999 to make rural water supply at sustainable. It is piloted in 200 districts. Limitations on success arise from the absence of guidance ad training opportunities appropriate expertise in some implementing organisations, particularly in knowledge of current gender and poverty-sensitives participation strategies. Similar deficiencies are seen in the organisations responsible for allocating funds and monitoring in all preconditions in place it is likely that only part of the funds will be used effectively.

ANM

In 1995, the Human Development Report focussed upon gender disparity high lighting that women receive unequal treatment all over the world. The need to integrate women into development without which no country can lay claim to development, was internationally proclaimed in the 1995 Beijing conference. Although there have been successes in improving the health of women and children worldwide, there remain an unfinished agenda of unnecessary, preventable deaths, illness and disability that disproportionately affects poor women and children especially in rural areas of developing regions of the world.

The World Health Organization estimates that more than 80% of world's population may rely on traditional medicine as its primary source of medical care including advice of medical care including advice and assistance during pregnancy, infant and child health, and maternal health keeping this in mind the early interventions to improve the health of women and children need to be integrated into the care provided by ANM.

In the governmental rural health set up the ANM is the health functionary closest to the community. ANM is found at sub-center alongwith the multipurpose health worker (M.P.H.W.) who deals mainly with malaria, sanitation and to a small extent family welfare. The domain of ANM usually consists of half a dozen villages – one of which is a sub-center village, visits to villages and houses, providing services, giving medicines, tendering advice to men, women and children, keeping touch with PHC/CHC and even district hospital, attending meetings, procuring essential supplies and performing other odd jobs. The present paper examines the role of ANM in reproductive and child health. At the same time an attempt has been made to understand and explore the problems faced by them. The importance of ANM in rural health has been highlighted. Health policy aimed at improving health should certainly include efforts to provide ANM in each and every village or some trained male and female volunteers from villages. It is these factors which are often overlooked in the planning finding and services to rural areas. Rural health programs must change from being dependent on demand to being based on active offer of preventive measures. The active offer must be sustained by non-standardized communication procedures with the aim of providing empowerment of involved people. ANM is the primary care givers in India. They have demonstrated bold leadership under extreme adversity. Consequently were empowered and involved.

CHAPTER-21

BIOMEDICAL WASTE MANAGEMENT

BIOMEDICAL WASTE MANAGEMENT

According to Bio-medical waste (Management and Handling) Rules, 1998 of India, "Bio-medical waste" means any waste, which is generated during the diagnosis, treatment or immunisation of human beings or animals or in research activities pertaining thereto or in the production or testing of biologicals, and including categories as mentioned in schedule I.

Definitions

In these rules unless the context otherwise requires :

1. **"Act"** means the *Environment (Protection) Act, 1986* (29 of 1986);
2. **"Animal House"** means *a place where animals are reared/kept for testing purposes;*
3. **"Authorisation"** means *permission granted by the prescribed authority for the generation, collection, reception, storage, transportation, treatment, disposal and/or any other form of handling of bio-medical waste in accordance with these rules and any guidelines issued by the Central Government.*
4. **"Authorised person"** means *an occupier or operator authorised by the prescribed authority to generate, collect, receive, store, transport, treat, dispose and/or handle bio-medical waste in accordance with these rules and any guidelines issued by the Central Government.*
5. **"Bio-medical waste"** means *any waste, which is generated during the diagnosis, treatment or immunisation of human beings or animal or in research activities pertaining thereto or in the production or testing of biologicals and including categories mentioned in Schedule I.*

6. **"Biologicals"** means *any preparation made from organisms or microorganisms or product of metabolism and biochemical reactions intended for use in the diagnosis, immunisation or the treatment of human beings or animals or in research activities pertaining thereto.*

7. **"Bio-medical waste treatment facility"** means *any facility wherein treatment disposal of bio-medical waste or processes incidental to such treatment or disposal is carried out.*

8. **"Occupier"** in *relation to any institution generating bio-medical waste, which includes a hospital, nursing home, clinic dispensary, veterinary institution, animal house, pathological laboratory, blood bank called by whatever name means a person who has control over that institution and or its-premises.*

9. **"Operator of a bio-medical waste facility"** means *a person who owns or controls or operates a facility for the collection, reception, storage, transport, treatment, disposal or any other form of handling of bio-medical waste.*

Treatment and Disposal

1. Bio-medical waste shall be treated and disposed of in accordance with Schedule I and in compliance with the standards prescribed in Schedule V.
2. Every occupier, where required, shall set up in accordance with the time-schedule in Schedule VI, requisite bio-medical waste treatment facilities like *incinerator, autoclave, microwave system* for the treatment of waste or ensure requisite treatment of waste at a common waste treatment facility or any other waste treatment facility.

Segregation, Packaging, Transportation and Storage

1. Bio-medical waste *shall not be mixed with other wastes.*
2. Bio-medical waste *shall be segregated into containers/bags at the point of generation in accordance with Schedule II prior to its storage, transportation, treatment and disposal. The containers shall be labeled according to Schedule III.*
3. If a container is transported from the premises where bio-medical waste in generated to any waste treatment facility outside the premises, *the container shall, apart from the lable prescribed* in Schedule III, *also carry information prescribed in Schedule IV.*
4. *Notwithstanding anything contained in the Motor Vehicles Act,*

1988 or rules thereunder, untreated bio-medical waste shall be transported only in such vehicle as may be authorised for the purpose by the competent authority as specified by the government.

5. No untreated bio-medical waste shall be kept stored beyond a period of 48 hours :

   Provided that if for any reason it becomes necessary to store the waste beyond such period, the authorised person must take permission of the prescribed authority and take measures to ensure that the waste does not adversely affect human health and the environment.

Prescribed Authority

1. The Government of every State and Union Territory shall establish a prescribed authority with such members as may be pacified for granting authorisation and implementing these rules. If the prescribed authority comprises of more than one member, a chairperson for the authority shall be designated.

Provided that the authority may entertain the appeal after the expiry of the said period of thirty days if it is satisfied that the appellant was prevented by sufficient cause from filing the appeal in time.

SCHEDULE-I
(See Rule 5)

CATEGORIES OF BIO-MEDICAL WASTES

Option	Waste Category Waste Class	Treatment & Disposal
Category No.1	**Human Anatomical Wastes** (Human tissues, organs, body parts.)	Incineration@/ deep burial*
Category No.2	**Animal Wastes** (Animal tissues, organs, body parts carcasses, bleeding parts, fluid, blood and experimental animals used in research, waste generated by veterinary hospitals, discharge from hospitals, animal houses.)	Incineration@/ deep burial*
Category No.3	**Microbiology & Biotechnology Waste** (Wastes from laboratory cultures, stocks or specimens of micro-organisms live or attenuated vaccines, human and animal cell culture used in research and infecti-	Local autoclaving micro-waving/ incineration@

	ous agents from research and industrial laboratories, wastes from production of biologicals, toxins, dishes and devices used for transfer of cultures.)	
Category No.4.	**Waste Sharps** (Needles, syringes, scalpels, blades, glass, etc. that may cause puncture and cuts. This includes both used and unused sharps.)	Disinfection by chemical treatment$/autoclaving, micro-waving and mutilation/shredding.#
Category No.5	**Discarded Medicines and Cytotoxic drugs** (Wastes comprising of outdated, contaminated and discarded medicines.)	Incineration@/destruction & drugs disposal in secured landfills.
Category No.6	**Solid Waste** (Items contaminated with blood, and body fluids including cotton dressings, soiled plaster casts, lines beddings, other material contaminated with blood.)	Incineration@ autoclaving/microwaving.
Category No.7	**Solid Waste** (Wastes generated from disposable items other than the waste sharps such as tubings, catheters, intravenous sets etc.)	Disinfection by chemical treatment,$ autoclaving/microwaving & multilation/shredding.#
Category No.8	**Liquid Waste** (Waste generated from laboratory and washing, cleaning, house-keeping and disinfecting activities.)	Disinfection by chemical treatment,$ and discharge into drains.
Category No.9	**Incineration Ash** (Ash from incineration of any bio-medical waste)	Disposal in municipal landfill.
Category No.10	**Chemical Waste** (Chemicals used in production of biologicals, chemicals used in disinfection, as insecticides, etc.)	Chemical treatment$ and discharge into drains for liquids & secured landfill for solids.

$ Chemicals treatment using at least 1% hypochlorite solution or any other equivalent chemical reagent. It must be ensured that chemical treatment ensures disinfection.
\#   Multilation/shredding must be such so as to prevent unauthorised reuse.
@   There will be no chemical pretreatment before incineration. Chlorinated plastics shall not be incinerated.
*   Deep burial shall be an option available only in towns with population less than five lakhs and in rural areas.

SCHEDULE-II

(See Rule 6)

COLOUR CODING AND TYPE OF CONTAINER FOR DISPOSAL OF BIO-MEDICAL WASTES

Colour Cording	Type of Container	Waste Category	Treatment options as per Schedule I
Yellow	Plastic bag	Cat.1, Cat.2, & Cat.3, Cat.6	Incineration/deep burial
Red	Disinfected container/ plastic bag	Cat.3, Cat.6, Cat.7	Autoclaving/ Microwaving/ Chemical Treatment
Blue/White translucent	Plastic bag/puncture proof container	Cat.4, Cat.7	Autoclaving/Micro-waving/Chemical Treatment and destruction/shredding
Black	Plastic bag	Cat.5 & Cat.9 and Cat.10 (Solid)	Disposal in secured landfill.

Notes:
1. Colour coding of waste categories with multiple treatment options as defined in Schedule I, shall be selected depending on treatment option chosen, which shall be as specified in Schedule I.
2. Waste collection bags for waste types needing incineration shall not be made of chlorinated plastics.
3. Categories 8 and 10 (liquid) do not require containers/bags.
4. Categories 3 if disinfected locally need not be put in containers/bags.

SCHEDULE-III

Label for Bio-Medical Waste Containers/Bags

BIOHAZARD SYMBOL   CYTOTOXIC HAZARD SYMBOL

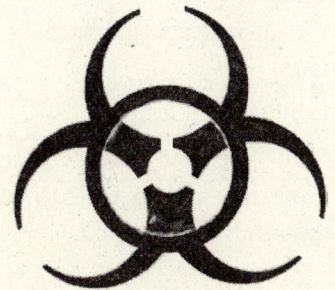
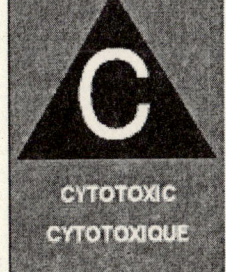

BIOHAZARD   HANDLE WITH CARE   CYTOTOXIC

Washable shall be non-washable and prominently visible.

BIOMEDICAL WASTES (BMW)

Wastes generated during diagnosis, treatment or immunization of human beings or animals or in research activities pertaining there to or in the production of biologicals, or it is that component of hospital waste & is hazardous to human health & environment if not properly managed or disposed off.

Categories of Biomedical Waste/Ministry of Environment & Forests

Category	Treatment & Disposal
1. Human anatomical waste	Incineration/deep burial
2. Animal waste	Incineration/deep burial
3. Microbiology & Biotechnology waste	Local autoclaving/micro-wave/incineration
4. Waste Sharps	Disinfection (Chemical treatment, autoclave microwave, mutilation/shredding)
5. Discarded medicines & Cytotoxic drugs	Incineration/destruction & drug disposal in secured landfills.
6. Solid Waste (Items contaminated with blood or fluids)	Incineration, autoclaving or microwaving.
7. Solid Waste (Items generated from disposable items other than sharps)	Chemical disinfection autoclaving/microwave multilation, shredding.
8. Liquid Waste	Chemical disinfection and discharge into drains.
9. Incineration Ash	Disposal in municipal landfill.
10. Chemical Waste	Chemical treatment and discharge into drains for liquids and secured landfill for solids.

- 85% – Non hazardous wastes.
- 10% – Infectious wastes.
- 5% – Non infectious wastes but hazardous.

Biomedical Waste Management

Collection and segregation of wastes :

- Prevents contamination of general waste by infectious waste.
- Store and dispose off infectious wastes under strict supervision.
  1. General waste : Black bag.
  2. Infectious waste (excluding sharps) : Red bag.
  3. Sharps : Strong puncture – proof containers.
  4. Human anatomical wastes : Yellow bag.
  5. Animal wastes : Orange bag.

In Hospitals :

i) Yellow bag – Human anatomical wastes, swabs, dressings, bandages, etc. (for incineration).

ii) Red bag – Plastics with human secretions, syringe, etc. (for autoclaving).

iii) Black bag – General wastes

Stored wastes : must be –

1. protected from H_2O, rain, wind.
2. kept non putrescent.
3. kept in locked dumpsters, sheds, other secure containers.
4. protected from animals, rag pickers, etc. wastes should not be stored for > 48 hrs.

Packaging :

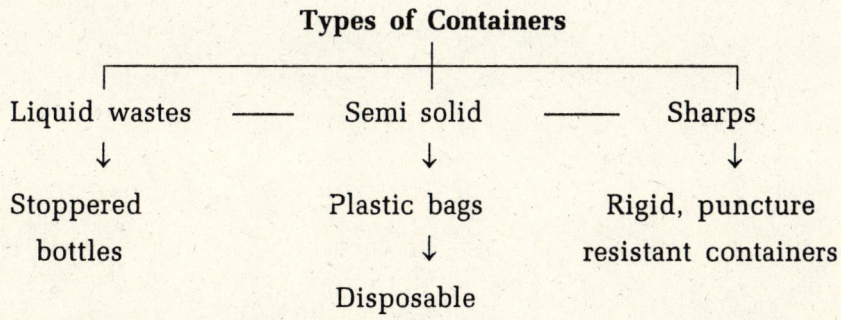

Containers must have biohazard and toxic hazard symbols.

Person collecting wastes :

1. Must wear masks, gowns, boot, gloves.

2. Made aware of hazards of materials handled.
3. Subjected to regular health check-ups.
4. Immunized.
5. Should report any injury they sustain at work.

CHAPTER-22

DISASTER MANAGEMENT

DISASTER MANAGEMENT

The high density of cities and human settlements make them particularly vulnerable to disasters and hazards. Not a week goes by without news of a disaster, natural or man-made, effecting huge losses on humans and the environment as a whole.

A disaster can be defined as "any occurrence that causes damage, ecological disruption, loss of human life or deterioration of health and health services on a scale sufficient to warrant an extraordinary response from outside the affected community or area".

A hazard can be defined as any phenomenon that has the potential to cause disruption or damage to people and their environment.

Disasters are becoming more complex, where a range of multiple factors in the social, cultural and natural spheres are increasing the risks associated with disasters.

The well known saying on health, of "Prevention is better than cure", can very much be applied to disaster management as well. It is increasingly becoming apparent that planning and preparedness, prevention, mitigation, response and relief, and recovery, to tackle disasters are critical in order to reduce the negative impacts and effects of such events. The role of communities and individual families in taking appropriate action to mitigate the impacts of disasters has been emphasized, as local governments and emergency services realize that response to an emergency situation can be hampered by the disaster itself, and relief can best be delivered by those closest at hand. Community based disaster management is now becoming an integral part of any local or national disaster management planning.

Lessons in disaster management are emerging, albeit unfortunately after a disaster has struck :

- **Build local community capacity**

  It is important to support and build local capacities for people to mitigate and prevent disasters, and cope with post-disaster impacts. Such capacities will also enable communities to cope better with those few disasters which are unavoidable.

- **Create partnerships and alliances**

  There are a number of organizations and groups that are involved, or need to be involved, in disaster management. It is important to build participatory alliances and partnerships among these entities in order to map out responsibilities and activities.

- **Share and exchange information**

  Knowledge embedded in different organizations and groups need to be recorded and shared among all of them, and used for different purposes. This is particularly true of universities and research institutions in the region where disasters occur. Regular learning opportunities are critical for communities to understand, experience and prepare themselves for a disaster.

- **Develop learning and decision-making tools**

Existing knowledge and understanding of disasters, man-made and natural has to be used to develop learning and decision-making tools that can be used for disaster mitigation, including the creation of disaster maps, mitigation plans etc.

Goals of Disaster Management :

(1) Reduce or avoid losses from hazards;

(2) Assure prompt assistance to victims;

(3) Achieve rapid & effective recovery.

Disaster management aims to reduce, or avoid, the potential losses from hazards, assure prompt and appropriate assistance to victims of disaster, and achieve rapid and effective recovery. The Disaster management cycle illustrates the ongoing process by which governments, businesses, and civil society plan for and reduce the impact of disasters, react during and immediately following a disaster, and take steps to recover after a disaster has occurred. Appropriate actions at all points in the cycle lead to greater preparedness, better warnings, reduced vulnerability or the prevention of disasters during the next iteration of the cycle. The complete disaster management cycle includes the shaping of public policies and plans that either modify the causes of disasters or mitigate their effects on people, property, and infrastructure. The mitigation and preparedness phases occur as disaster management improvements are made in anticipation of a disaster event. Developmental considerations play a key role in contributing to the mitigation and preparation of a community to effectively confront a disaster. As a disaster occurs, disaster manage-ment actors, in particular humanitarian organizations, become involved in the immediate response and long-term recovery phases. The four disaster management phases illustrated here do not always, or even generally, occur in isolation or in this precise order. Often phases of the cycle overlap and the length of each phase greatly depends on the severity of the disaster.

- **Mitigation** – Minimizing the effects of disaster.
  Examples : building codes and zoning; vulnerability analyses; public education.
- **Preparedness** – Planning how to respond.
  Examples : preparedness plans; emergency exercises/training; warning systems.
- **Response** – Efforts to minimize the hazards created by a disaster.
  Examples : search and rescue; emergency relief.
- **Recovery** – Returning the community to normal.
  Examples : temporary housing; grants; medical care.

Sustainable Development

Developmental considerations contribute to all aspects of the disaster management cycle. One of the main goals of disaster management, and one of its strongest links with development, is the promotion of sustainable livelihoods and their protection and recovery during disasters and emergencies. Where this goal is achieved, people have a greater capacity to deal with disasters and their recovery is more rapid and long lasting. In a development oriented disaster management approach, the objectives are to reduce hazards, prevent disasters, and prepare for emergencies. Therefore, developmental considerations are strongly represented in the mitigation and preparedness phases of the disaster management cycle. Inappropriate development processes can lead to increased vulnerability to disasters and loss of preparedness for emergency situations.

Immediately following disaster there is possibility of transmission of communicable diseases e.g. gastro-enteritis, acute respiratory infections, etc. which need proper vaccination, medical care, nutrition, safe water, proper food, basic sanitation along with personal hygiene and vector control.

Mitigation

Mitigation activities actually eliminate or reduce the probability of disaster occurrence, or reduce the effects of unavoidable disasters. Mitigation measures include building codes; vulnerability analyses updates; zoning and land use management; building use regulations and safety codes; preventive health care; and public education.

Mitigation will depend on the incorporation of appropriate measures in national and regional development planning. Its effectiveness will also depend on the availability of information on hazards, emergency risks, and the counter measures to be taken. The mitigation phase, and indeed the whole disaster management cycle, includes the shaping of public policies and plans that either modify the causes of disasters or mitigate their effects on people, property, and infrastructure.

Preparedness

The goal of emergency preparedness programs is to achieve a satisfactory level of readiness to respond to any emergency situation through programs that strengthen the technical and managerial capacity of governments, organizations, and communities. These measures can be described as logistical readiness to deal with disasters and can be enhanced by having response mechanisms and procedures, rehearsals, developing long-term and short-term strategies, public education and building early warning systems. Preparedness can also take the form of ensuring that strategic reserves of food, equipment, water, medicines and other essentials are maintained in cases of national or local catastrophes.

During the preparedness phase, governments, organizations, and individuals develop plans to save lives, minimize disaster damage, and enhance disaster response operations. Preparedness measures include preparedness plans; emergency exercises/training; warning systems; emergency communications systems; evacuations plans and training;

resource inventories; emergency personnel/contact lists; mutual aid agreements; and public information/education. As with mitigations efforts, preparedness actions depend on the incorporation of appropriate measures in national and regional development plans. In addition, their effectiveness depends on the availability of information on hazards, emergency risks and the countermeasures to be taken, and on the degree to which government agencies, non-governmental organizations and the general public are able to make use of this information.

Humanitarian Action

During a disaster, humanitarian agencies are often called upon to deal with immediate response and recovery. To be able to respond effectively, these agencies must have experienced leaders, trained personnel, adequate transport and logistic support, appropriate communications, and guidelines for working in emergencies. If the necessary preparations have not been made, the humanitarian agencies will not be able to meet the immediate needs of the people.

Response

The aim of emergency response is to provide immediate assistance to maintain life, improve health and support the morale of the affected population. Such assistance may range from providing specific but limited aid, such as assisting refugees with transport, temporary shelter, and food, to establishing semi-permanent settle-ment in camps and other locations. It also may involve initial repairs to damaged infrastructure. The focus in the response phase is on meeting the basic needs of the people until more permanent and sustainable solutions can be found. Humanitarian organizations are often strongly present in this phase of the disaster management cycle.

Recovery

As the emergency is brought under control, the affected population is capable of undertaking a growing number of activities aimed at restoring their lives and the infrastructure that supports them. There is no distinct point at which immediate relief changes into recovery and then into long-term sustainable development. There will be many opportunities during the recovery period to enhance prevention and increase preparedness, thus reducing vulnerability. Ideally, there should be a smooth transition from recovery to on-going development.

Recovery activities continue until all systems return to normal or better. Recovery measures, both short and long term, include returning vital life-support systems to minimum operating standards; temporary housing; public information; health and safety education; reconstruction; counseling programs; and economic impact studies.

Disasters in India

Indian Subcontinent : among the world's most disaster prone areas.
- 54% of land vulnerable to earthquakes.
- 8% of land vulnerable to cyclones.
- 5% of land vulnerable to floods.

> 1 million houses damaged annually + human, social, other losses.

Earthquakes

- 12% land is liable to severe earthquakes (intensity MSK IX or more).
- 18% land is liable to MSK VIII (similar to Latur/Uttarkashi).
- 25% land is liable to MSK VII (similar to Jabalpur quake).

Biggest quakes in : Andamans, Kuchchh, Himachal, Kashmir, N. Bihar and the North East.

Wind and Cyclones

- 1891-1990 : 262 cyclones (92 severe) in a 50 km wide strip on the East Coast.
- Less severe cyclonic activity on West Coast (33 cyclones in the same period).
- In 19 severe cyclonic storms, death tool > 10,000 lives.

In 21 cyclones in Bay of Bengal (India + Bangladesh) 1.25 million lives have been lost.

Foods

- Floods in the Indo-Gangetic-Brahmaputra plains are an annual feature.
- On an average, a few hundred lives are lost millions are rendered homeless.
- Lakhs of hectares of crops are damaged every year.

The latest disaster witnessed by the world was Tsunami on 26 Dec., 2004.

National Policy

Objectives

The objectives of India's National Policy for natural disaster reduction is to reduce :

- Loss of Lives.
- Property damage.
- Economic disruption.

Goals

- Creating Public Awareness about Safety from disasters.
- Amending/Enacting legislation for safety from hazards.
- Planning development areas with safety from hazards.
- Protection of habitations from adverse hazard impacts.
- Constructing new buildings safe from hazards.
- Retrofitting existing buildings for improving hazard resistance.

Legislation Needed

- Amendments to town/country planing acts and Master plan area development rules.
- Land use zoning in hazard prone areas and establishing techno-legal regimes.
- Incorporation of safety requirements in building bye-laws of local bodies/panchayats – applicable to new buildings and extensions of old buildings. Empowering local bodies to exercise control.
- Legislation to upgrade hazard resistance of critical buildings for use and safety of large number of people – schools, hospitals, cinemas, congregation halls, water tanks, towers, telephone exchanges, fire stations, headquarters of police and administration.

Health Sectors and Disaster Management

1. All buildings where health services operate in **disaster**-prone areas must carry out vulnerability and risk assessments of the structures and essential hospital services.
2. Appropriate **mitigation** measures must be taken in the design and construction of new health facilities or the remodeling and expansion of existing establishments in accordance with an integrated **disaster mitigation** plan.

3. Non-structural **mitigation** or intervention measures must be included in plans for maintenance, inspection, remodeling, and upgrading existing **hospitals**.
4. Risk reduction specifications must be met as part of the procedures for acquiring, operating, and maintaining hospital equipment and systems.
5. Hospital **disaster** preparedness plans must be reviewed to take into account hospital vulnerability.
6. Design and building codes must be enforced in the design and construction of health facilities. They must aim not just to protect the lives of their occupants but also to ensure the uninterrupted operations of the facility after a **disaster** has struck.
7. Health care administrators, medical staff, builders and maintenance personnel must be made aware of the standards to be met for buildings entrusted to withstand the impact of potential national **disaster**.
8. **Hospitals** must keep up to date information and floor plans to their buildings, architectural, engineering and technical design in a safe and accessible place.

SAMPLE QUESTION PAPER-I

Attempt All the questions. Parts I, II and III should be answered in separate answer-books.

PART – I

1. Outline the organisation and structure for delivery of Primary Health Care in India. (10)

2. Write short notes on :
   (a) Prevention of water-borne diseases. (5)
   (b) Air pollution in urban areas. (5)

PART – II

3. Describe the magnitude of the problem of (P.E.M.) Protein Energy Malnutrition in India. Discuss management of a child suffering from grade III PEM. (10)

4. Write short notes on :
   (a) Trained birth attendant. (5)
   (b) National Health Policy, 2002. (5)

PART – III

5. Briefly describe principles of health education. Discuss, with suitable examples, I.E.C. activities in the prevention of H.I.V./A.I.D.S. (10)

6. Write short notes on :
   (a) Components of R.C.H. programme in India, highlighting the differences from C.S.S.M. programme. (5)
   (b) Geriatric health services in India. (5)

SAMPLE QUESTION PAPER-II

Attempt All the questions. Parts I, II and III should be answered in separate answer-books.

PART – I

1. Discuss National Acute Respiratory Infection Control Program. Describe the role of health worker in the same. (10)

2. Write short notes on :
   (a) Surveillance. (5)
   (b) Carrier state. (5)

PART – II

3. Define epidemiology. Explain briefly various steps in the investigation of an outbreak of food poisoning. (10)

4. Write short notes on :
   (a) Sampling. (5)
   (b) Concept of positive health. (5)

PART – III

5. Discuss epidemiology of coronary artery disease. Describe various levels of prevention for its control. (10)

6. Differentiate between :
   (a) Cross sectional and Longitudinal studies. (3)
   (b) Case fatality rate and proportional mortality rate. (3)
   (c) Pie chart and Bar chart. (4)

SAMPLE QUESTION PAPER-III

Attempt All Questions.
Parts I, II and III are to be answered in separate answer-books.

PART – I

1. Explain the following with examples :
   (a) Causal association. 3
   (b) Notification. 3
   (c) Healthy carrier. 3
   (d) Opportunistic infection. 3
   (e) Eradication. 3

2. Write short notes on :
   (a) Sample registration scheme. 5
   (b) Criteria for screening of a disease. 5

PART – II

3. How will you investigate and control an outbreak of gastroenteritis in a hostel? Write in brief. 10

4. Write short notes on :
   (a) Indicator of water quality. 5
   (b) Normal distribution curve. 5

PART – III

5. Enumerate the types of viral hepatitis. Discuss the prevention and control of Hepatitis 'B'. 10

OR

Discuss the Modified Plan of Operation for Malaria Control.

6. Discuss briefly :
   (a) Syndromic approach for S.T.Ds. in males. 5
   (b) Effect of air pollution on health and measures taken for its reduction in Delhi 5

SAMPLE QUESTION PAPER-IV

Attempt All Questions
Parts I, II and III are to be answered in separate answer-books.

PART – I

1. Describe the epidemiology of road accidents in India. Discuss measures for their prevention and control.   10

2. Write short notes on :
   (a) Measures to combat biological warfare.   5
   (b) Biomedical waste management in a P.H.C.   5

PART – II

3. Describe programme strategy and your role as P.H.C. medical officer in National leprosy eradication programme.   10

4. Write short notes on :
   (a) Normal curve.   5
   (b) Enhanced Malaria Control Project.   5

PART – III

5. Briefly describe management and health education for the following :
   (a) A five-year old child with diarrhoea.   5
   (b) A nine-month old boy with A.R.I.   5

6. Differentiate between :
   (a) Cluster testing and contact tracing.   3
   (b) Relative risk and Attributable risk.   3
   (c) Analytical and Experimental studies.   4

SAMPLE QUESTION PAPER-V

Attempt All Questions
Parts I, II and III *are to be answered in separate answer-books.*

PART – I

1. What are the main components of R.C.H. Program? Discuss health problems of adolescents and strategies to improve them. 10

2. Write short notes on :
   (a) Ergonomics. 5
   (b) Sickness absenteeism. 5

PART – II

3. Enumerate diseases associated with micronutrient deficiency. Describe measures for their prevention. 10

4. Write short notes on :
   (a) Community Needs Assessment. 5
   (b) E.S.I. Act. 5

PART – III

5. Describe briefly your role at Primary Health Centre in :
   (a) Drug supply. 5
   (b) Organizing pulse polio immunization program. 5

6. Draw suitable labelled diagrams to explain :
   (a) Natural history of disease and levels of prevention. 4
   (b) Age pyramid in India. 3
   (c) Demographic cycle. 3

SAMPLE QUESTION PAPER-VI

Attempt All Questions
Parts I, II and III are to be answered in separate answer-books.

PART – I

1. Discuss briefly :
   (a) Benefits provided to the beneficiaries under E.S.I. act. — 5
   (b) Functions of male multipurpose worker. — 5

2. Write short notes on :
   (a) ABC analysis — 3
   (b) Risks and benefits of oral contraceptives. — 4
   (c) Rehabilitation of child suffering from poliomyelitis. — 3

PART – II

3. Discuss in detail the planning of R.C.H. services for population catered by a community health centre. — 10

4. Discuss briefly :
   (a) Role of cultural factors in health and disease. — 5
   (b) Health hazards of air pollution. — 5

PART – III

5. Enumerate causes of Protein Energy Malnutrition (P.E.M.) in under five children. How will you manage a child suffering from P.E.M. grade-II. — 10

6. Write short notes on :
   (a) Asbestosis. — 4
   (b) Demographic cycle. — 3
   (c) Sand fly. — 3

FINAL QUESTION PAPER
1990-PREVENTIVE & SOCIAL MEDICINE
BHMS (PART-I)
GROUP-A

Answer four questions of which Q. No. 8 is compulsory

1. What are the common causes of infant mortality in our country? Suggest measures for its reduction. 5+15

2. What is primary Health care? Discuss the role of Primary Health centre in providing health services to the community of India. 5+15

3. Discuss the epidemiology of Japanese Encephalitis in India with its preventive and control measures. 20

OR

Discuss the salient features of National Leprosy eradication programme. Do you think leprosy can be eradicated by 2000 A.D.? Give reasons for your answer. 10+2+8

4. What is "Potable Water"? What are the water borne diseases? How they can be prevented in a municipal town of West Bengal? Give details. 5+5+10

5. As a medical officer of Primary Health centre you observe number of malnutritional cases. How you will asses such nutritional deficiency cases in P.H.C. area? 20

6. Name the different methods of F.W. planning (briefly) suitable for rural India. What is demographic cycle? 10+10

7. Discuss in details the benefits provided in E.S.I. and its draw backs. 20

8. (A) Write short notes on any two of the following : 5×2

   i) Levels of prevention of a disease; ii) Statistical averages; iii) Biological Treatment of Sewage; iv) Balanced Diet.

   (B) Fill in the blanks :

   i) The period of time necessary for the development of the in the insect is called ii) are substances which are used to kill microorganisms outside the human body.

FINAL QUESTION PAPER
1991-PREVENTIVE & SOCIAL MEDICINE
BHMS (PART-I)
GROUP-A

1. (A) Put a tick mark (✓) on the correct answer (Any Five) 2×5

   i) Birth rate of India is 10/20/25/30. ii) Vector of Filaria is Culex fatigans/Anopheles stephensi/Aedes/Anopheles minimus. iii) World Health day is observed every year on 1st March/7th April/14th July/22nd December. iv) Bagassosis is caused by inhalation of dust from sugar cane/iron/cotton fibre/silica. v) Hepatitis is caused by virus/bacteria protozoa/helminth. vi) Incubation period of Diptheria is usually 5 days/15 days/20 days/22 days.

   (B) Fill in the blanks :

   i) Levels of prevention of a discaso are ..... ii) Types of carrier may be...... iii) DPT vaceiners are given to prevent ...... iv) Vegetable sources of protein in our daily diet are ....

2. Describe the general principles of control of a communicable disease. 20

3. What is a "balanced died"? Prepare a balanced diet chart for a pregnant woman. 5+15

4. Describe in detail any field visit that you think most important. Give reasons. 15+5

5. What are the common causes of maternal mortality in rural areas? Suggest measures for its reduction. 5+15

6. What is the difference between : (Any Four)

   a) Epidemic & Endemic; b) Cross infection & Cross Ventilation; c) Chlorine demand & Residual chlorine of a volume of water; d) Presumptive coliform count & Presumptive treatment of Malaria; e) Medical benefit & Sickness benefit under ESI ACT. f) Crude Birth Rate & General fertility rate.

GROUP-B
Answer any one question. The figures in the margin indicate full marks.

7. Discuss the concept of the Health and disease. How can you apply your knowledge of organon of medicine for prevention of disease? 5+5+10

8. Is it possible to prevent and control tuberculosis with the help of potentised homoeopathic medicine? Justify your statement with reasons. 20

9. Is preventive medicine compatible with homoeopathy in theory and practice"? Discuss. 20

FINAL QUESTION PAPER
1993-PREVENTIVE & SOCIAL MEDICINE
BHMS (PART-I)
GROUP-A

Answer four questions, of which question No. 1 is compulsory

1. (A) Fill up the blanks – any four of the following :
   (a) Disease agents are; (b) Sources of Iron in our diet; (c) Disease transmitted by Mosquito are; (d) Write 5 goals to be reached by 2000 AD; (e) Water borne disease are; (f) Manifestation of Vit-a deficiency are

   (B) Write short notes on any four of the following :
   (a) Comprehensive Health Care; (b) demographic Cycle; (c) Conventional contraceptives, (d) Oral Rehydration salt; (e) Potable Water; (f) Maternity Benefit.

2. Mention the common causes of materal Mortality in rural India, Suggest measures for reduction of such mortality. 5+15

3. Define "Malnutrition". Mention the common Nutritional Disorders in India. Suggest measures for prevention of any one of them. 3+5+12

4. Define "Epidemiology". What is "Epidemiologial Triad"? Write briefly the different steps of Epidetric Investigation of a disease. 3+3+14

5. Discus different level of prevention of disease. Which of the level you think most important give reason. 5+15

6. Write briefly the various Methods of presentation of statistical data. 20

GROUP-B
Answer any one question

7. Is preventive Medicine compatable with Homoeopathy in theory and practice? Discuss. 20

8. Discuss prophylaxis and Vaccination critically from Homoeopathic point of vision. 20

9. Discuss the concept of Health and disease. How can you apply your knowledge of organon of Medicine for prevention of disease? 4+4+12

FINAL QUESTION PAPER
1994-PREVENTIVE & SOCIAL MEDICINE
BHMS (PART-I)
GROUP-A

Answer any Four questions

1. (A) Give a tick mark for the correct answer :   1×5
   i) B.C.G. is a killed vaccine True/False. ii) Disinfection means killing of spores True/False. iii) Beri Beri is due to Vit B deficiency – True/False. iv) Kala-azar is spread by sand-fly-True/False. V) Acute Anterior Polimoelitis is a water-boune disease True/False.

   (B) What do you mean by (Any Five)   3×5
   i) Quarantine and isolation. ii) Vector and Vital layer. iii) Fomites and Carrier. iv) Active Immunity and active surveillance in Malaria. v) Balanced Diet and dietary cycle. vi) Incubation period and extrinsic Incubation period. vii) Epidemic and Endemic.

2. Name the diseases under eradication programme. Outline the salient components of any one them.   5+15

3. Explain "Levels of prevention of Diseases" with reference to Tuberculosis. 20

4. What are the diseases spread by mosquito ? Outline the various measures for control of mosquitoes.   5+15

5. Write notes on any Two of the following diseases.   10+10
   a) Rabies; b) Plague; c) Sexually transited diseases.

6. Mention in brief the components of school health services.   20

7. What are the common cause of maternal mortality in our country? Suggest briefly the measures adopted for its reduction.   20

8. Outline the measures to be adopted for control of diarrhoea diseases in rural areas.

GROUP-B
Answer any one question

9. What is social medicine? What is preventive/medicine? Write the scope of prophylactic treatment in homoeopathy.   5+5+10

10. Describe the General principles laid down by Hahnemann for prevention and control of communicable diseases.   20

11. Is it possible to prevent and control Tuberculosis with the help of potentised homeopathic medicine? Justify your statement with reasons.   20

FINAL QUESTION PAPER
1995-PREVENTIVE & SOCIAL MEDICINE
BHMS (PART-I)
GROUP-A

Answer any four questions of which No. 1 is compulsory

1. (A) Choose the most appropriate answer :   2×5
   i) Incubation period of polliemyclitis is 2 days/10 days/14 days/28 days.
   ii) Population of India is 80 million/850 million/8000 million.
   iii) Target for reduction of infant mortality rate by 2000 A.D. to 60/75/100.
   iv) Blidt's spot is a sign of deficiency of Vit A/Vit B_1/Vit C.
   v) Attenuated virus are the content of Triple angigon/Moasles vaccine/B.C.G. vaccine.

   (B) Write short notes on <u>any two</u> of the following :   5×2
   a) Definitive Host & Intermediate host. b) Quarantine & Isolation c) Demographic cycle and cyclical trend of a disease/Pestourization and sterilization.

2. "Name three National Disease Eradiation programme" and mention the salient features of <u>any one</u> of them.   8+12

3. What is balanced diet? Write a chart of balanced diet for a pregnant women. 5+15

4. What is maternal mortality rate? Suggest measures for reduction of maternal mortality in our country.   3+17

5. Write short answers on the following (any two) :   10×2
   a) Medical Termination of Pregnancy (M.T.P.) Act, 1971 b) Primary Health Care
   c) Census d) Levels of prevention of disease.

6. What is Immunity? Write in detail the Immunization Schedule followed under National Programme under one year age.

GROUP-B
Answer any one question

7. What is "Genus Epidemicus"? Describe the scope of "Genus Epidemicus?. In preventing and controlling of epidemic of measles. State clearly how you will arrive at "Genus Epidemicus".   5+8+7

8. Does homoeopathy corroborate the popular law view "Preventive is better than cure"? If so, how? If not why not? Justify your answer citing and example of Helminthic infection.   20

9. Discuss prophylaxis and vaccination critically from homoeopathic point of view.   20

FINAL QUESTION PAPER
1996-PREVENTIVE & SOCIAL MEDICINE
BHMS (PART-I)
GROUP-A

Answer any four questions of which No. 1 is compulsory

1. (A) Choose the most appropriate answer :   2×5
   - i) Immunisation schedule starts from 4 weeks/6 weeks/8 weeks/within months;
   - ii) Breast feeding should be started within ½ hour of birth/1 hour of birth/6 hours of birth/12 hours of birth;
   - iii) In Measles rash appears after 4th day of fever/6th day of fever/7 days of fever/along with fever;
   - iv) Night blindness is a symptoms of deficiency of Vit. B_1/Vit A/Vit C.
   - v) The most sensitive demographic indicator is maternal mortality rate/infant mortality rate/death rate/neonatal mortality rate.

   (B) Write short notes on <u>any two</u> of the following :   5×2
   - (a) Surveillance in malaria;
   - (b) Levels of prevention;
   - (c) Health of all by 2000 A.D.;
   - (d) Multidrug therapy in leprosy;
   - (e) District tuberculosis centre.

2. Enumerate national nutritional programmes. Discuss in brief I.C.D.S. Programme.   8+12

3. Discuss the 3 tire system of health care delivery in rural India.   20

4. Name some water born disease. What are the method by which these can be prevented.   5+15

5. What are the causes of infant mortality? Suggest measures for reducing the high infant mortality in India.   8+12

6. Write short answers on the following (any two) :
   (a) Medical benefits of E.S.I; (b) Intra-uterine contraceptive devices; (c) Voluntary Health Organisation (d) Balanced diet.

GROUP-B

7. Discuss the role of early diagnosis and treatment in preventing epidemics with specific examples. Where and how would like to apply the principles of homoeopathy medicine in controlling epidemics.   10+10

FINAL QUESTION PAPER
1997-PREVENTIVE & SOCIAL MEDICINE
BHMS (PART-I)
GROUP-A

Answer any four questions of which No. 1 is compulsory

1. (A) Complete the following sentences with the most appropriate answer :
   i) Defluoridation of water can be done by the technique of permutit/ Walgondn;
   ii) Reden 1 Walker coefficient is related to yellow fever/disinfection/ standard deviation.
   iii) Incubation period of staphylococcal food poisoning is 1 to 6 hours/12 to 24 hours/24 to 48 hours.
   iv) Hepatitis B is spread by Serum/Water/Air.
   v) Humidity is measured by anemometer/densitometer/psychrometer.

   (B) Write short notes on <u>any two</u> of the following : 5×2
   i) Pastourisation of milk; ii) Kata thermometer; iii) Endemic Goitre; iv) Personal hygine;

2. What are the dictory sources of Vitamin A? Describe the measures taken to prevent blindness due to Vitamin A deficiency. 20

3. Enumerate the currently available methods for family planning. Describe briefly the method of use and the problems associated with intra-utering contraceptive devices (IUCD). 8+12

4. What diseases are transmitted by sandflies ? Describe the epidemiology and measures for control of Kala-azar. 5+15

5. Who are the beneficiaries of ICDS (Integrated Child Development Services) scheme? Describe in brief the different services that are available under this scheme. 5+10

6. Describe the process of purification of drinking water suitable for a large metropolis like Calcutta. 20

7. Name five important zoonotic diseases. Describe the measures taken for prevention of rabies following a dog bite.

8. Write brief note on any two of the following :
   i) Epidemiological triod; ii) Functions of WHO; iii) Sanitary latrine.

GROUP-B

9. What is genus epidemicus? State clearly you will arrive at 'Genus Epidemicus'. Describe the scope of genus epidemicus in preventing and controlling epidemic cholera. 5+5+10

10. Describe the principle laid down by Hahnemann for prevention and control of communicable diseases.

11. What measures you would take as a Homoeopath for preventing an out break of Gastroenteritis in thickly populated area. Mention five medicines with their indications. 10+5×2

FINAL QUESTION PAPER
1999-PREVENTIVE & SOCIAL MEDICINE
BHMS (PART-I)
GROUP-A

Answer Q. No. 1 and any three from the rest

1. (A) Give two examples of each of the following :   2×5
   i) Good dietary sources of Vitamin A
   ii) Milk borne diseases
   iii) Insecticides
   iv) Statistical averages
   v) Disease transmitted by culex Mosquito

   (B) Write short notes on any two :   5×2
   i) Rehabilitation. ii) Pneumoconiosis. iii) Overcrowding.

2. Describe the advantages of breast feeding and disadvantages of bottle feeding.   10+10

3. What are the sources of vital statistics? Describe briefly how census helps in this process.   10+10

4. What are different methods of contraception available of the female partner? What are the desirable and undesirable side-effects of hormonal contraceptives   10+10

5. Give a brief account of benefits available under ESI scheme.   20

6. What methods are available for disposal of refuse? Describe a method suitable for rural areas.   10+10

7. How is an outbreak of food poisoning differentiated from an outbreal of cholera?   20

8. Name different National Programmes in Nutrition. Describe any one of them.   5+15

GROUP-B

9. What is meant by immunisation? Describe the scopes of immunisation in Homoeopathy.   8+12

10. What is preventive Medicine? Describe the Scope of preventive medicine in Homoeopathy.   8+12

11. What measures you would take as a Homoeopath for prevention an outbreak of gastroenteritis in thickly populated area. What are the instructions given by Hahnemann for controlling of epidemic diseases?   10+10

BIBLIOGRAPHY

Man and Medicine : Towards Health for All
References
1. Jaggi, O.P (1973) Indian System of Medicine, Atma Ram and son.
2. Kishore, Jugal (1974) Swart hind, 18, 36.
3. Martin F.M (1977) Lancet.
4. Roemer, M.I (1972) Public Health No. 48, Geneva.
5. WHO–UNICEF (1978) Health for All, Sr. No. 1.
6. Carlson, R.J (1975) The End of Medicine, Wiley.
7. Morley, David, et al (1984) Practising Health for All, Oxford University Press.
8. WHO (1970) World Health, May 1970.
9. Mahler, H (1977) World Health, Nov. 1977.
10. WHO (1976) WHO Chronicle, 30 (1) 8.

Concepts of Health and Disease
References
1. Evang, K (1967) In Health of Mankind, Ciba Foundation.
2. WHO (1979) Health for all, Sr. No. 2.
3. Sartovrivs, N (1983) Bull. WHO, 61 (1).
4. Dubos, R (1969) WHO Chro. 23:499.
5. Carlos, M (1978) Bull PaHo. 12:7.
6. WHO (1984) Techa Rep., Sr. No. 706.
7. WHO (1976) Chr. 30(1) 16.
8. WHO (1984) World Health, May 1984.
9. Soper F.L (1962) AMJ Public Health, S2 : 724:745.
10. WHO (1973) Techn Rep., Ser. No. 533.

Principles of Epidemiology
References

1. A Dictionary of epidemiology, JM Lart, editor, Oxford University Press, New York, 1995.
2. Greenberg, R.S (ed) Medical Epidemiology, Norwalk Applet on and Lange, 1993.
3. San Risser, PhD/Will Risser, MD. PhD–Randomized Clinical Trial, WWW.legacy.csom.umn.edu/WWW.pages faculolt/vweekwerth/F02.
4. WHO (1981) Health for All, Sr. No. 4.
5. WHO (1968) Techn. Rep., Sr. No. 389.
6. WHO (1972) Techn. Rep.
7. Vassey MP and P.H Strasser (1980) Lancet.
8. Hoover, R.N and P.H Strasser (1980) Lancet.
9. Doll, R and Peto (1976) Brit. Med J.
10. Lee an et al (1969) J. Nati. Cancer Inst.

Principles of Epidemiology and Epidemiologic Method
References

1. Acheson, RM (1978) Brit. Med. J.2.
2. Langmvir, AD (1975) Int. J. Epi. 4.
3. WHO (1967) Techn. Rep., Sr. No. 365.
4. Rooks, J.B et all (1979) JAMA 242, 644-648.
5. Weser, J.K. etal (1983) Lancet, 1:1027-31.
6. Susser M.W (1977) AM. J. CPI los : 1-15.
7. Adour K.K. et al (1979 JAMA, 233 : 5 27-539.
8. Speirs, A.L (1962) Lancet, 1:303.
9. Doll, R and A. B. Hill (1956) Brit. Med. J., 2 : 1071.
10. Editorial (1977) Lancet, 2, 747.

Nutrition and Health
References

1. Survey of Infant Mortality, Registrar General's Office Report, 1979.
2. Alphones, K.J. : Kottayam, Kerala's first literate town. *Times of India*, December 17, 1993.
3. Bhat, R. : The private health care sector in India. In : Paying for India's Health Care : Berman, Peter and Khan, M.K. (Eds), Sage Publications, New Delhi/Newbury Rock/London, 1993.
4. Viswanathan, H. and Rodhe, J.E. : Diarrhoea in rural India. A nationwide study of mothers and practitioners, New Delhi, Vision Books, 1990.
5. Ghosh, S. : The female child in India – A struggle for survival. N.F.I. Bulletin, 8(4), 1987.
6. Bang, R., et al : High prevalence of gynaecological diseases in rural Indian women, Lancet, January, 85-88, 1989.
7. Wasserheit, G.N., et al : Reproductive tract infections in famiy planning population in rural Bangladesh. Studies in Family Planning, Volume 20(2) March-April 1989.
8. Koening, M.A., Fauvean, V., Chowdhary, A.I., Chakraborty, J. and Khan, H.A. : Maternal mortality in Matlab, Bangladesh, 1976-85. Studies in Family Planning, 19(2), March-April, 1988.
9. Registrar General's Report. Occasional Paper No. 5, 1988.
10. Shanti Ghosh – Child Survival and Safe Motherhood – The hard Road ahead.
    WWW.nutrition foundation of India.com
11. Donald P. Kotler, M.D. – Basic assessment of Nutritent status.
12. WWW.rjlsystems.com/Oocs/Nutritions.Pdf
13. James W.P.T. (1982) – Medicine international.
14. Rodricks, J.V. (1976) Food Nutritions C.F.A.O.
15. Morris, J.N. et al (1977) Brit. Med. J.
16. National Nutrition, Hyderabad (1977) Ann. Rep.

17. WHO (1976) Techn. Rep., Ser. No. 705.
18. WHO (1977) Techn Rep., Ser. No. 612.
19. WHO/FAO (1955) Techn. Rep., Ser. No. 197.
20. WHO (1978) Bull. W.H.O., 56 (4) 519.
21. WHO (1963) Techn. Rep., Ser. No. 53.